Business Mastery

Fourth Edition

A Guide for Creating a Fulfilling,
Thriving Business and Keeping it Successful

by

Cherie M. Sohnen-Moe

Business Mastery[4]

A Guide for Creating a Fulfilling, Thriving Business and Keeping It Successful

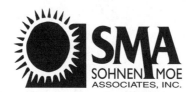

Published by Sohnen-Moe Associates, Inc.
3900 W Costco Dr #168-367
Tucson, AZ 85741-2999
520-743-3936 • 800-786-4774
www.sohnen-moe.com • www.businessmastery.us

Publisher's Cataloging-in-Publication
     (Prepared by Quality Books, Inc)

Sohnen-Moe, Cherie.
     Business mastery: a guide for creating a fulfilling, thriving business and keeping it successful / by Cherie Sohnen-Moe.—4th ed.
          p. cm.
          Includes bibliographical references and index
          Preassigned LCCN: 2007906959
          ISBN-13: 978-0-9621265-7-4
          ISBN-10: 0-9621265-7-8
1. Small business-Management--Handbooks, manuals, etc. 2. Healing--Practice--Handbooks, manuals, etc.   I. Title.

HD62.7.S64 2007   658.02'2
                    QBI07-600281

Editors: Sheri Piper, Melissa B. Mower and Beth Mayer
Cover Design: Umanga deSilva
Clip art provided by: ClickArt © 1996, 1995, 1994, 1993 T/Maker Company; Clip Art © 1990-1997, RT Computer Graphics, N.M.; Corel Draw!5 ©1994, Corel Corporation
Printed in the United States of America

Table of Contents

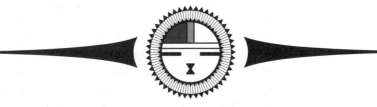

Preface

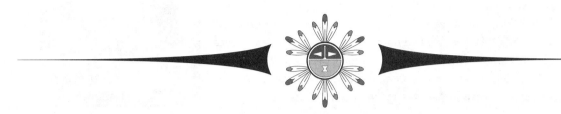

Introduction

Mastering business is like bringing a rainbow down to earth. It is about taking dreams, principles, goals and ideals and turning them into something real that you and others can see and appreciate. In the approach taken in this book, business mastery is not about taking steps one-two-three and you're there. Instead, this approach asks you to recognize that many colors fill the rainbow of success, and you blend these colors into the shades that best suit you.

For the past two decades, *Business Mastery* has supported business owners in all realms to reach new levels of success. This book is written specifically for wellness professionals. If you're a massage therapist, chiropractor, counselor, acupuncturist, homeopath, Rolfing® practitioner, nutritional consultant, naturopath, herbalist, Reiki practitioner, esthetician, psychiatrist, Polarity therapist, physician, aromatherapist, personal trainer, reflexologist, physical therapist, yoga instructor, or a practitioner of any of the numerous allied healthcare professions, this book is for you!

This edition of *Business Mastery* includes updated information and new topics of interest. You can find valuable bonus material on the *Business Mastery* website (www.businessmastery.us), such as resource books, website links, forms and information on select topics. To make it easy to find these extra resources, each chapter of the book has a corresponding section on the website. Please visit the site regularly as we plan to continually update it. I hope you find this edition of *Business Mastery* even more valuable and fun to use.

While most wellness practitioners ultimately work for themselves, many practitioners start their careers as an employee or augment their private practice by taking a part-time job. Since the previous edition of *Business Mastery* was published, the job market has expanded considerably. Thus, you'll find two chapters chock-full of information on navigating your way through the job market and finding your ideal job.

Business Mastery takes an in-depth look at how to build and maintain a successful practice. Depending on your level of business experience and expertise, you may find that you only need to concentrate on certain sections of this book. Some of the topics may not be relevant to you now, yet may become so in the future. These business skills are fundamental to your success—whether you work for someone else or are self-employed. Whatever path you choose, you can count on *Business Mastery* to help make your dreams a reality.

I wish you great happiness, health, prosperity, success and balance!

About The Author

Cherie Sohnen-Moe is an author, business coach and international workshop leader. She has been a successful business owner since 1978. Before shifting her focus to education and coaching, she was in private practice for many years as a massage and holistic health practitioner. She has served as a faculty member at the Desert Institute of Healing Arts (DIHA) and the Arizona School of Acupuncture and Oriental Medicine (ASAOM), and is an adjunct professor at Clayton College. Cherie is the author of *Present Yourself Powerfully,* and co-author of *The Ethics of Touch.* She has written more than 100 articles that have been published in more than 15 national and international magazines.

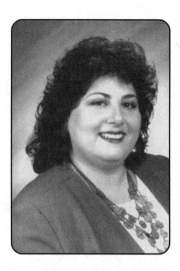

Cherie holds a degree in psychology from the University of California, Los Angeles. She has received the Distinguished Service Award and the Professional Achievement Award from the American Society for Training and Development (ASTD), and the Outstanding Instructor Award at DIHA. She lives in Tucson, Arizona with her husband, Jim, and their dog, Cinder.

Cherie is dedicated to assisting people reach the success they desire: personally, financially and professionally.

Acknowledgments

So many people have supported me in making this book a reality. Much of the material for this book has been developed and refined over the past 30 years in my coaching practice, in courses and seminars I've facilitated, and through my own process of personal and professional development.

The 4th edition has been a team effort! It has been a pleasure to work with the following people whose writings, reviews, research and editing have enriched and added clarity to this project: Jada Ahern, Ben Benjamin, Nikki Charns, C. Diane Ealy, Reagan Hatch, Andrea Kartch, Kathy Lynn Lee, Whitney Lowe, Jon Lumsden, Virginia Mahoney, Beth Mayer, Jim Moe, Shaye Moore, Daz Moran, Melissa Mower, Terri Osborne, Ravensara Siobhan Travillian, Neil Wilkinson and Jan Zobel. I give special appreciation to Sheri Piper for her outstanding editorial assistance throughout the project, and to Umanga deSilva for her beautiful cover design and creative interior book layout.

Many people were involved in the previous editions of *Business Mastery*. I am grateful for the content suggestions, editing assistance, artistic creation, inspiration and general support I received from Dominick Angiulo, Margaret Avery Moon, Simi Aziz, Barb Baun, Terry Belville, Phyllis Bloom, Barbara Buchanan, Jacque Dailey, Robert Decker, Rich Foster, Julie Goodwin, Janice Hollender, Helene Jewell, Jamie Lee, Maryanne LaBrash, Mark Moseley, Nancy Parker, Christine Rosche, Bob Sexton, Helen Sohnen, Karen Wilhelmsen, Tracy Williams and Kalyn Wolf. Thank you all!

I acknowledge all of my friends who encourage me to pursue my dreams and keep me laughing. Most of all I am so thankful for my wonderful husband, Jim. He has assisted in every phase of this book. His unconditional love and total support for whatever I choose to do has given me the courage to follow my heart.

How to Use This Book

No matter where you are in your career, if you're willing to take a new look at your life and challenge some of your old thought patterns, you'll find that reading this book from beginning to end is an incredibly valuable process.

Business Mastery has been designed to follow a pattern—the chapters build upon each other. You may need to read a specific chapter and then go back to the beginning of the book. For instance, if you're considering going into partnership, proceed directly to Chapters 9 and 10. Maybe you've been in practice for a while now; you have a business plan, you know what you want out of life, and you still aren't accomplishing your goals. In that case you may want to start with Chapter 3, Success Strategies.

Some sections include aspects of business that may not pertain to you—such as product sales, group practice, employees or working for someone else. Just review them (someday, you may decide to incorporate those areas) and complete the sections that are appropriate to *your* career path.

This isn't a book to sit and read in one evening. It is filled with numerous exercises and soul-searching questions. It may take a while to complete this manual. One way to make this more manageable (and less overwhelming) is to allot a specific amount of time each day to work through the book. This isn't a book to read and put on a shelf. *Business Mastery* is a handbook—a resource tool for you to use regularly. It will help you create the success that you truly deserve!

What's in a Name?

For consistency and simplicity, the term practitioner is used throughout this book to refer to all types of wellness professionals. Although some scenarios refer to specific professions, they are relevant to almost every field. It wasn't feasible to include specific examples for each type of practice—otherwise this book would have contained many thousands of pages. It is my hope that everyone can easily relate to the examples provided.

The term client is used instead of patient throughout this book, primarily to recognize that the relationship between a practitioner and client is a partnership. This approach assures that the best interests of the client are served. It also honors the client's role as active participant rather than a passive recipient of wellness services.

Traditionally, the male pronoun has been used generically to refer to women as well as men. As our culture and language have evolved, an enlightened approach to pronoun use aims to refer to all persons equally. As the English language lacks neutral pronouns to accomplish this task, the solution chosen is to alternate the use of the female and male pronouns throughout the *Business Mastery* book.

Create a Business Journal

One of the first activities is to create a business journal, in which you can keep your responses to the exercises, your business plan and samples of your marketing materials (you can put cards and brochures in plastic sleeves). Even if you do the written work on computer, you may want to keep printed copies in the notebook.

Online Workbook

Get the most out of the *Business Mastery* book by doing the exercises and regularly referring to them. We've made it easier by creating the *Business Mastery Workbook,* which includes all of the written exercises and checklists from this book. To download your free copy, go to www.businessmastery.us/workbook.php.

Special Note for Students

Program durations vary from school to school: from several months to several years. Sometimes the business course is taught midway and other times near the end of the program. Some schools include 15 hours of business education, others 100. To download a checklist of action steps to prepare you for success by the time you graduate, visit www.businessmastery.us/student-checklist.php.

Continuing Education Units

You can obtain Continuing Education Units (CEUs) for each chapter. Our courses are recognized by many organizations, and we're approved providers for the National Certification Board for Therapeutic Massage and Bodywork and the Florida State Department of Health. If you're interested in using this material for CEUs, please call 800-786-4774 or visit www.businessmastery.us.

Special Note for Teachers

We offer a multitude of free teaching resources to schools requiring *Business Mastery:* a 70-page guide on the Art of Teaching; Lesson Plan Builders (goals, objectives and activities) for each chapter; 600[+] Slides and Handouts; a Test Bank; and 16-, 36- and 70-hour Syllabi with full daily lesson plans.

Pictograph Glossary

The following icons signal tips, resources and exercises.

 Exercise: Most of the exercises involve writing. This is your cue to get out your business journal or go to your computer.

 Idea: Quick tips or suggestions for other ways to utilize the information.

 Publication Resources: Books, magazines and other publications with more information on specific topics.

Internet Resources.

Sohnen-Moe Online Resources: at www.businessmastery.us.

Inspirational Quotes.

 Step Forward: Lets you know where you can find related information in a subsequent section.

Step Back: Reminds you to refer to an earlier section.

Part I

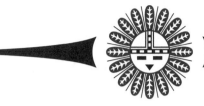

Set a Strong Foundation

As you work to make your career dreams a reality, Part I of *Business Mastery* explores how to set a strong foundation. It prepares you to make decisions about your career based on a clear sense of who you are and what you want to accomplish.

Chapter 1 looks at ways to increase your self-awareness and to make self-knowledge into a powerful ally for the work ahead of you. It also provides practical insights into career opportunities in the wellness field, as well as exercises to help you begin to locate your place in this exciting field.

Chapter 2 helps you transform the insights you gained from Chapter 1 into the activities of goal setting, strategic planning, and follow-through. These three key activities form the common denominator among successful people in all fields. This chapter assists you in developing a mission statement and goals—and translating them into activities vital to the daily, weekly, and monthly growth of your business. We then look at how savvy business people use strategic planning to create a roadmap to success.

Chapter 3 helps you define what success means to you, and supports you in a fearless examination of roadblocks that may stand in your way. You'll also find tips on how successful people manage their time, track results and handle risks wisely.

Chapter 4 looks at how to ensure that your career lasts for the long term and grows as you do. It identifies time-tested ways to enhance career longevity and avoid burnout. The chapter also explores ways to develop a strong support system to help you stay on track and true to your vision.

Getting Started

• First Steps •

Achieving success in the business world while staying true to the principles of healing and service to others may at times seem like a paradox. The business world is often portrayed as being heartless, as indeed it can be if you don't know the rules. The exciting thing is that once you do learn the rules, you can choose which ones you want to incorporate in your life and determine how to circumvent the ones you don't like.

Many people who choose a career as a wellness practitioner don't enjoy the business facets and thus don't take the time to learn the rules for success. Unfortunately, that attitude rarely leads to success. On the other hand, those who take the time to master basic business knowledge and build solid career skills often enjoy a smooth road to success and prosperity.

To do the work you love, it's crucial to develop the business savvy that gives you the knowledge, tools and insights you need to make informed career choices—choices that best support your financial and professional growth. Always remember why you chose your profession and stay grounded in the experience of the difference you make.

Rachel Naomi Remen, M.D., wrote an inspiring article in the Spring 1996 issue of *Noetic Sciences Review*, titled "In the Service of Life." She states:

> *Service rests on the basic premise that the nature of life is sacred, that life is a holy mystery which has an unknown purpose. When we serve, we know that we belong to life and to that purpose. Fundamentally, helping, fixing and service are ways of seeing life. When you help, you see life as weak, when you fix, you see life as broken. When you serve, you see life as whole. Lastly, fixing and helping are the basis of curing, but not healing. Only service heals.*

What lies behind us and what lies before us are tiny matters compared to what lies within us.
— Oliver Wendell Holmes

Self-Awareness is Key ✴

A journey of a thousand miles begins with a single step.
— Lao Tzu

Communication Styles and Personality Types

www.myersbriggs.org
www.discprofile.com
www.enneagraminstitute.com
www.similarminds.com

One of the most important traits that successful people have in common is the dedication to knowledge. Knowledge is power. Self-awareness is the foundation of that knowledge. So before you even begin to create or update a plan for your career or business, it's vital that you assess your current state.

The first step is to get a clear picture of your own personality style and unique quirks. You can easily do this by taking a personality quiz in any of several books (or on many websites) about personality types or social styles. What book or system you choose to work with isn't as important as finding material that rings true for you. The best books on personality types and communication styles offer a balance of conceptual and practical information, and include plenty of stories about how differences play out in day-to-day interactions.

It is extremely difficult to get to your destination if you don't know where you are. Include the personal aspects of your life as well as the professional ones. You are a whole being and your career is only one—albeit a very significant—part of your life. This chapter contains several activities designed to assist you in assessing yourself, exploring career options and visualizing your future.

Wheel of Life Exercise

Figure 1.1 is a completed example of an exercise called the "Wheel of Life." Its purpose is to support you in evaluating your life. Imagine that the center point (A) is the least desirable state and the outside of the circle (B) is the most desirable state. Look at each category. Take a moment to think about where you are right now. Where is that in relation to where you want to be? Then mark along the line for each of the 10 categories where you feel you are right now. Finally, connect the dots. Do you have a balanced wheel or does it look like a starburst? Keep in mind that it's very difficult to smoothly roll through life when your wheel (life) isn't balanced.

You also might mark the "spokes" with an arrow in the direction that you see that particular spoke going. For example, if you're in school, then the education dot is an arrow pointing to the outside. If there is no particular activity in that spoke, then just put a dot.

Consider this wheel from two points of view. First, notice any categories that are proportionately nearer the center than others. Those are the areas on which you need to concentrate on improving. The object is to bring more balance to your wheel. The second aspect is to enhance all the categories so that they're toward the outside (most desirable) of the circle.

Another way to utilize this tool is to make a Wheel of Life that represents your ideal life situation. On a blank Wheel of Life write activities on each spoke that enable you to grow or maintain your position in each area of your life.

I recommend that you do this exercise every few months. It is a great way to chart your progress!

Figure 1.1

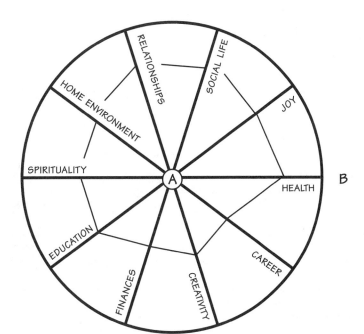

www.businessmastery.us/
forms.php#busman
to print a blank copy of
the Wheel of Life.

Personal Assessment

Write a biographical sketch spanning your birth to the present. Include personal and family information as well as career details.

List the following:
- Your major accomplishments
- Your talents and abilities
- The three things you do best
- Your challenges
- Obstacles you've overcome
- Three things you do the least well
- Three things for which you want to be remembered
- Memories you treasure most
- How you would like others to describe you
- Three things you want to accomplish in your life

Career Assessment

Describe the current state of your career or business experience. Include length of time in your field, average yearly income and number of clients.

List the following:
- What are the three attributes of your practice of which you are the most proud?
- What is working well?
- What isn't working well?
- What changes would you like to see occur?
- What would you like people to say about your business?

Assessment for Students

Highlight your previous job experience, education and background that can contribute to your success in this career field.

List the following:
- Which previous jobs have you most enjoyed?
- Which previous jobs have you least enjoyed?
- Do you feel comfortable reporting to others?
- Do you like to manage your own time or prefer someone else setting priorities and schedules?
- What kinds of clients do you prefer to work with?
- Do you enjoy or genuinely dislike paperwork?
- Do you like performing a variety of business tasks each day and week?
- How many hours do you work or want to work each week?
- Do you prefer to spend the majority of time working with clients?
- Do you have marketing experience? Do you enjoy it?
- Do you offer other services besides your primary training? What other modalities/ knowledge do you want to learn?
- Are you a disciplined, self-starter with an interest in running a business? What life experience has given you the opportunity to know this about yourself?
- Do you enjoy researching or teaching?
- Do your family and friends support your career goals?
- Who has given you career guidance already or might be a mentor for you?

Why Clarify Your Values?

A satisfying and balanced life occurs when your values are in synchrony with the way you live your life and run your business. Invest the time in exploring your values. After all, they're the major conscious and unconscious influences on the decisions you make throughout your life. Many conflicts in one's life, both professional and personal, arise because there is a clash of values either within oneself or with others.

Questions to Clarify Your Personal Values

My Ideal Life
- What would I do with my life if I could do anything? Why?

Happiness
- The people I know who seem to be happy are happy because...
- I am happiest when I am...
- What is my most treasured memory? Why?

Relationships
- The most admirable things about me are...
- When I look at my home life, the activities that are of the most worth are...
- The things I most value in a relationship are...
- Who and what have been major influences in my values development?
- Who are the most important people in my life? What could I do to improve those relationships?

Core Values
- What values are most important to me?
- What are the character traits I deem essential?
- What is the greatest accomplishment of my life? What do I hope to do that is as great or even better?
- If I only had one year to live, I would concentrate on...
  Am I doing those things now? If not, why?

Questions to Clarify Your Professional Values

My Work Life
- My attitudes and beliefs about wellness are...
- My attitudes and beliefs about my profession are...

Professionalism
- How do my values enhance my professionalism and affect my work with clients?
- What are the most meaningful attributes of an effective practitioner in my field?
- Which of my personal values conflict with professional rules of conduct?
- Which of my personal values conflict with laws or regulation?

Core Values
- What are the most important personal characteristics for someone in my field?
- What are the key professional characteristics for someone in my field?
- When I look at my work life in perspective, the activities that have the most worth to me are...

✳ Exploring Career Paths ✳

Contact your professional associations for current industry trends and statistics.

Employment in the complementary and alternative medicine (CAM) fields is expected to increase by 48.8 percent from 2002 to 2012. According to survey data released in 2004 by the National Center for Health Statistics, 36 percent of U.S. consumers are using some form of CAM. The breakdown of CAM usage is as follows:

> 18.9% took herbs and herbal medicines
> 11.6% did deep breathing exercises
> 7.6% meditated
> 7.5% had chiropractic care
> 5.1% practiced yoga
> 5.0% received massage
> 3.5% participated in diet-based therapies

Complementary and Alternative Medicine use among adults

www.cdc.gov/nchs/data/ad/ad343.pdf

Additionally, it's estimated that the U.S. public spends more than $30 billion annually in out-of-pocket expenses for the services of professional CAM healthcare providers which include chiropractic, acupuncture and massage/bodywork practitioners. In view of these trends, the career outlook for wellness practitioners is bright.

The rapidly expanding career opportunities are due to a constellation of factors: a widening interest in stress management and preventive wellness; the public's disillusionment with the high cost of prescriptions and traditional medical care; and a fast-growing population of baby boomers age 55 and over looking for ways to cope with the physical challenges and stress associated with aging.

Most wellness practitioners love what they do. How could one not love a career where you can help people reduce stress, improve their health, get in touch with themselves and feel better so quickly? What is not so often mentioned is the high percentage of graduates who fail to become successful in their careers. Although the causes are many, most failures are rooted in a lack of business savvy.

At first glance, it may seem that acquiring advanced technical skills and a high degree of expertise are sure ways to success. However, this is only one part of the equation. Other key factors for success are business savvy and strong interpersonal communication skills. Without this solid foundation, your career and technical skills cannot flourish.

Fundamental interpersonal skills include creating rapport and building relationships; developing a soothing and inspiring manner with clients; setting appropriate personal and professional boundaries; and creating a safe space for clients. Develop awareness of and adhere to high standards of professionalism. These skills serve you well whether you run your own business or work for someone else.

Figure 1.2 provides a brief overview of career paths for wellness practitioners. Keep in mind that the specific venues listed under Employee and Self-Employed can overlap.

Figure 1.2

The Wide World of Holistic Wellness . . .

Employee (Full-time or Part-time)

Spas
    Day Spa
    Dental Spa
    Destination Spa
    Resort Spa
    Luxury Hotel Spa
    Cruise Ship Spa
    Medical Spa

**Holistic Healthcare Clinic or
Wellness Center**

Specialty Clinic/Center
(e.g., all acupuncture, all massage therapy)

Hospital or Medical Clinic
    Medical Center
    Orthopedic Physician's Office
    Physical Therapy Clinic
    Rehabilitation Center
    Sports Medicine Clinic

Self-Employed

Private Practice
    Home Office
    Private Office in a Professional Building
    Room in Another's Practice
        (e.g., Chiropractor's Office)
    On-site / Outcalls
    Fitness Center / Gym / Health Club
    Corporate Wellness Program
    Day Spa
    Dental Spa
    Hospital
    Hospice
    Personal Practitioner for a Celebrity
        or Professional Athlete
    Salon

Group Practice
    Holistic Healthcare Clinic or Wellness Center
    Medical Clinic

Next, we explore some effective ways to sharpen your career focus and look at the pros and cons of self-employment versus working for someone else. The more information and insights you have into possible career paths, the better prepared you are to make choices best suited to your unique personality and goals.

Why Clear Career Focus Is Essential ❋

It is the commonest of mistakes to consider that the limit of our power of perception is also the limit of all there is to perceive.
— C.W. Leadbeater

Douglas Helmer, Ph.D., author of *The Massage Therapy Career Focus Workbook*, says that if you ask an aspiring somatic practitioner what she wants to "do," she'll usually give you her job title. For example, "I'm training to be a massage therapist," or, "I'm learning to be an acupuncturist." Probe any deeper and these same aspiring wellness providers are often stuck for an answer. If you ask them where they want to work, you'll often get, "I don't know." Ask who they want to treat and the response is usually, "I'm not sure." Ask them if they want to be an employee or work on their own, and you'll most likely hear, "I haven't decided." Finally, ask if they think not knowing the answers to these questions is a problem, and most reply, "It's not a problem, and there's lots of time to figure that out after graduation." Unfortunately there simply isn't "lots of time" to make these vital career decisions. Practitioners who arrive at graduation day without a crystal clear vision of some basic parameters that define a preferred career are likely to land up in the "Did Not Stay in the Profession After Two Years" column.

The Massage Therapy Career Focus Workbook points out that the career focus parameters can be as simple as knowing the answers to the journalist's five W's & one H: Who? What? When? Where? Why? How? Looking for an easy way to sharpen your career focus? Take a few minutes to reflect upon the questions in the Five W's and One H chart (Figure 1.3).

Figure 1.3

The Five W's and One H

Who:
Who do you want to work with? or, Who—that is, what type of client—do you want to work on? Young people? Elderly people? Athletic people?

What:
What do you want to provide to your clients? What kind of treatment? What kind of outcome do you desire? What kind of environment will you provide?

When:
When do you want to work? Strictly 9-5? Do you want your weekends free? Do you have a preference or are you flexible?

Where:
Where do you want to work? Are you looking for a spa/resort setting? Clinical? On-site?

Why:
Why do you want to work in a certain area or focus? Is it to communicate more effectively? Do you want to build your referral network? Is your main goal to help people?

How:
How do you want to care for your clients? How will you approach your clients? Will you approach the whole client or their specific condition? Will you actively work with them so they learn to care for themselves or passively so they'll depend on you for future treatments?

Career Tracks

The two primary career tracks are to work for a company or be self-employed. Within those two paths are a number of possibilities. Some people kick-start their careers by working at a spa or clinic, others take part-time jobs to augment their private practices, some choose a private practice right away, and there are those who prefer to only work for others.

Another consideration is the amount of time you want to work. Some people want to work full time while others choose to permanently work in their field on a part-time basis (they either have another career, are raising a family, or want to pursue other interests).

The information in this section assists you in determining which options best fit your overall goals and personality. Specific details on how to set up a private practice or work for a company are covered in Chapters 7 through 10.

According to the International Spa Association (ISPA), approximately 32 percent of massage practitioners work in spas.

Employment

Working as an employee provides many potential benefits such as the possibility of walking into a full practice with little marketing; providing a larger scope of services for your clients' well-being; starting out with a ready-made professional image; reduced paperwork (there's usually an office manager); the ability to focus on hands-on work; access to better and more varied equipment and supplies; excellent built-in referral base; and office staff that does the scheduling, places confirmation calls and handles financial transactions.

Think about yourself. Do you enjoy working as part of a team? Do you enjoy focusing primarily on client well-being? Do you prefer the convenience of an office support staff and less paperwork? Do you like the idea of someone else handling marketing and business logistics?

Do you like working within an established structure? Working in these settings also requires conforming to a set image, policies and procedures. You might need to alter your style and scope of practice to align with the company's vision and schedule.

Take a few moments to review the following chart (Figure 1.4) that highlights the pros and cons of working for an employer. It may provide some new insights as you consider your career path.

Chapter 8
for details on resumes, job interviews and being an employee.

Figure 1.4

Employment Pros and Cons

Pros of Working for an Employer	Cons of Working for an Employer
• Possibility of walking into a full practice with little marketing • Providing a larger scope of services for your clients' well-being • Starting out with a ready-made professional image • Being part of a team with clear and established boundaries • Reduced paperwork (there is usually an office manager) • Ability to focus on hands-on work • Access to better and more varied equipment and supplies • Excellent built-in referral base • Office staff that does the scheduling, places confirmation calls and handles financial transactions • You can receive discounts on services and products • Use of the facilities • Employee benefits can include health insurance, paid vacations, paid sick days, pension plans, profit sharing and reimbursement for continuing education	• Lack of control over the scheduling • Rarely get to choose your clients • Possibly needing to alter your treatments in terms of style, modalities and length • Conforming to a set image, policies and procedures • There is no guarantee your shifts will be filled • Potential to get booked for a specific service even if it isn't clear that you're proficient in that technique or if contraindications are present • In spas there is little chance to mark progress or make lasting connections because clients don't return very often • Possibly required to perform other services when not doing your primary service • Expectation to promote services and products regardless of whether you like them • Sharing a treatment room with other practitioners

Self-Employment ● ●

Private practice is the most prevalent option for wellness practitioners, although not everyone is well suited for this type of enterprise. It takes a certain personality type to be truly successful in one's own business. Successful business owners are inventive and follow through with their plans. They respect money. They possess considerable expertise in their particular career field and have broad experience in several others. They have very good verbal and written communication skills and are usually considered very personable. They are positive thinkers, determined, self-disciplined, service oriented and persistent—they don't quit!

Think about yourself. Do you possess these qualities? In most instances (unless, for example, you have a partner with a lot of business acumen), it's not enough just to have talent, you need to manage the "business." Many small businesses that don't succeed are examples of this problem—talent without proper business skills.

Some of the advantages of being self-employed are having a potentially flexible schedule, being independent, being your own boss and the possibility of receiving tax advantages. Frequently you're more creative and experience increased personal satisfaction and a greater sense of achievement. Self-employment may also offer you a better opportunity to contribute to others.

Disadvantages of being self-employed are the long hours—usually 10 to 14 hours per day, six to seven days a week. As a business owner, not only are you working with clients, you're also actively marketing and managing your practice. In the beginning, you may need to devote two to three hours in business promotion and development for every hour of client interaction. Sometimes the start-up costs are greater than you've anticipated, just printing business cards and mailing notices adds up. You may also experience a deep sense of "aloneness." The income is usually not steady and there are financial risks. Finally, the statistics for success for small businesses aren't exactly inspiring.

According to a 2006 study by the U.S. Small Business Administration (SBA), two-thirds of new companies survive at least two years and about 44 percent continue for at least four years—instead of the more often cited (but inaccurate) statistics that claim that one out of five (20 percent) businesses are successful after five years.[1]

Though the odds are improving, these statistics can still seem quite depressing. At the very least they're cause for concern. The two major reasons for failure are mismanagement and undercapitalization. Mismanagement is generally a result of poor planning, not realistically evaluating strengths and weaknesses, failing to anticipate obstacles, improper budgeting and lacking the necessary business skills. Undercapitalization is not having enough start-up capital or needing to take draw (salary) before the business is firmly established.

Take a few moments to review the chart that highlights the pros and cons of self-employment (Figure 1.5). This career path presents some unique challenges. The chart may help you realistically assess if you have what it takes to run a business.

The U.S. Small Business Administration is a wonderful source of information. The people are friendly and do their best to assist you. The following (revised) questions and worksheets are from their Management Aids MP12.

According to the SBA, niche health and fitness are hot markets for small businesses.

Chapter 12
for specifics on the actual running of a business.

Self-Employment Assessment

- Are you willing to take the risks in being self-employed?
- Do you know how much credit you can get from your suppliers?
- Do you know where you're going to get your start-up funding?
- Have you talked to a banker about your plans?
- If you need/want a partner with money or skills that you don't have, do you know someone who is qualified and appropriate?
- Have you talked to a lawyer about your business?
- Does your family support your plan to be in business?
- Could you net more money working for someone else?

Under each question, check the answer that says what you feel or comes closest to it. Be honest with yourself.

Are you a self-starter?
- ❏ I do things on my own, nobody has to tell me to get going.
- ❏ If someone gets me started, I keep going all right.
- ❏ I don't prefer to put myself out until I have to.

How do you feel about other people?
- ❏ I like people. I can get along with just about everybody.
- ❏ I have plenty of friends—I don't need anyone else.
- ❏ Most people irritate me.

What type of work do you prefer?
- ❏ I prefer a balance of hands-on and mental work.
- ❏ I prefer to focus primarily on client well-being and hands-on work.
- ❏ I prefer to do the least amount of work possible.

Can you lead others?
- ❏ I can get most people to go along when I start something.
- ❏ I can give the orders if someone tells me what we should do.
- ❏ I let someone else get things moving. Then I go along if I feel like it.

Can you take responsibility?
- ❏ I like to take charge of things and see them through.
- ❏ I'll take over if I have to, but I'd rather let someone else be responsible.
- ❏ There's always some eager beaver around wanting to show how smart he is. I say let him.

How good an organizer are you?
- ❏ I like to have a plan before I start. I'm usually the one to get things lined up when the group wants to do something.
- ❏ I do all right unless things get too confused. Then I quit.
- ❏ I get all set and then something comes along and presents too many problems. So I just take things as they come.

How good a worker are you?
- ❏ I can keep going as long as I need to. I don't mind working hard for something I want.
- ❏ I'll work hard for a while, but when I've had enough, that's it!
- ❏ I can't see that hard work gets you anywhere.

Can you make decisions?
- ❏ I can make up my mind in a hurry if I have to. It usually turns out okay, too.
- ❏ I can if I have plenty of time. If I have to make up my mind fast, I think later I should have decided the other way.
- ❏ I don't like to be the one who has to decide things.

Can people trust what you say?
- ❏ You bet they can. I don't say things I don't mean.
- ❏ I try to be on the level most of the time, but sometimes I just say what is easiest.
- ❏ Why bother if the other person doesn't know the difference?

Can you stick with it?
- ❏ If I make up my mind to do something, I don't let anything stop me.
- ❏ I usually finish what I start—if it goes well.
- ❏ If it doesn't go my way right away, I tend to quit.

How good is your health?
- ❏ I never run down.
- ❏ I have enough energy for most things I want to do.
- ❏ I run out of energy sooner than most of my friends seem to.

> **Suggestion:** Before you fill out this checklist, photocopy it for use in your journal or go to www.businessmastery.us to print a copy.

Self-Employment Checklist Scoring Key

After completing the Self-Employment Checklist, count the checks you made beside the answers to each question. How many checks are beside the first answer? The second answer? The third answer?

If most of your checks are beside the first answer, you probably have what it takes to run a business. If not, you're likely to have more trouble than you can handle by yourself. Find a partner who is strong on the points in which you experience challenges. If many checks are beside the third answer, not even a good partner could shore you up.

At this point you still may be uncertain about being self-employed or working for someone else. The next section on Your Ideal Future assists you in discerning what you really want in your life and career.

Figure 1.5

Self-Employment Pros and Cons

Pros of Self-Employment

- You determine the client screening procedures
- Control over standards and scope of practice
- You choose your target markets
- Freedom to determine your image
- Potential for unlimited income
- Opportunity for creativity
- Flexible schedule
- Tax write-offs

Cons of Self-Employment

- Potential for loneliness and isolation
- You take all the risks
- Potential cash flow problems
- Initial funding of the business
- Safety risks are increased if you work alone or provide on-site services
- Might need to delay financial expenditures such as expensive equipment
- You are the one responsible for making certain everything is done
- Responsibility for administrative and logistical activities
- You are responsible for getting and retaining clients
- The only "employment benefits" you receive are the ones you pay for yourself
- No true paid vacations, holidays or sick days

❋ Your Ideal Future ❋

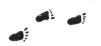

Chapter 3, Pages 43-44

for information on how visualization works.

Creative visualization is a powerful tool for career success. This section stimulates your imagination to visualize and manifest your ideal future. Allow yourself the freedom to state your desires, dreams and goals. Remember, this is about your IDEALS, not necessarily what you think is realistic. We forge some of these dreams into goals in the next chapter. Make any notes in your business journal.

Visualizing Your Life and Career Success

Envisioning your life is one of the most enjoyable aspects of long-range planning. This is where you let your imagination range free. Put aside any concerns about whether your vision is realistic or attainable. If you have any negative thoughts about your ability or worthiness to have this life, acknowledge those thoughts and continue with the exercise. Encompass all areas of your life, including your career, environment, relationships, finances, education, spirituality, health and social life. If you prefer to visualize with your eyes closed, you may want to have a friend read you these questions, or you could make an audio tape of the exercise—leaving ample time for thought between questions.

Your Ideal Life

- *Imagine that you're living the life of your dreams right now. Describe where you live: Where do you reside—what city, state or country? What type of home do you live in? How is it furnished? What is the ambiance? Think about yourself: What do you look like? What are your attitudes toward life? How do you nurture yourself? How do you feel about yourself? Contemplate your relationships: Who are your friends? How do you interact with your family? How do you impact others? What are the important characteristics of your romantic relationship? What is your social life like?*

- *Now think about your career: What is your profession? What are your responsibilities and activities? What type of business atmosphere do you have? Who are your co-workers? What are your business relationships like? What is your financial status?*

- *Reflect upon your personal growth: What activities do you engage in to take care of your well-being? How are you furthering your education? What do you do to foster your spirituality? How do you spend your leisure time?*

- *Lastly, consider any other areas that are important to you: What do you do to make certain these things happen? What are your attitudes about them?*

In summary, the question to ask yourself is: "If I could be anywhere doing anything, where would I be and what would I be doing?" Be sure to note any realizations in your journal. Sometimes what's important are the qualities of life and not necessarily the specific activities. For instance, your future vision might not have "looked" dramatically different from your current status, but perhaps it "felt" different. Maybe you were more relaxed, energetic and happier. The following exercise continues to add depth to your visualization.

Your Ideal Career

1. Where do you want to practice? What city, state or country?

2. Do you want to travel as part of your career? ❑ Yes ❑ No ❑ Maybe If yes, where?

3. How many hours per week do you want to work? Doing what specifically? In addition to client interaction, include the other business-related activities such as marketing, bookkeeping, networking and planning.

4. What type of work location do you want? Do you want to have a private office or work at a medical facility? Do you want an office in your home? Would you rather just do outcalls? Or would you prefer a combination of the above?

5. What type(s) of people do you want to have as clients?

6. Which professions could provide referrals to your business?

7. For which professions can you be a good source of referrals?

8. What benefits do you want your business (or employer) to offer (e.g., health insurance, paid vacations, retirement fund)?

9. Do you want to work as an employee or run your own business?

If you plan to be self-employed, also answer the following questions:

10. Do you want to have multiple locations? ❑ Yes ❑ No ❑ Maybe If yes, where?

11. Do you want any associates? ❑ Yes ❑ No ❑ Maybe
    How many? What would they do?

12. What type of business atmosphere do you want?

13. How much do you want the net business profit to be annually? $ _____

14. How much money do you want for your salary/draw after taxes? $ _____

15. Describe your ideal office/location in detail including external features, the style of decorations, equipment and ambiance.

If you plan to work for someone else, answer the following questions:

16. What is the lowest fee or percentage you will accept? $ _____ or _____ %

17. List at least five places or people for whom you'd like to work.

18. Describe the ideal business agreement. What would you like your employer to offer? What are you willing to provide?

Now comes the difficult part—determining whether you're on the path to making your dreams become reality and ascertaining what you're willing to do to have your life be that of your dreams. It is perfectly okay to not work on everything at once—actually you will probably drive yourself (and those around you) crazy if you attempt to change too many things too quickly.

You may also find that you aren't willing to take some of the required steps to achieve an aspect of your dream. Give yourself permission to set your own boundaries and priorities. This is where dreams differentiate from goals. And thus, Chapter 2.

*Courage is very important.
Like a muscle, it is
strengthened by use.*
— Ruth Gordon

Life Planning

• Goal Setting •

Now that you have assessed your current status and envisioned your ideal work life, it's time to add substance to them by setting clear purposes, priorities and goals for your life and your practice. As you work through this chapter, keep in mind that you may need to revisit it several times to work through all of the exercises. It takes time and patience to anchor your dreams into practical, everyday steps that lead to completed goals. Do not get discouraged if at times it seems overwhelming. Just take a break to re-energize, and come back to your goal setting when you're ready. Keep in mind that goal setting is a lifelong practice.

Goal setting is the means of turning your dreams into reality. Many people imagine great things, yet very few accomplish their dreams. Dreams are similar to wishes: they are things we fantasize about, yet we do little to make certain they occur (but we're certainly ecstatic when they do). Goals are dreams to which you commit and take action to ensure their attainment.

Goal setting is tied into the *reticular activating system (RAS)*. The RAS is a cluster of nerve cells in the brain stem between the myelencephalon (medulla oblongata) and mesencephalon (midbrain) that regulates alertness and attention. It is also believed to be the center of arousal and motivation. Our senses (particularly sight) are constantly flooded with a vast amount of stimuli, yet we're consciously aware of only a fraction of that data. Most of that information is unnecessary for our well-being, so it gets screened. In essence, we have programmed directional signalers (or in some cases, blinders) in our brains. Although this may seem like an oversimplification, it's indeed how it functions.

For example, recall the last time you decided to get a new car. You finally chose the model and color, and it seemed like everywhere you went, you saw "your car." Of course all those people didn't just go out and purchase those cars when you did. Those cars were already on the road. You just hardly noticed them before because they weren't significant to you. This is the magnificence of goal setting. By establishing clear goals, you're programming your brain to be aware and notify your conscious mind of the information and opportunities that YOU DESIRE.

The future belongs to those who believe in the beauty of their dreams.
— Eleanor Roosevelt

The inability to actualize goals is usually related to unclear goals, lack of commitment, conflict or negative conditioning. Very few people write goals, and of those who do, most don't always write their goals in a way that easily produces results. Sometimes they claim to want something, but what they really want is what that something represents. Occasionally conflicts exist in relation to the achievement of their goals. The attainment of one goal may preclude the fulfillment of another, or the consequences may not be viewed favorably by their immediate family or colleagues.

Setting Realistic Goals ⬟

If you have built castles in the air, your work need not be lost; that is where they should be. Now put foundations under them.
— Henry David Thoreau

The first step is to set aside some time to think about your goals and put them into writing. It may be helpful to review your written goals to be sure that they reflect your true desires—not what your spouse, parent, boss or peers think you should want.

Sometimes it can be tempting to set unrealistic deadlines or goals that are dependent on other people. It is also easy to get caught up in a flurry of goal writing and generate pages and pages of goals, then hardly accomplish anything. At other times, we may get so bogged down in details that we lose sight of the big picture.

As you can see, setting realistic goals is often a balancing act. It requires careful thought. While you reach for your greatest potential, it's important to ground your dreams in step-by-step actions that help you achieve your goals.

The Power of Goals ● ●

The purpose of life is a life of purpose.
— Robert Byrne

Whitney W. Lowe

Bend, Oregon

Whitney Lowe has been setting goals for more than a decade. He is a very self-disciplined person, and once he learned about goal setting, he took to it right away. He sets goals because, "I have found this to be an important part of the planning process as well as the process of measuring my success. When I set goals, it's the first step in giving me direction about how to get where I want to go. Once the goal is established, I can work backwards from there until I have identified all the smaller steps that are necessary to accomplish that goal. Unless some of the bigger goals are broken down into these smaller steps, it's very difficult to get started working on them. I feel that I have accomplished some very large tasks, such as getting a book finished and constantly meeting production deadlines for my bimonthly research newsletter. I have also set goals for myself in relation to my massage practice that are just as important. For example, I have found when I set small goals for studying and reviewing topics of anatomy, kinesiology or pathology, it was much easier to accomplish this study, and I really looked forward to it."

Purpose, Priorities and Goals ✳

Purpose ● ●

You need a context for your goals, something to connect them. Otherwise they become chores, and most people do almost anything to avoid chores. **Purpose** provides that context. Purpose is very general—it's a direction, a theme. You can never actually complete a purpose; it's an ongoing process. Take a moment and think about what is really meaningful to you. Is there a common thread—one statement that encompasses your ideals, values and dreams? You may have a purpose for your life and purposes for every major area of your life.

What you get by achieving your goals is not as important as what you become by achieving your goals.
— Zig Ziglar

Overall Life Purpose Examples ● ● ●
- I make a positive difference.
- I am happy.
- My life is an expression of love and joy.

You may find your life purpose shifting over time, becoming more refined. Remember, it isn't written in stone, though in most instances your priorities and goals are more likely to change, and not your life purpose. One of the most significant features of having a distinct life purpose is that it becomes easier to resolve any conflicting goals when you know the direction for your life.

Career Purpose Examples ● ● ●
- My career supports myself and others in being happy and healthy.
- I make a healthy difference.
- My career is a source of joy and prosperity.
- I am innovative and successful in my career.
- My career is a joyous expression of who I am.

Priorities ● ●

Priorities are general areas of concern. They are less vague and not so all-encompassing as purposes, yet not as specific as goals. Priorities are statements of intention that are connected with values.

General Life Priorities Examples ● ● ●
- My relationships are nurturing and fun.
- I am creative in all that I do.
- Each and every day I learn something new.
- My body is a manifestation of health and beauty.
- My communications are open and honest.

Career Priorities Examples • • •

- My career is fulfilling and provides me with the income that I desire.
- I enjoy my work.
- I regularly participate with other colleagues.
- I continually expand my knowledge and skills.
- I am creative in my work.
- My work environment is nurturing and professional.

Goals • •

Goals are very specific things, events or experiences that have a definite completion, and you can objectively know when you've achieved them. Effective goals have the characteristics found in the acronym of SMARTER:

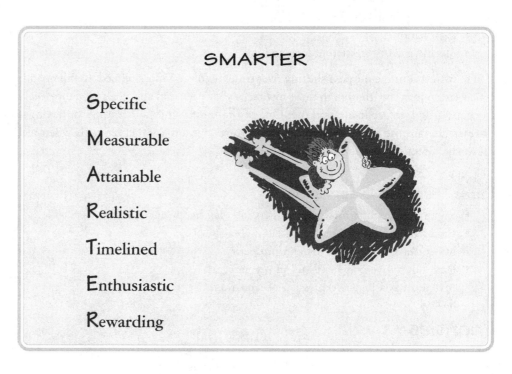

SMARTER

Specific

Measurable

Attainable

Realistic

Timelined

Enthusiastic

Rewarding

Career Goal Examples • • •

- I earn at least $40,000 per year.
- I have a wonderful music system in my office.
- I keep my client files current.
- I invest at least five hours each week in marketing.
- I review my business plan every three months.
- I read at least one business-related book each month.
- I am an active member of two business groups.

The secret of success is constancy to purpose.
— Benjamin Disraeli

If one advances confidently in the direction of his dreams, and endeavors to live the life which he has imagined, he will meet with a success unexpected in common hours.
— Henry David Thoreau

Goal Setting Techniques

1. Always state your goals in the positive PRESENT TENSE. If you write in the future, they may remain in the future—never attained.
2. Personalize your goals: use a pronoun (e.g., I, we, they, "your name") in every sentence.
3. Make your goals real: something you know you can accomplish on your own without help or without someone waving a magic wand over you.
4. Do not use the terms "try," "will," "not," "never," "should," "would," "could" and "want."
5. Include deadline dates whenever possible.
6. Have fun!

Effective goal setting is the groundwork for success. I advocate that you have written goals in addition to any other techniques you employ. The written word is so powerful! By inscribing your intentions, you say to yourself and the world that you know you deserve to have these things happen. Sometimes people are afraid to write down their goals because they don't think they can achieve them, and thus they don't want a written reminder of their failures.

Failure, per se, doesn't really exist in goal setting. Usually when you don't accomplish a goal it's due to setting an inappropriate deadline, having inaccurate information, experiencing blocks, encountering conflicts, not really wanting the goal or being unwilling (or unable) to do what's required to accomplish the goal. Having written goals can only serve to support and teach you, enhancing your self-knowledge.

One of the ways to magnify the power of your goals is to involve as many of your senses as possible (particularly sight, touch and sound) in the process. In addition to writing, you may want to use a variety of methods from visual illustration to audio recordings to physical representations.

Great things are not done by impulse, but by a series of small things brought together.
— Vincent van Gogh

Make a Collage ••

Collages are a wonderful way to visually create your goals. To make a collage, get a large piece of poster board (22" x 28" is available in many colors at art supply stores). Set aside a couple of hours, get comfortable, put on some nice music, make yourself a cup of tea, get a stack of magazines, a pair of scissors and some glue, and prepare to have a fantastic experience! (By the way, this is a lot of fun to do with friends.) The next thing to do is to decide the purpose of your collage—be it a representation of your whole life, your career, the next six months or even just one major goal. Keeping your purpose in mind, go through the magazines and cut out pictures and words that appeal to you. Let your intuition be your guide. The items you choose may not be what you had anticipated. Don't worry about finding the "perfect" pictures or words. They may be very abstract or elicit a certain emotion. Remember, this is a representation of your dreams and goals.

Give yourself a time limit for cutting, or else you may find yourself there for days. After you've cut out plenty of pictures and words, glue them onto the poster board. You also may want to write some goals or affirmations on the board. Then spend some time with your collage—allow yourself to experience the full impact. Finally, hang your collage in a place where you can see it every day.

Create a Picture Book • •

Picture Books are a combination of a collage and a picture book. Instead of gluing the pictures and words to paper or poster board, you pin them on a bulletin board. This technique makes it easy to literally shift your goals—put them in different perspective, add more goals and take them down once they've been achieved. The supplies needed are a large, three-ring binder, a set of at least eight dividers, notebook paper, scissors, glue and magazines. Use the dividers to arrange the categories of your goals (e.g., health, finances, education, marketing). Follow the same directions for the collage, except glue the pictures and words by category onto notebook paper and then put the sheets in the binder. You can write your goals next to the pictures. The advantages of a picture book are that you can carry it with you and you can easily add more pages to it. The disadvantage is that you may not look at it as frequently as you would a collage.

The more frequently you review your goals, the more likely you are to achieve them.

Record Your Goals • •

Audiotape Recordings of your goals are very effective. Write out your goals before you tape them, following the suggested Goal Setting Techniques. If possible, use a high-quality recording system. The beauty of taping your goals is that you can listen to them at any time. It can be particularly beneficial to listen to your tape while sleeping for the subliminal effects. An interesting alternative is to have someone who is a positive authority figure, role model or mentor record some of the goals. Experiment!

You have to know what you want to get it.
— Gertrude Stein

Build a Miniature Replica • •

Physical Representations are excellent tools for depicting your goal(s). The idea is to create a three-dimensional object that you can see and touch. This can be very powerful. It makes you really "look" at what you say you want. Generally it's a time-intensive endeavor, but it can be well worth it, particularly for the goals that are very meaningful to you and the ones you find difficult to achieve.

For example, if one of your goals is to remodel your office, you may want to build a miniature version of your office with all of the proposed changes. Get samples of the paint or wallpaper and put them on the walls. Make (or buy) miniature furniture. Create it as closely as possible to your plans. If one of your goals is to exercise regularly, you may want to make a sculpture of yourself exercising. If you cannot easily recognize yourself, attach a photo of your face to the sculpture.

Pay attention to details. Make your replica as realistic as possible. Don't let a (perceived) lack of artistic proficiency limit your creativity in visualizing and expressing your goals. Be inventive and have fun!

The inclusion of scent adds another potent dimension. For example, if you've been telling yourself for the last few years that you'd really like to take a winter vacation in the mountains and you still haven't left the city, it may be that you need to make that goal more tangible. You might want to design a model of the desired location. Start by making a mini-mountain. Then construct a little cabin, and inside it put pictures of yourself and whomever else you want for company. Make some pine trees (using real pine needles if possible), and put pine essence on the trees. Now, every time you walk by your mountain, you see it, touch it, take in a deep breath and smell the pine trees....

Writing your Goals • •

Written Goals are a powerful visual (and actually auditory) declaration of your intentions. The two most commonly used methods for goal setting are outline format and mind mapping. The **Outline** technique is very effective for logical thinkers. When you use the outline format (see Figure 2.1), you write your purpose and your priorities, and list the specific goals under each priority.

The **Mind Mapping** approach is excellent for visually-oriented thinkers. In mind mapping (see Figure 2.2), you actually write the purpose in the center of a page, attach spokes to the circle onto which you list the priorities, and extend lines off of each spoke onto which you write the specific goals. Another mind-mapping option is to draw an image in the middle of a page (such as an office filled with clients or a stack of money). Then add related images as well as written priorities and goals.

You may find it helpful to use a combination of these two goal setting methods. Post your major goals in a prominent place where you can see it, (although not in your clients' view). One of the benefits of having written goals is that it's much easier to track progress. The other major advantage of writing your goals is you can cross them out when they're completed—this contributes to feelings of accomplishment, reward and acknowledgment.

Opportunity is missed by most people because it is dressed in overalls and looks like work.
— Thomas Edison

Figure 2.1

Outline Format Example

Purpose: My career is an expression of who I am.

Priority 1: I continually expand my knowledge and skills.

Priority 1 Goals: Each month I meet with colleagues to share business experiences.

> I read at least two business magazines each month.
> I take a public speaking course before my second year in business.

Priority 2: My work environment is professional and nurturing.

Priority 2 Goals: I paint my office by July 1.

> I have a wonderful music system in my office by August 15.
> I clean my office every week.

Priority 3: My career provides me with the income I desire.

Priority 3 Goals: I earn at least $40,000 this year.

> I take a three-week vacation this winter.
> I increase my client retention rate by at least 20 percent.

Figure 2.2

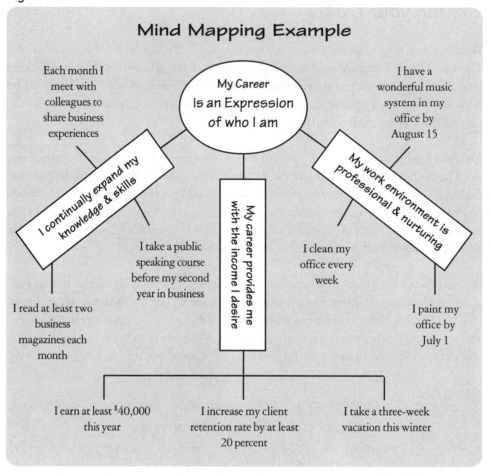

Mind Mapping Example

My Career is an Expression of who I am

Each month I meet with colleagues to share business experiences

I continually expand my knowledge & skills

I read at least two business magazines each month

I take a public speaking course before my second year in business

My career provides me with the income I desire

I clean my office every week

I have a wonderful music system in my office by August 15

My work environment is professional & nurturing

I paint my office by July 1

I earn at least $40,000 this year

I increase my client retention rate by at least 20 percent

I take a three-week vacation this winter

When setting goals use the format with which you feel the most comfortable and proves to be the most effective. It is important to have written goals in addition to any other format, particularly for your career. You may want to use some of the other methods as a means of positive reinforcement or visualization. What is crucial is the way you actually state your goals and the individual steps necessary to accomplish them. Keep your goals SMARTER, follow the suggested goal setting techniques and, most importantly of all, be sure they're YOUR goals. Setting goals can be creative and exciting. If you tend to use mainly one method, experiment with other techniques. Use as many of your senses as possible. Goal setting is a necessary component of success, but it doesn't have to be a burden. Remember, the purpose of setting goals is to make your dreams become reality.

Clarifying Your Life Vision •

Before you even begin to consider developing or enhancing your practice, it's imperative to set a strong foundation by clarifying your life's purpose, priorities and goals. Then you can more effectively create your other plans. The following exercise guides you in writing your purpose, priorities and goals for your overall life—with a focus on your career for the next five years, three years, one year and six months. Your Wheel of Life and the previous exercises in this chapter and Chapter 1 can serve as guides.

Life Planning

Take a few deep breaths, relax and let your dreams and goals express themselves. Let them guide your mind, heart and hands. For now, don't worry about "how" you write them. Let your creativity flow. You can always go back later and rephrase your statements. Start by clarifying your life purpose. Review your Personal Assessment Exercises from Chapter 1. Think about your values, ideals and dreams. Create a statement that reflects the essence of your life. Next, think about the aspects of life that are meaningful to you, and create priorities for those areas. Be sure to include all areas on the Wheel of Life. Then identify your life goals. Repeat this process for your five-year, three-year, one-year and six-month plan.

Overall Life Plan

My purpose in life is...
My major priorities in life are...
My major goals in life are...

Five-Year Plan

My purpose for the next five years is...
My major priorities for the next five years are...
My major goals for the next five years are...

Three-Year Plan

My purpose for the next three years is...
My major priorities for the next three years are...
My major goals for the next three years are...

One-Year Plan

My purpose for the next year is...
My major priorities for the next year are...
My major goals for the next year are...

Six-Month Plan

My purpose for the next six months is...
My major priorities for the next six months are...
My major goals for the next six months are...

Planning Reflection Exercise

Now that you've taken the time to clarify your purposes, priorities and goals, it's time for reflection. Ask yourself the following questions:

- What do I need to change in my life to accomplish these things?
- What help from others do I need to achieve success in these areas?
- Who are the people that can help me?
- What problems do I anticipate when acting on these goals?
- What will I achieve if I complete these goals?

Ranking Goals ✳

Congratulations! You now have written your intentions for your life and created your purposes, priorities and goals for your career. Having built this foundation puts you miles ahead of the general public and well on your path to success. Just writing some of your goals may be all the planning you need to do.

Not all goals or activities carry the same ultimate value. Some goals have a higher intrinsic worth, while others require more immediate action. This holds true whether you're planning your life, month, week or day. Review your goal lists and rank them with an "A," "B" or "C." The "A" goals are the ones that are the most crucial for you to attain—the ones you can commit to right now. The "B" goals have importance to you, but aren't as significant as the "A" goals. The "C" goals are ones that would be nice if they actualized, but you are not ready to commit to accomplishing them at this moment.

The next step in ranking your goals is to arrange them in terms of time priority. Start with your "A" goals. Make sure all goals have assigned target dates for completion. Then numerically rank each goal according to time priority (1 being the highest). Using the Sample Career Goals (see page 16), your time priority list might look like this:

> 7. *I earn at least* $40,000 *per year.*
> 5. *I have a wonderful music system in my office.*
> 2. *I keep my client files current.*
> 6. *I review my business plan every three months.*
> 1. *I invest at least five hours each week in marketing.*
> 4. *I read at least one business-related book each month.*
> 3. *I am an active member of two business groups.*

✳ Strategic Planning ✳

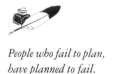

People who fail to plan, have planned to fail.
— George Hewell

We've all heard the cliché, "If you want to get something done, ask a busy person." This is because busy people have learned (often by necessity) how to plan and organize their lives. We can incorporate those skills into our lives so that we do not become overwhelmed or miss opportunities.

Some goals may be very complex and require numerous sub-steps to be accomplished. This process of "divide and conquer" (i.e., breaking down a difficult problem into manageable chunks) is what strategic planning is about. Beware! This is also the stage that many people neglect to do and therefore become overwhelmed.

Let's say that your vision is to: work with 25 clients each week; practice in an office space with other wellness practitioners; share a secretary who handles all the paperwork, bookkeeping and scheduling; and net $45,000 per year. Of the many goals necessary to manifest this vision, the goal we use to illustrate the strategic planning process is to increase weekly clientele bookings from 15 to 25 clients within six months. See Figure 2.4.

Strategic planning is a layered system: start with your major goal, analyze it, and break it into smaller goals and steps. You may find that some of the smaller steps need to be refined further. I recommend that you make a master list of the activities required to achieve the major goal and use separate sheets for each project. In the strategic planning illustration, several of the goals need to have their own project sheet because of the many steps required to attain the goal (e.g., getting interviewed and doing the cooperative marketing projects). Other goals are more straightforward and self-explanatory, such as reading three business books and doing daily affirmations. If you experience any resistance or difficulty with any of your goals, break the goal down into as many specific steps as possible.

The most elaborate plan isn't going to create results if it isn't implemented. Transfer your goals and items from strategic planning sheets to a calendar, or create a simple tracking document on your computer (calendar programs make planning much less cumbersome). Refer to it often. It takes time, but long-term planning is time well invested. The clarity you acquire and the organization you create always save you at least the amount of time spent in actual planning.

Luck is a matter of preparation meeting opportunity.
— Oprah Winfrey

Figure 2.3

Action Steps for Strategic Planning

1. List the current date and target date for accomplishing the goal.
2. Identify the major goal.
3. Describe the existing situation.
4. List the benefits of achieving the goal.
5. Brainstorm possible courses of action.
6. Choose the best solution.
7. Outline an action plan.
8. Determine potential challenges and solutions.
9. Identify required resources.
10. Outline action steps and target date for each step.

Figure 2.4

Strategic Planning Example

Today's Date: February 15   **Target Date:** August 15

Goal: I work with at least 25 clients per week.

Situation Description: I have been in practice for almost two years. I had a corporate account with ABC Electronics, but the company relocated. Now I am averaging only 15 clients per week.

Benefits of Achieving This Goal: I can meet my lifestyle needs, pay off my school loans, take a vacation and start a savings account.

Possible Courses of Action:

1. Get a part-time job at a clinic.
2. Hire an agent.
3. Actively market my practice.

Best Course: The most appropriate long-term solution is to actively market my practice, which could also include securing another corporate account.

Proposal Outline: To have 25 clients per week, I need a base of 100 active clients: five weekly, 15 biweekly, 40 monthly and 40 occasional. I design a creative, fun marketing plan that includes increasing client retention.

Advantages: By augmenting my client list, I increase the odds of achieving my goal. Once my base is established, I won't have to put in as much effort into getting new clients because I incorporate client retention techniques.

Potential Conflicts/Disadvantages:

1. I don't really like marketing.
2. I'm not sure what to do.
3. There's a new company (with four therapists) offering corporate massage.

Solutions:

1. Do clearing exercises. Remind myself that marketing is simply sharing who I am and what I do. Do some of my marketing activities with colleagues.
2. Read books and magazines. Take marketing classes. Work with a business coach. Invest five hours per week on marketing.
3. Affiliate myself with the corporate massage company. Or determine what my differential advantage is and pursue other accounts.

Action Required to Begin: Review my client files to determine massage frequency. Set aside at least two hours to outline my marketing plan.

Resources Needed: Time, paper, pencils and files. Ideally, samples of other therapists' marketing plans.

There is no such thing as an inappropriate goal, just a faulty time frame.

Specific Steps to Achieve This Goal	Target Date
I receive weekly massages	Starting 2/15
I finalize my marketing plan (vision, goals and analysis)	2/28
I invest five hours per week to marketing for new clients	Starting 3/1
I attend at least two networking functions monthly	Starting 3/1
I do daily affirmations	Starting 3/1
I invest two hours per week in client retention	Starting 3/1
I do thorough intake interviews and treatment plans with all my clients	Starting 3/1
For each of the next six months I add 10 new clients to my client base	Starting 3/1
I distribute at least 150 business cards monthly	Starting 3/1
I do weekly client follow-up through calls and cards	Starting 3/1
I review and update my marketing plan monthly	Starting 3/1
I redesign my brochures	3/20
I sponsor a Massage-a-thon for my favorite charity	3/20
I join a business support group	3/30
I send a letter containing some type of incentive to non-current clients	3/30
I secure at least one corporate massage account	4/30
I distribute at least 100 brochures monthly	Starting 4/1
I make at least one corporate massage proposal/presentation monthly	Starting 4/1
I do at least two presentations/demonstrations monthly	Starting 4/1
I contact at least two allied wellness practitioners monthly	Starting 4/1
I send a welcome packet to all new clients	Starting 4/1
I read at least three business books	4/1, 6/1, 8/1
I send a newsletter to my clients	4/20, 7/20
I participate in at least two cooperative marketing projects	5/15, 7/15
I have a booth at the Wellness Expo	5/20
I develop a summer special for current clients	5/25
I get interviewed by the local paper	5/31
I am a featured guest on two radio programs	6/2
I host a chair massage booth at the Annual Street Fair	6/15
I appear on four television programs	6/30
I continue to add four new clients each month	Starting 9/1

Strategic Planning

www.businessmastery.us/
forms.php#busman
for blank copies of the
Strategic Planning sheets.

Figure 2.5

Strategic Planning Benefits

- You're less likely to forget a major step.
- Creative ideas and brainstorming come easier.
- Goals become clarified and more real.
- You gain a better overall picture.
- You realize that some steps may require more immediate action than others.
- You gain knowledge of what is necessary to accomplish the goal.
- A more accurate timetable is developed.
- A written description of your intentions is a self-motivational tool.

The method of the enterprising is to plan with audacity, and execute with vigor; to sketch out a map of possibilities; and then to treat them as probabilities.

— Bovee

Planning helps renew enthusiasm, especially if a goal is tough to accomplish. Whenever you reduce a goal to its component parts, the small steps toward reaching it are less overwhelming and more possible. You gain confidence with each little step forward.

• Follow-Through •

Creating your life to be what you desire is a lifelong process. Putting your goals into writing is the first step. To increase the potential of achieving your goals you need to rely on a variety of skills and everyday activities:

- Identify and clear obstacles.
- Take time to develop a strategic plan.
- Prioritize your daily activities.
- Track your goals.
- Develop a daily practice of using visualization and affirmations.

A knowledge of the path cannot be substituted for putting one foot in front of the other.

— M.C. Richards

So far we have covered methods for self-exploration, goal setting and strategic planning. Tracking goals and prioritizing your activities are techniques to assist you in staying on target. These topics, along with useful tools for achieving your goals, such as visualization, affirmation, clearing techniques and some newly developed techniques to transform negative subconscious beliefs, are examined in Chapter 3.

Success Strategies

• What Is Success? •

"Thriving on chaos" is a phrase that Tom Peters has made common in the marketplace, and is also an apt description of how many of us lead our lives. But what is the price of our success through chaos? Have we excised ourselves (and our families) from our lives? It is easy to get enmeshed in our projects—telling ourselves that we will take time off next weekend, or maybe next month, well, at least sometime this year....

Quite often we have conflicting ideas of what it means to be successful and our requirements for success may vary greatly in the personal, business and social realms. What does success really mean to you? Are you successful only if you earn a certain amount of money, perform miracles in your work, look a particular way, are in a perfect relationship, drive a great car or live in the right neighborhood? In other words, what are your values? Is success a "thing" to achieve or a way of being?

In the book *Lead, Follow, or Get Out of the Way*, Jim Lundy describes success as the achievement of predetermined goals.[1] This means any goal! The key word is "predetermined." For instance, you may have accomplished something (possibly even something major) that you hadn't really intended or even given much thought to and somehow the victory seemed hollow. Most likely that feeling was because you hadn't previously claimed it as a goal. Achievements are so much more fulfilling when they're planned. Thus, success is really a process—one that involves setting and achieving goals.

People are always blaming their circumstances for what they are. I don't believe in circumstances. The people who get on in this world are the people who get up and look for the circumstances they want, and, if they can't find them, make them.
— George Bernard Shaw

Figure 3.1

Typical Success Markers

- Gross income a business generates
- Profit or salary
- Number of years in practice
- Number of years in current job
- Scope of practice
- Total client base
- Number of clients seen each week
- Number of hours worked
- Amount of leisure time enjoyed
- Number of associates and employees
- Office location, square footage or ambiance
- Prominence on a local, national or international level

Identify Your Success Markers

List your success markers. Refer to the values exercises in Chapter 1 and explore how your values relate to your success. Identify what's truly important to you in terms of your overall life and then determine your career success markers. Only you can determine what success is for you—although others might attempt to influence you. As the saying goes, "One person's junk is another's treasure."

Self-Management •

There is truly an art to being successful in the business world while staying balanced. It would be simple if our lives weren't filled with meaningful activities. That just isn't the case. Most of us have a career or business, a family, social activities and civic responsibilities. All of these are important. At times we may feel as though we're jugglers in a circus—keeping everything going, yet not fully enjoying any one aspect. So, what can we do? We certainly can't create a 30-hour day.

The key to success is self-management. Self-management is artfully directing your life so that you easily and joyfully accomplish what you desire. It is about taking personal responsibility for every facet of your life and increasing personal productivity while staying true to yourself. See Figure 3.2 for some of the components of effective self-management.

Figure 3.2

> ## Effective Self-Management Components
>
> - Knowing your values and living them
> - Clarifying your purpose
> - Setting priorities and goals
> - Managing your time effectively
> - Taking business risks wisely
> - Staying inspired
> - Balancing your personal and professional life
> - Overcoming barriers to your success
> - Committing to lifelong learning and professional development

• Barriers to Success •

Nothing in life is to be feared. It is only to be understood.
— Marie Curie

To make the road to success a bit easier to travel, we take a look at some common barriers and what you can do to overcome them. Barriers to success can take varying shapes in our everyday lives and show up at the most inopportune times. Perhaps you've met the "Inner Critic," who stands ready to deliver a hefty dose of self-doubt or unhelpful criticism. Or you may find yourself enjoying a career success moment and the next day you make some odd blunder that casts a shadow on what you previously accomplished. Perhaps you find yourself coming up with incredibly creative ways to procrastinate. If any of these scenarios sound familiar, rest assured you aren't alone. These barriers to success and others are familiar to most successful professionals. They have wisely taken the time to understand the most common barriers and found effective ways to overcome them. Most barriers to success have their roots in negative conditioning. The good news is that you can change this conditioning.

Attitudes, Beliefs and Perceptions •

Your attitude, not your aptitude, will determine your altitude.
— Zig Ziglar

Attitude plays a critical role in determining the difference between self-sabotage and success. Attitude is how one decides to approach something. Attitude is a choice. Attitude is the "lens" that colors how we view life experiences. All too often when we encounter something new or challenging we automatically have a negative attitude about it. But if we choose to look at the new situation objectively and decide to stay open to learn more about it, our attitude already changes from a negative one to a positive one that is willing to adjust to the new circumstances.

Our attitudes stem from our beliefs. Ron Dalrymple, author of *The Inner Manager*,[2] states the following about false beliefs:

> "As children, we are conditioned to believe many things and to adopt the arbitrary attitudes, emotions and behaviors of others. The delusions become our accepted reality. History is filled with examples of humankind's false beliefs, misperceptions and misguided behavior. Many of us limit and constrict ourselves daily with such notions. All of it's unnecessary."

> "Perhaps the greatest thing to discover in life is that our potential for creativity, accomplishment and success is far greater than our imaginations allow. Motivational psychologists tell us if we can conceive it and believe it, we can achieve it. The power of thought, fueled by focused, positive emotions and consistent behavior, produces results of immense proportions. We must learn how the mind truly works and how we can best work with it, to get the most out of life and out of our practices."

While the ability to cultivate and maintain a positive attitude is a key to success, developing clear perception also keeps you on track to achieve your goals. Perception is much like attitude, although it's not always about choice. When we are faced with something new or challenging, we can choose to have a positive attitude toward it but that doesn't mean that we automatically perceive it for what it is.

One of the wonders of life is the ability of people to "see" things in a different light. For instance, if you interview 10 people who have witnessed an event, you likely get 10 different depictions. Our perceptions are affected by our history, beliefs and physiology. This is why it's vital to get feedback from trusted advisors. It is so easy to get tunnel vision and believe that your perception is the **absolute** truth.

How to Avoid Self-Sabotage ✴

If you find yourself slipping into negative self-talk, repeating errors and not learning from past mistakes, procrastinating or surrounding yourself with inappropriate people, chances are a subtle undercurrent of self-sabotage is at work. Other common indicators of self-sabotage are blaming others for your misfortune or expecting failure.

The Inner Critic ● ●

Often the inner critic, that internal voice that tells us we're not good enough or that points out our faults and imperfections, becomes a formidable barrier to our success. This voice usually results from well-intended adults telling us as children what mistakes we were making. Unfortunately, when we internalized these comments as children, we had no filter in place to pick and choose which ones were useful and which ones weren't. So as adults, we are left with the whole bag. The inner critic can remind us to slow down when we are impatient. But it can also generate feelings of inadequacy as it nitpicks at everything we do, contributing to our barriers rather than our successes.

Page 48
for techniques to dissolve problems.

Perception Exercises
www.grand-illusions.com/opticalillusions

www.sandlotscience.com

Human beings can alter their lives by altering their attitudes.
— William James

Establishing a Helpful Relationship with Your Inner Critic[3]
by C. Diane Ealy, Ph.D.

Begin to take control of your inner critic by getting an image of it. What does it look like? You may need to close your eyes to see this image. Give yourself time for the picture to develop. What does the voice sound like? What does the critic feel like? Conjure up as vivid a picture of it as you can.

Now start a dialogue with it. You may want to conduct this discussion in writing, out loud (you probably ought to be alone if you choose this option), or inside your head. Acknowledge the positive things your inner critic can help you accomplish: more patience, increased attention to necessary details, making time for relaxation. Explain that it interferes with your progress when it criticizes you without compassion and at times when you are creating or otherwise making forward progress. This is the aspect of the inner critic that you want to be free of and it needs to understand this. If it thinks you are trying to destroy it completely, it will fight hard for its life. You will have an extremely difficult task in trying to quiet it. So clearly explain to it that you want to keep the beneficial aspects and mute the destructive ones, that there's a time for it to speak and a time to be silent.

To accomplish this separation, ask your inner critic to be quiet when it starts nagging. When you hear its voice, simply saying "stop" may be enough to quiet it. You may mentally hold up a stop sign or put your hand out in a motion that says "stop." Initially, you will probably have to use more force than simply asking for silence. You may have to imagine putting it on a shelf, outside of your office, or even outdoors. (I used to put mine into a brown burlap bag, tie it with a drawstring, then put it outside.) Always remind your inner critic you will invite it back when you need it.

During your communication with your inner critic, be respectful. After all, it thinks it's being helpful to you. Once you point out how it gets in your way and how it can benefit you, it will become increasingly helpful. Transforming your inner critic into an inner helper takes time, so be patient with yourself and with it. You will be rewarded with an inner voice that is a helpful guide, or editor, or whatever you need.

Negative Conditioning ● ●

People are greatly influenced by events that have happened to them throughout their lifetime. Often we allow (subconsciously or consciously) our past mistakes, incompletions and even our successes to obstruct the creation and accomplishment of new goals. We are not always aware just how much impact our past has on our present and future.

We are a product of our experience. To cope with emotionally painful and difficult life events, it's common to respond with what is popularly referred to as "survival skills." The resulting beliefs and behavior tendencies, which may work well in the short term, can sometimes get in the way of living a happy and productive life. For instance, conclusions formed in the past may have been based upon false information or useful for a situation that was only valid at that time. Just because particular actions were effective in past situations doesn't mean they will work equally well in the future. Simply stated, it's extremely difficult to be creative and spontaneous when shouldering the burden of the past.

Releasing negative thought patterns is not always easy, but the results of doing so are worth the effort. When you're detached from those past beliefs and attitudes, you can replace them with new supportive thoughts that contribute to having your life be the way YOU want. Frequently, this clearing stage is overlooked (or worse, considered irrelevant or too time-consuming) and people attempt to move directly into repatterning. This is one reason why setting goals, writing affirmations, visualizing your goals and listening to motivational recordings don't always work.

Tap Into Your Inner Power ● ● ●

Sometimes lingering conflicts and negative conditioning need to be unearthed, acknowledged and accepted before they can be replaced. For clearing to be truly effective, it must take place on all levels: mental, emotional, physical and spiritual. The clearing process requires recognizing that a block exists and being willing to go through whatever it takes to fully release it, even if that means re-experiencing the buried negativity and pain.

Many people have used clearing techniques to pave the way to career success. Some well-known techniques include psychotherapy, bodywork/massage, yoga, rebirthing, some forms of martial arts, energy balancing, water flotation tanks, transpersonal counseling, hypnotherapy, meditation, cognitive therapy, psychic work and written/verbal clearing exercises. Sometimes professional help is needed to break free from limiting beliefs rooted in the subconscious mind. This is particularly true if you find yourself bumping up against the same old behaviors and habits, confronting the same old thorny issues. Counselors trained in such methods as PSYCH-K and Emotional Freedom Techniques specialize in this type of personal growth work. Based on new discoveries regarding the body's subtle energies, these techniques have proven highly successful for many.

You may choose one or more techniques depending upon the issue. All of them aim to empower you to realize your deepest desires and to achieve career success. You may respond better to one type of clearing technique than another. Experiment!

If you bring forth what is inside you, what you bring forth will save you.
— The Gospel
        according to Thomas

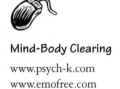

Mind-Body Clearing

www.psych-k.com
www.emofree.com

Sentence Completions Clearing Technique ● ● ●

An example of one technique for releasing old thought patterns is called *sentence completions*. This clearing process is designed to elicit conscious and unconscious thoughts, attitudes, beliefs and feelings so that they can be recognized and released, thus enabling you to be more free to achieve what you really desire.

You can do these exercises alone by writing or verbally with a partner. If you want to do it verbally, have your partner ask you the questions and you let your answers come out uncensored. Your partner's role is to keep you moving through the process.

The directions for this exercise are: Designate one page for each question. At the top of the first page, write down the first question. Answer the question with the first thoughts that come to your mind. Don't try to figure out the "right" answers, as there are none. Let your thoughts and feelings come out uncensored.

Continue to list your thoughts. Fill the whole page. It isn't necessary to write complete sentences. Occasionally reread the question and list any new or different thoughts. Some of your answers may not make sense and that's okay. When you think that the list is finished, go over it again. Add any additional thoughts. For instance, with the clearing sentence of, "The Things that are important to me are..." responses might be:

Doing what I want	*Friends*
Success	*Tacos*
Feeling good about myself	*Money*
Having fun	*Movies*
Making a difference in the world	*Traveling*
Being healthy	*Happiness*

Remember, it might not make sense—but if that's what's there, respect it.

Notice any unconscious defense mechanisms that may occur to distract you such as thoughts (e.g., the other things you really ought to be doing, how hungry you are, how silly this exercise is), daydreaming, falling asleep or going blank. If you're experiencing these defenses, stop briefly, acknowledge to yourself what is happening and then continue with the exercise.

Do this same procedure for each question. It is common to find that some of your answers are the same or quite similar for different questions. Do not restrict any of the answers that come up.

The following sentence completions exercise is designed to assist you in removing obstacles to fulfilling your dreams. Go to your business journal. Set aside 21 pages and follow the preceding instructions.

It's not whether you get knocked down. It's whether you get up again.
— Vince Lombardi

Sentence Completions

1. The things I've wanted to accomplish, but haven't are...
2. The projects I've begun, but never completed are...
3. The communications I've withheld are...
4. The goals I've put off are...
5. The things for which I haven't forgiven myself are...
6. The things for which I haven't forgiven others are...
7. The things that are important to me are...
8. Some of my major goals in life are...
9. I see myself as...
10. Others perceive me as...
11. If I could do anything I want and earn money doing it, I would...
12. Money, to me, is...
13. The people and circumstances that influence my success are...
14. Having a successful career means...
15. The ways my career supports me in achieving my life goals are...
16. The ways my career limits me in achieving my life goals are...
17. Regarding my career, things I don't want to ever have to do are...
18. Regarding my career, the things I really enjoy are...
19. The things I am afraid would happen if I achieve my goals are...
20. The ways I would have to change to achieve my goals are...
21. The things I am really willing to do to achieve my goals are...

After you have made your lists, review them one more time, add any other thoughts that come to mind and then take in a deep breath, exhale and release your past and any energy associated with it by shredding or (preferably) burning the lists.

Procrastination • •

Even if you're on the right track, you'll get run over if you just sit there.
— Will Rogers

"Never put off until tomorrow what you can do today!" is the aphorism which makes every procrastinator cringe. Everyone has experienced putting off various duties, tasks and responsibilities until the last possible minute (or longer). If this becomes a habit, it can be detrimental. According to business experts, this is the most common symptom of self-sabotage for a small business owner.

Procrastination brings to mind words such as lazy, unproductive and inefficient, yet procrastination is not necessarily a negative state. In fact, it's simply a signal that it's time to evaluate the status of the task in question and discover the reason(s) why it's staying at the bottom of the "to-do" pile.

The reasons for procrastination are numerous. Perhaps one of the most common is setting such high, perfectionistic expectations for performance that accomplishing the task appears overwhelming, if not impossible. It is easy to set yourself up in this manner—to never feel quite good enough, continually dissatisfied with your performance even though you got the job done. The delayed project then becomes a representation of your fear of failure and inadequacy.

Perfectionists believe that "adequate" or "sufficient" performance simply is not good enough. "Adequate" and "inadequate" come to mean the same thing. Put these three words—perfection, adequate and inadequate—in their proper perspective. Nothing is inherently wrong in having high standards but they need to be evaluated to determine if they're realistic. Perfection is impossible. To do a job adequately is to do what is needed. Inadequate means not meeting minimal requirements. If you feel fear about some task that you have to do, it could be that you're setting perfectionistic standards for yourself that are difficult to meet.

The main challenge for many perfectionists is that they believe that perfectionism is highly desirable. They see no reason to break their addiction to trying to be perfect. What they often fail to realize is that they're paying a high toll for maintaining their perfectionism. Creativity suffers greatly. In *The Woman's Book of Creativity*, Dr. Ealy notes that being tied to perfectionism sabotages creativity. "Creativity and perfection, like oil and water, don't mix. Expressing ourselves creatively requires us to assume risks, make mistakes, experiment with the unknown and take leaps of faith. These activities occur only when we're energized by a spirit of adventure and curiosity."[4]

Oftentimes people can convince themselves that a task is critical when it isn't. It is prudent to evaluate whether a task is actually necessary. You must evaluate and rank your tasks (this may take the assistance of a consultant). If the task is not something that you want to do and it isn't really necessary, then maybe you can take yourself off the hook.

Possibly you've agreed to do a certain task or activity that you really didn't want to do. If this is the case, it may not be too late to renegotiate. If you frequently find yourself having difficulty saying "No!" and procrastinate as a result, learn how to set limits and boundaries.

Sometimes procrastination is brought on by a lack of information. If you expect yourself to do a task without having the necessary knowledge, even the most routine task can become daunting. Before you begin a project, map out the technical, informational and functional requirements. Once you have determined what supplies, information and other resources are needed to complete the task—obtain them and begin your project. Being organized can make any task more palatable and run more smoothly. Additionally, give yourself permission to ask for the help you need. Asking for help can provide you with the energy and support to accomplish the task.

When procrastination simply comes down to having to do a task that must be done but is loathsome, or you're feeling a lack of creativity, here are some techniques that may help you move on: reframing; task breakdown and simplification; and delegation. Figure 3.3 gives a brief overview of each technique.

Putting off an easy thing makes it hard, and putting off a hard one makes it impossible.
— George H. Lonmer

Some men have thousands of reasons why they cannot do what they want to, when all they need is one reason why they can.
— Mary Frances Berry

Figure 3.3

Overcoming Procrastination

Reframing
Find an alternative way to view the project at hand. This may be done by creating a more pleasant environment to work on the task, such as listening to enjoyable music, sitting in a comfortable chair, sipping on your favorite beverage or involving another person (preferably with a good sense of humor) in the task.

Put the task into perspective. For example, let's say you've five marketing calls to make, but you have been putting them off for weeks, telling yourself that you aren't good on the phone, you hate to do marketing and you would rather just see your clients. At this rate the calls won't get done. Reframe the situation by asking yourself why you're making these calls. Remind yourself what you hope to accomplish and consider how these calls bring you closer to your goals. Reframing the situation and focusing on how doing a task may bring you closer to having what you want in your life can definitely bring more energy to tasks you have been avoiding.

Task Breakdown
Clarify action items and a timeline for a project by setting clear goals with target dates. This is basically taking things one step at a time and keeping them as simple as possible.

Delegation (or subcontracting)
Delegate tasks to colleagues or employees. Explore the possibilities. Determine if there are portions of the task (if not the whole thing) that can be done more easily and effectively by someone else. Consider trading tasks with a colleague. Remember that when you delegate or trade, you aren't handing over total responsibility for the finished product. You still need to oversee the tasks to assure their completion.

Never put off a task until tomorrow if you can delegate it today.
— Helen Reynolds

Genius is one percent inspiration and 99 percent perspiration.
— Thomas A. Edison

Procrastination isn't only a personal issue, it affects associates and staff as well. If you've discovered that you're a perfectionist, it can be extremely difficult to accurately gauge others' performance. You may be setting standards so high that not even you could attain them. Are you projecting your own perfectionism? Are you creating an atmosphere where people are afraid to take risks? Is it safe for your co-workers or employees to make mistakes?

If this is indeed the situation, discuss it with your associates and staff. Let them know that you're aware of your tendencies and address methods to improve working conditions. You need to set new standards—they can still be high, but not out of reach. If you can come to an agreement, everyone wins—you're happy, the people you work with won't feel as pressured and the company gets higher quality work from the staff.

Procrastination in self and others is an issue that most people have to deal with at some point in their lives. Procrastination is a symptom. The important thing to remember is to listen to yourself. Find out what is behind the behavior. Evaluate the dynamics. Then you can alleviate the procrastination by making the necessary changes—be they internal or external.

Figure 3.4

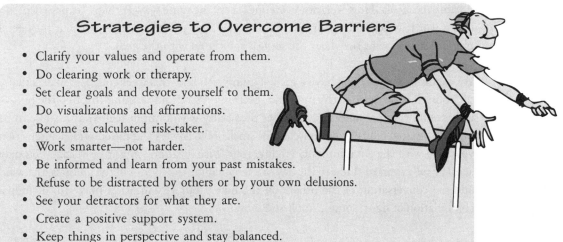

Strategies to Overcome Barriers

- Clarify your values and operate from them.
- Do clearing work or therapy.
- Set clear goals and devote yourself to them.
- Do visualizations and affirmations.
- Become a calculated risk-taker.
- Work smarter—not harder.
- Be informed and learn from your past mistakes.
- Refuse to be distracted by others or by your own delusions.
- See your detractors for what they are.
- Create a positive support system.
- Keep things in perspective and stay balanced.

❋ Tools for Actualizing Goals ❋

Now that you've made friends with your inner critic and learned how to avoid the pitfalls of negative conditioning and procrastination, it's time to explore two simple yet powerful tools for success: affirmations and creative visualization. Many successful people, from astronauts to Olympic athletes, have used these techniques to achieve daily success and high performance. We'll also look at some useful tips for breaking through blocks to creativity and dissolving thorny problems. All of these techniques are easy to learn and use. No special equipment needed!

Creative Visualization ❋

Creative visualization has inspired many people and accelerated their ability to change their lives and accomplish their goals. Yet for others it has been a source of frustration. A popular saying goes "If you can't see it, you can't get it." That statement is true, but only in its purest sense.

According to successconsciousness.com, creative visualization is:

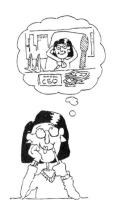

> "...the ability to use the imagination, see images in our minds and make them come true. If we add concentration and feelings, it becomes a great creative power that makes things happen. Used in the right way, visualization can bring changes into our lives. The thought is the matrix or blueprint; the feelings provide the energy, the 'electricity.'"

Creative visualization can help you stay inspired, energized and on track to achieve your dreams and goals. However, not everyone "sees" the same way. Perhaps "experience" is a better word. When some people envision a goal they don't actually see it, but they get a physical sensation or they hear the sounds associated with the goal.

For example, let's say you have a goal of going on a hike this weekend. You may actually see yourself waking up in the morning, getting dressed and walking through the hills—fully seeing the surroundings. Another possibility is you might feel what it's like to be hiking: the stretching of your muscles, the smell of the flowers and the emotional interaction you have with the environment. Finally, your "visualization" might be verbal. You may actually talk yourself through the day or even imagine the sounds of the animals, the wind and the conversation of the others on the hike. Your visualization may also include a combination of sight, sound, smell and sensation.

Creative Visualization:
Use the Power of Your
Imagination to Create What
You Want in Your Life
by Shakti Gawain

Indeed, the more senses you incorporate into your visualizations, the more powerful they become. You can visualize in your head, use the methods described under Goal Setting Techniques in Chapter 2, or create your own process. Another option is to carry a picture of the goal. For example, if you want a new car, have someone take a picture of you sitting in the exact model you desire or cut out a picture of the car from a brochure (and possibly glue on a picture of your face in the driver's seat). It isn't necessary to "visualize" in any specific way. What works for one person may not for another. Do what works best for you.

Fortunately, creative visualization is such a powerful tool that practicing five minutes a day can balance out hours, days, or even years of negative patterning. Be patient. Even a few minutes a day will bear much fruit.

Affirmations •

You are never given a wish
without also being given
the power to make it true.
You may have to work for
it, however.
— Richard Bach

An affirmation is a positive declaration that something is already so. It can be general or very specific. It is a constructive thought that you deliberately choose to place in your consciousness to produce a desired result. The purpose of writing or saying affirmations is to support you in actualizing your dreams and goals by replacing negative self-talk with positive self-talk.

When you create affirmations, you're in essence planting a seed for new beginnings. Avoid becoming attached to the specific details of "how" the affirmation will manifest. As with goal setting, always state your affirmations in the positive present tense and personalize them. Choose affirmations that feel good to you. What works for one person may not work for you. Affirmations can be used in many ways to produce powerful results. Experiment with some of the following suggestions.

Doubt, resistance and physical discomfort are natural side effects of the affirming process. If you notice these feelings while you're creating an affirmation, don't fight them. Accept them, acknowledge them and allow their expression. Sometimes these feelings are signals of deep conflicts that may require more (or other types) of clearing.

Affirmations are most effective when the path is clear of resistance. In *Law of Attraction*, author and Neuro Linguistic Programming trainer Michael J. Losier suggests another way to steer clear of resistance when using affirmations. Instead of stating affirmations in the positive tense, which can stir up feelings of "That's just not true," Losier suggests that you simply rephrase affirmations to state that you're "in the process" of creating what you want. For example, "I am in the process of growing a successful and prosperous business that supports my clients' sense of well-being and happiness."[5]

If you want to find out more about the connection between energy, our thoughts and the world of 'matter' around us, Losier suggests taking a look at the movie *What the Bleep Do We Know!?*,[6] a lively and sometimes humorous look at the world of quantum physics.

If you're a skeptic and this all sounds like New Age fluff, you may want to browse through a short book, *The Hidden Messages in Water*.[7] It introduces the work of renowned Japanese scientist Masaru Emoto, who has discovered through his high-speed photography of water crystals that molecules of water are affected by our thoughts, words and feelings. The many color photographs speak volumes about the power of our words and thoughts.

Figure 3.5

Keep in mind the power of your thoughts as you work with your favorite affirmations.

Affirmation Techniques

- Read your affirmations at least three times per day.
- Write each affirmation 10 to 20 times in succession.
- Write your affirmations while speaking them aloud to yourself.
- Write your affirmations in the first, second and third person.
  For example: *"I, Sue, am healthy." "You, Sue, are healthy." "She, Sue, is healthy."*
- Write your affirmations and tape them up (or use Post-it® notes) around your home, car and office. Put them on the telephone, the refrigerator, your desk, mirrors, doors, over your bed and on the dashboard.
- Make bookmarks with your affirmations on them.
- Record your affirmations on tape and listen to them as you drive, exercise and before you go to sleep.
- Meditate on your affirmations.
- Stand in front of a mirror and look at yourself while saying your affirmations.
- Take turns saying and accepting affirmations with a friend.
- Make flash cards with your affirmations and carry them with you.
- Design or buy clothes with affirmations on them.
- Sing or chant your affirmations.

www.businessmastery.us/ clear-negative-energy.php for an exercise to help discharge negative energy associated with affirmations.

Affirmations

Mind, Body and Spirit

My life is a continual expansion of joy and aliveness.
Everything I need is already within me.
I trust my intuition.
My life is filled with laughter and love.
I am the master of my life.
I fully love and accept myself as I am.
I live up to my own highest ideals.
I communicate clearly and effectively.
I am a radiant, powerful being.
I am happy!
I am vibrantly healthy.
My life is a joyous adventure.
I am creative in all that I do.
My relationships are nurturing and fun.
I am aligned with the divine plan of my life.
I appreciate the good in my life.
I am in an exciting, romantic relationship.
I allow people to support me and they do.

Career and Finances

My career is fulfilling and prosperous.
The more abundance I have, the more I have to share.
I am well-organized.
I am true to myself.
My creativity is flowing and focused.
I am a dynamic public speaker.
My career supports me in being who I am.
I have the time, energy, wisdom and money to accomplish my goals.
Every dollar I circulate returns to me multiplied.
I see the opportunities in life.
I manifest my power with integrity and love.

Breaking Old Habits

A lot of habitual beliefs and behaviors can sabotage your efforts to be successful. You may want to experiment with a fun and easy technique known as cross-lateral movement to break through blocks, increase your creativity and generate useful ideas for your business. As Dr. Ealy explains in *The Woman's Book of Creativity*[8], a cross-lateral movement cuts across an imaginary line splitting the body in half vertically. This happens when you swing the right arm across the body to the left side. These movements stimulate the learning centers of your brain while breaking up routine. They are designed to help the left and right hemispheres of the brain "talk" to each other more clearly so that you get the benefit of clear and creative thinking.

Experience firsthand the benefits of this technique by taking a few moments to do the following exercise.

Basic Cross-Lateral Exercise

Give yourself plenty of room and take off your shoes. Start by standing up and swinging your left foot over your right. Then swing your right foot over your left. Repeat this action many times, establishing a rhythm. Now add your arms, swinging in the opposite direction from your legs. Establish your rhythm. Next follow your feet with your head so both are moving in one direction while your arms are going in the opposite direction. If you lose the pattern, stop everything, then start with the feet and build the movement.

To add interest, imagine yourself eating a favorite food, watching a colorful sunset and petting your cat all at the same time. Have fun using images that are entertaining and relaxing for you. Maintain this movement and imagery for five minutes. Add music if you like. You may be pleasantly surprised to find yourself breathing vigorously and wanting to sit down after five minutes yet at the same time feeling exceptionally alert mentally.

Note: Cross-lateral movements can elevate your pulse, so pace yourself appropriately.

You can use this exercise for many issues. If you want to generate some new ideas for your business, set that intention before beginning the movements. As soon as you finish, begin writing what comes. If you're dealing with a specific problem, regardless of the type, embrace the problem then dance with it, using cross-laterals. Notice what has happened to it after you finish the movements. If you're engaged in a task that requires a lot of sitting, get up periodically and do some cross-lateral movements. You will find that you have increased your energy level and are mentally alert with ready access to your creativity. Have fun with this exercise!

Creative minds have always been known to survive any kind of bad training.
— Anna Freud

Dissolving Problems ●

We all slip into negative thoughts from time to time. Sadness and anger are normal experiences. The key is to acknowledge these thoughts and feelings and then let them go. Sometimes this is an easy task and other times it's Herculean. Sentence completions exercises are an excellent method for releasing energy associated with negative conditioning. If you're having difficulties with a specific problem, first take an honest look to see if you're truly willing to resolve the problem. If you are, put aside approximately two hours and do the following clearing exercise.

Dissolving Problems

Take some notebook paper and write the following questions on the top of each sheet of paper, putting one question on each piece of paper and keeping them in the order given. Spend at least five minutes per page actually doing the exercise.

- What is the area you're having difficulty with? Describe in detail.
- What are your fears and attitudes regarding your problem?
- What aren't you getting?
- What are you getting that you don't want?
- What are you getting that you do want?
- Regarding this problem, how have you been trying to resolve it?
- Regarding this problem, what do you think you should be doing?
- What is it that you want?
- What is it that you should want?
- What are the benefits of not resolving this problem?
- What would you have to give up to resolve this problem?
- What would you have to realize to resolve this problem?
- What are you holding on to or protecting in regards to your problem?
- Who or what is limiting you?
- By solving this problem, what new problems will be created?
- What is it that you *really* want?
- What are the specific things you will do to resolve this problem?

● Time Management Principles ●

Time management isn't about which appointment book you use. It is really about how well you use your time. It is based on realizing how much your time is worth and choosing activities that are the highest priority for you to achieve your goals. Time can either be an asset or a liability; it all depends on your attitudes. You can't alter time, only your attitudes and behaviors relating to time. Your attitudes toward time are influenced by conditioning and by your self-esteem.

What Is Your Attitude Toward Time?

- What thoughts and feelings do you have concerning time?
- How did your family relate to time?
- Do you respect yourself by taking the time to take care of yourself?
- Do you view time as your friend or your enemy?

As you work to develop your time management skills and discover new ways to boost your personal productivity, you find many benefits.

Figure 3.6

Effective Time Management Benefits

- Doing the same work in less time.
- Increasing personal productivity.
- Earning more money.
- Decreasing frustration and stress.
- Having more time for planning.
- Devoting more time to your family.
- Spending more time with hobbies and recreation.
- Improving your health.
- Experiencing increased joy and success.

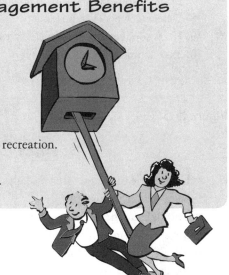

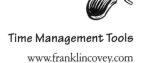

Time Management Tools
www.franklincovey.com

The Pareto Principle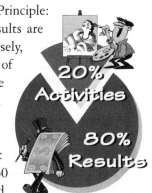

The fundamental basis of time management is the Pareto Principle: The Pareto Principle states that 80 percent of your results are produced by 20 percent of your activities. And, conversely, 20 percent of your results are produced by 80 percent of your activities. Time management techniques are effective because most people spend a lot of time in activities that are not an efficient use of their time. These percentages vary for individual cases, but the principle holds. The more you learn to focus on these 20 percent activities and turn them into 40 percent or even 60 percent, the more productive, prosperous and balanced you become.

Figure 3.7

Top 10 Time Management Tips

1. Do your most challenging work during your peak performance cycles.
2. Group similar activities together.
3. Discourage interruptions.
4. Learn to say "no."
5. Track important data and activities.
6. Avoid procrastination.
7. Respect your body's and mind's cycles.
8. Delegate whenever possible.
9. Keep supplies stocked and easy to access.
10. Take a quick stretch break every 20 minutes.

Figure 3.8

Plan Like a Pro

- Invest at least 10 minutes in daily planning.
- Focus on "A" goals first.
- Throughout the day ask yourself, "Is this the best use of my time?"
- Set specific times for taking and returning phone calls.
- Set a schedule and follow it.
- Review your master goal list at least once per week.
- At the end of the day, create the next day's goals and activities list.

Types of Time Needed to Run a Business

If you decide to become a business owner and intend to achieve optimal results, remember that you need to allot time for varied tasks. You need time to plan, work with clients, manage the business, continue your education, market your practice, communicate, develop ideas, take care of yourself and have fun. Investing at least 10 to 15 minutes in daily planning is crucial to managing your time wisely.

A common pitfall is to create an incredible to-do list, then let it fall to the wayside as everyday distractions pull you this way and that. Like a road map, the list gets you where you're going if you consult it as you navigate your day. If you ignore the road map, chances are you will take some unproductive detours. Another common pitfall is taking too rigid an approach to following your daily or weekly "to-do" list. This tends to create extra stress when unavoidable "sidetrips" require you to adjust course and take a more flexible path through your day.

When you have a clear purpose and have identified priorities, goals and plans of action, you don't get so overwhelmed, even when the unexpected appears at your doorstep. You know what you have to do, the order in which to do it and when it needs to be done. Sometimes people imagine things to be far more complicated than they really are. Recognize that there are different types of time you need and the amount of time spent in each category may vary from day to day.

Set a regular schedule for your business. Decide what days and what hours you will work. You may want to do this on a weekly or monthly basis. Once you've made your schedule, stick to it. Even if you don't have the time slots filled with clients, you can always do other business activities. It can be so tempting to look at your appointment book, not see anything scheduled for the afternoon and decide to go play. Occasionally this is fine, just be careful it doesn't become a habit.

Work Smarter—Not Harder

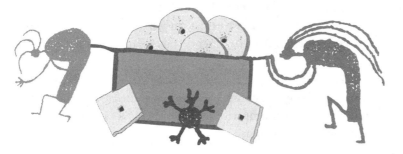

The time you spend in planning is always well-invested. When you first start planning, it may seem to take a long time; after doing it on a regular basis, you can plan your day very quickly. Remember, planning is to ultimately simplify your life—not make it more complicated.

The basis of productive planning is effective goal setting. The major element in planning (especially daily planning) is ranking. After you have written your daily plan, evaluate it. Decide which activities absolutely must get done today and rate them as Imperative. Review the other items and indicate the ones that need to be done very soon by labeling them as Important. Mark the rest of the activities (the ones that it would be nice if you accomplished them, but they're not of major significance) as being Desirable.

A year from now you will wish you had started today.
— Karen Lamb

Chapter 2, Page 28
for more information on
prioritizing goals.

Managing Business Logistics ••

We often forget to schedule appropriate time for the day-to-day tasks such as doing laundry, making phone calls, supervising staff (if you have any), keeping files and purchasing supplies. All of these activities take time, often a lot more than anticipated.

Another aspect of managing your business has to do with respecting yourself and time in relation to bartering (or trading) services. Barter is usually a supplemental method of obtaining products and services that you prefer to not purchase with cash. The downside is that some people get so into bartering that they never earn any money. Be very clear about your reasons for trading. Before you do any type of bartering, ask yourself if you would spend money on that product or service if you had the cash. If not, don't trade. Also remember that in most countries barter is considered taxable income.

There is a fundamental difference between working harder and working smarter.

Working with Clients ••

The majority of your time is spent providing client services. Your ability to effectively schedule appointments greatly impacts your success and your stress level. Allot sufficient time between clients while not having large blocks of unproductive time. You may discover that you need to schedule an extra half hour for new clients and some ongoing clients who regularly need additional time. You may need a longer recuperation time after certain clients. Sometimes staying within the allotted session time can be difficult when you don't have anything else scheduled immediately after the session. While having the flexibility to extend a session is nice, be careful to respect the time boundaries of yourself and your client. The longer you're in practice, the more adept you become in judging how much time is necessary to spend with clients and between sessions.

One way to simplify scheduling is to set up a standing appointment with regular clients. For example, you may have a regular client scheduled for 10 a.m. each Wednesday. Both you and your client agree that this appointment stays in place each week unless the client calls to cancel. This approach creates a sense of comfort and ease for both practitioner and client.

Daily Plan
www.businessmastery.us

If you work as an employee of a spa, group practice or medical center, you may have little control over scheduling client sessions. However, in some cases, you can communicate scheduling preferences to an appropriate staff member who may agree to accommodate you whenever possible.

Professional Development ••

Continuing education is necessary to your career growth. Find ways to broaden your knowledge, particularly in the areas of interpersonal skills, product knowledge, technical skills and business skills. Some ways to do that are: reading magazines and books; taking classes; attending seminars; watching videos; and networking.

It is also helpful to be assessed periodically. This can be done by your clients and by colleagues. Some practitioners have every client fill out a form for every session and others go through this process only once or twice per year. Feedback is essential for your professional growth. This concept can seem a bit scary—the idea of being evaluated does have some ego risk involved, but how are you going to know which areas to enhance if no one tells you? Remember, knowledge is power. Since most work in this field is very individualized, it's recommended that you obtain as many evaluations as possible to get broader, more objective feedback. Many practitioners find evaluations highly beneficial. They are also a good way to get your clients more involved in their treatment.

Getting assessed by your colleagues is essential. They can give you the kind of technical feedback that a client probably would not know. Again, it isn't necessary to be evaluated every time you work with your peers, but do it regularly. You can also make it fun. Your purpose is not to "find fault" but to support each other in achieving excellence. This can be an enjoyable and cost-effective way to grow professionally.

Idea Development ● ●

Developing ideas is one of the most exciting and creative aspects of any business. Always be open to new opportunities. Brainstorm ways to streamline your procedures. Find methods to reduce your effort by diversifying your practice (e.g., hire employees, sell products or subcontract out work to other practitioners and take a percentage of the fees). Create ways in which you work with more than one client at a time (e.g., offer group sessions, give seminars and publish articles and books). The possibilities are legion!

Marketing ● ●

Marketing your practice is vital to your success. This is the aspect of business that most wellness practitioners neglect. When you first start your practice, you may spend more hours marketing than actually working with clients. Then, even when your business seems to be established, you still need to actively market yourself. People move, change practitioners and try alternate methods of self-improvement. You can't rely on your clients to bring you more new clients. Marketing is necessary during all phases of your business. I have known several very successful practitioners whose businesses appeared to fall apart overnight. They were not marketing themselves well; they hadn't noticed the changes that were occurring until it was too late. So they had to "start all over again." You can avoid this through regular marketing. It is critical that you invest at least 15 percent of your work time in marketing.

Having Fun ● ●

When your desire for success is strong, having fun can easily get pushed to the bottom of the list or get neglected altogether. It tends to be one of the least planned aspects of life. People are inclined to leave their enjoyment to chance. Remember to balance your professional goals with your personal goals. Be sure to include fun in your life EVERY DAY!

The future has a way of arriving unannounced.
— George F. Will

He who every morning plans the transactions of the day, and follows out that plan, carries a thread that will guide him through the labyrinth of the most busy life.
— Victor Hugo

Personal Wellness ● ●

Taking care of yourself is imperative, yet many people put themselves last. It is so easy to get caught up in your business and being there for others, that literally no time is left for you. Take care of yourself mentally, physically, emotionally and spiritually. Make sure that every day you do at least one thing just for yourself. Respect your needs and wants. Create a support system for your business and personal life. Caregivers have a tendency to not allow themselves to be care-receivers. Don't let yourself fall into that syndrome. Allot as much time as needed to take care of you.

Chapter 4, Pages 65-68

for information on self-care and stress.

One of the major factors that influences your time is stress. If you do not handle stress productively, you can waste hours of time each day—not to mention time lost due to stress-related illness. Make certain that you exercise regularly, follow a healthy eating plan and receive regular wellness care (e.g., massage, acupuncture, chiropractic). Take a quick stretch break every 20 minutes. Allot a five-minute break every two hours to more thoroughly stretch your muscles, do some deep breathing, exercise your eyes and revitalize yourself.

High Priority Activities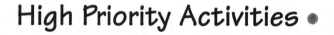

High priority activities are the "20 percent" that produce 80 percent of your results. Before you can begin to increase the time spent in those important activities, you must identify them. The following exercise is designed to assist you in clarifying your high priority activities. The objective of this exercise is to begin concentrating your time and energy on items you've rated as being the most crucial to your success. You may be surprised at what you discover.

High Priority Activities

Make a copy of the High Priority Activities form found on www.businessmastery.us/forms.php#busman, or draw three columns on a piece of paper, with the center column the widest. Label the left-hand column "Importance," the middle column "Activity" and the right-hand column "Time Spent." Think about the activities involved in your business. List at least 10 of the most important things you do in the center column. In the left-hand column, rate them in the order you think is most important to your success. In the right-hand column rate them in the order of how much time you spend in each activity.

The more you focus on your high priority activities, the more productive you are. You may also discover some conflicts. If this happens, refer to your purpose, priorities and goals. They usually provide direction. Sometimes you have to make difficult decisions and either delegate the other activities, simplify them or eliminate them. It is also recommended that you show your list to a colleague. You might have overlooked something or you need to switch some of your priorities—and it's usually easier for someone else to be objective.

• Tracking •

Frequently, in business, we have no idea why things are going the way they are, including when they're going well. Was it that last ad? Could it have been that interview in the newspaper? Maybe it was the new brochure? Or was it due to extending office hours on Thursday? Even though it isn't always possible to know for certain the exact action that generated the desired results, you greatly increase your knowledge and optimize your efforts by tracking the important components.

Tracking can help you anticipate potential problems so that you can take the appropriate steps to avoid them and modify the direction of the trend more to your liking. Tracking is dynamic in nature; it focuses on the way things change—the "motion" of business.

Tracking is a documentation of items, such as marketing activities, client profiles, appointment bookings and income levels, to identify trends. It is important to closely monitor a broad range of activities because your appointment book, checkbook and accounting journal don't always tell the whole story. A lot of critical data is not included in those books and if you use them as your major reference point for judging your success, you may find yourself in a predicament. Oftentimes things are not as they appear.

Results! Why, man, I have gotten a lot of results. I know several thousand things that won't work.
— Thomas A. Edison

For example, imagine that you have been fairly well booked and have had a satisfactory level of income for the last few months, so you haven't been putting much attention into marketing. Then the next month goes by and you discover (to your dismay) that your client load has decreased and your income level has significantly dropped. You don't quite understand how this could happen—after all, everything seemed to be going so well.

You decide to carefully review your books and find that you've only had three new clients in the last two months, four clients have completed their work with you and the time between sessions for the rest of your clients has been substantially increasing. Had you been keeping track of that kind of information on a summary sheet or a graph, you could have noticed the trend earlier and taken action (e.g., done some type of marketing) to rebuild your clientele. In any business, particularly one that's small, one slow month can be devastating.

Identifying seasonal trends is another helpful way to approach tracking. For instance, by tracking key business indicators, you may notice that for the last three years, your business dropped dramatically every October. Using that information, you can decide to increase your advertising and promotion in August and September, or you may just choose to take advantage of the slow period and plan a vacation for October. Conversely, it wouldn't be judicious for you to plan a vacation during your peak period.

Statistics are no substitute for judgment.
— Henry Clay

Tracking is also quite beneficial in determining which advertising media and promotional events have been most effective.

A tip for becoming more proficient at time management is to keep a log of how you spend your time. Track all of your activities for several weeks—include everything , such as time spent on telephone calls, dealing with interruptions, taking breaks, working with clients and so on. Tracking shows you where your time is being well spent or wasted.

Tracking Key Business Indicators ✸

What is the best method for tracking key business indicators? You might use graph paper, computerized spread sheets, custom-designed forms or simple notebook paper. Make the forms very clear and as straightforward as possible to fill out. Also, be certain to design your client forms so they provide you with information (e.g., how they heard about you), demographics and session notes for your tracking sheets. You may want to make charts and post them on the wall or put your tracking forms into a notebook. As you can see, tracking methods are varied and the best method depends on what works easily for you.

Experiment with tracking activities on a daily, weekly, monthly or quarterly basis. Consistency is essential, particularly when tracking the results of marketing campaigns, since it often takes several months to discern those results. Additionally, you may discover that the results were due to a combination of factors. Thus the measurable benefits of tracking are derived from the knowledge you develop over the long run.

Tracking is an essential component in making a business plan work. First you must decide what you want to track. The following list of items, your business plan and your high priority activities are excellent places to begin. This data provides you with the information you need to assess the progress of your long-term goals and strategies. It will also enhance your decision making for future marketing campaigns and general business direction.

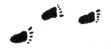

Chapter 13, Pages 268-270

regarding When to Alter Your Course.

Figure 3.9

Useful Items to Track

- Client demographics
- Total number of clients
- Number of clients per day
- Types of clients
- Session time spent per client
- Time spent per client in adjunct support
- Time between sessions
- Type of techniques utilized
- Number of sessions per client
- Average cost of total treatment plan
- How your clients heard about you
- Referrals generated by specific marketing campaigns
- Time spent in all business activities
- Total income (e.g., daily, weekly, monthly)
- Total expenses

Sample Tracking Forms ✳

Studies show that tracking in itself increases your productivity. It is an excellent way to keep yourself motivated, evaluate your status and help you determine the most appropriate areas in which to invest your time and money to build your practice. As with daily planning, it usually takes a little while to become adept at tracking. After you have experimented with various forms, you will discover the ones that are most appropriate for your needs and then it won't take you very much time at all to track (see Figures 3.10 and 3.11).

Invest the time required for tracking—it's an information-rich and inspiring tool to help you run a productive and profitable business.

Figure 3.10

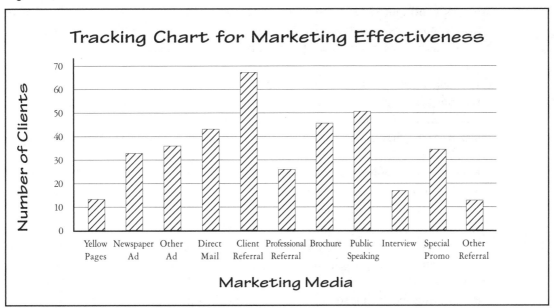

Figure 3.11

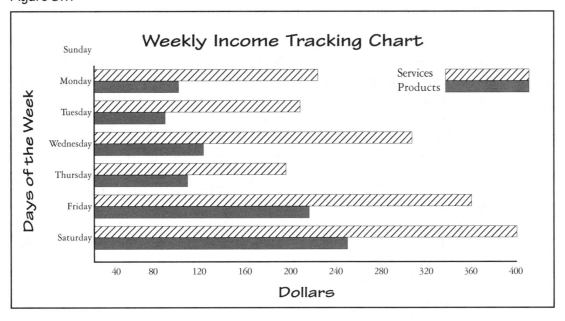

• The Art of Risk-Taking •

Two commonly heard truisms are "nothing ventured, nothing gained" and "no guts, no glory." Taking risks is an integral part of life and especially true in business. It is the doorway to success. The art of risk-taking is knowing how to take smart risks. There is a difference between being a risk-taker and a daredevil. Taking risks is not about blindly jumping into any situation. To become proficient in taking risks it's vital that you understand the components of risk-taking, learn how to minimize your potential losses and strengthen your risk-taking abilities.

The two major elements that influence your ability to successfully manage risks are the level of comfort you have in experiencing new or unusual situations and your self-esteem. Think about the source of your self-confidence. To what degree do you base it upon your opinions and values? How much do you look to others for validation? Is your behavior mainly motivated by external factors such as social approval and material consequences, or by internal considerations such as your beliefs and feelings?

In terms of self-esteem, the primary discomfort in taking risks stems from the fear of rejection. In considering your ability to feel confident in novel circumstances, the fundamental discomfort is usually due to inexperience. People take the safer routes so often that they haven't developed a bank of experiences from which to draw. Reflect upon your childhood. What messages were you given regarding the safety of your environment? How did your family deal with crises? What behaviors did you learn to adopt? You can alleviate a lot of anxiety by keeping your expectations realistic and embracing the opportunities for new experiences.

Risk-takers are achievers. They are not content with the status quo. They prefer action to inaction and follow through on their goals with little hesitation. They are exhilarated by challenges rather than intimidated by them and proceed despite their fears. They also carefully evaluate risks and develop strategic plans of action. They distinguish facts from their emotions, which enables them to handle crises well and empowers their decision-making process. Risk-takers have a strong commitment to being and producing the best.

Another factor that impacts people's freedom to take chances is finances. Most people are overly concerned with money. The truth is that most successful business owners have failed at least once before finally making it. Again, you're the best judge of what's appropriate. You are the only one who can determine whether a risk is worthwhile. If you're considering taking a risk that has monetary ramifications, allot the time to thoroughly evaluate the possibilities. One step you can take now is to reduce your debt as much as possible. Often what is more scary than the possibility of losing money is the potential for losing face.

Developing your skill in taking risks is a lifelong process. As you go through life, the stakes just seem to get higher. Build your repertoire of risk-taking experiences so that you successfully manage risks. By drawing upon your past experiences to see the similarities to the current situation, you can better determine an effective solution. Put yourself in situations that require you to exercise your creative problem-solving abilities. Start with low-risk situations, gradually increasing your confidence level so you feel more comfortable taking greater risks.

Ideals are like stars; you will not succeed in touching them with your hands. But like the seafaring man on the desert of waters, you choose them as your guides, and following them you will reach your destiny.
— Carl Schurz

Don't play for safety; it's the most dangerous thing in the world.
— Hugh Walpole

Figure 3.12

The Do's of Risk-Taking

- Have a life plan with clear goals.
- Make sure the risk is aligned with your life plan.
- Evaluate the potential gains and losses.
- Ask questions and research the situation.
- Know your strengths and limitations.
- Brainstorm several alternatives.
- List potential conflicts and solutions.
- Set a realistic timetable.
- Be flexible.
- Trust your intuition and instincts.
- Follow through and give it your best.
- Review and possibly revise your strategy.
- Ask for support.
- Acknowledge the people who give you support.

The Don'ts of Risk-Taking

- Be unrealistic.
- Be a perfectionist.
- Deny your feelings.
- Ignore or minimize problems.
- Mistake emotions for facts.
- Rush.
- Procrastinate.
- Blame others for your mistakes.
- Give up too soon.
- Be afraid to cut your losses and move on.
- Trust blindly.
- Risk just to prove yourself to others.
- Combine too many risks at once.

Exploring Taking Risks

The continual enhancement of your self-image is vital in cultivating risk-taking behaviors. Begin with positive self-talk. Fill your mind with thoughts about your potential. Become grounded in the knowledge that you are your own source of power and that this power is honorable. Expect to succeed. Release some of your conditioned apprehension and fear by doing the following clearing exercise.

Think about a situation that makes you feel uneasy. Imagine what is the very worst thing that could possibly happen. Then evaluate the situation. Is it really that bad? Are your fears justified? Finally, visualize yourself being comfortable and confident while in that risky situation.

Your attitudes about the world can greatly influence your facility in taking risks. Be enthusiastic about the present and future. Expand your view of life. Focus on the prospects for success and joy. Don't become immersed in the potentials for disaster. Accurately evaluate what would really happen if you were to take a risk and not succeed. Remember that success lies in taking action.

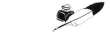

Never test the depth of the water with both feet.
— Kevin Coyne

✳ Motivation ✳

Motivation is about satisfying desires and needs. The major theories of motivation are often described as behavioral, cognitive, psychoanalytic, social learning, social cognition and humanistic. Listed below is a brief overview of each theory:

- The **Behavioral** point of view is based on observable behavior and states that biological responses to stimuli direct behavior (e.g., the famous Pavlov's dog experiments).
- The **Cognitive** approach is founded on the belief that making meaning is key to motivation and focuses on the impact of the structure and function of information processing.
- **Psychoanalytic** theory presumes that all action or behavior is a result of internal, biological instincts (e.g., Freudian analysis).
- **Social Learning** suggests that behavior can be motivated by an individual observing the consequences that others experience from their behaviors.
- **Social Cognition** proposes that the environment, an individual's behavior and the individual's knowledge, emotions and cognitive development influence each other to determine motivation.
- The **Humanistic** view focuses on personal growth and interpersonal relationships, believing that people behave out of intentionality and values.

Abraham Maslow is one of the most well-known researchers in the field of humanistic motivation. His original hierarchy of motivational needs had five divisions. Recently, psychologists have taken his notes and modified the hierarchy to the following eight levels: **physiological** (satisfaction of hunger, thirst and sex); **safety** (security, shelter and stability); **social** (belongingness and love); **esteem** (self-respect, power, competence, approval, recognition and prestige); **cognitive** (knowledge, understanding and exploration); **aesthetic** (symmetry, order and beauty); **self-actualization** (find self-fulfillment and realize one's potential); **transcendence** (connect to something beyond the ego or help others in their self-actualization). Maslow contends that people aren't compelled to reach a level until the needs of the level below are satisfied. Thus it's extraordinarily difficult to be motivated toward self-actualization or transcendence if your safety or esteem needs aren't met.

TRANSCENDENCE
SELF ACTUALIZATION
AESTHETIC
COGNITIVE
ESTEEM
SOCIAL
SAFETY
PHYSIOLOGICAL

Maslow's Modified Hierarchy of Motivational Needs

So if you find that you just can't motivate yourself to do a particular task, find out what other needs you have that are not being met. You must appeal to the needs and desires that are the strongest at any given moment. Once you have satisfied those other needs, it's easier to complete the specific task.

Motivation Techniques •

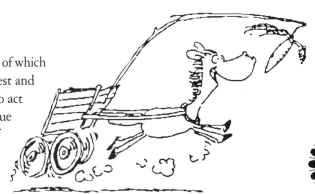

The two most common motivators are fear and incentive, both of which have serious shortcomings. Fear motivation is the oldest, easiest and universally least effective means of motivation. It forces you to act out of fear of the consequences. Parents frequently use this technique with young children. The primary limitation of this style of motivation is that most people (particularly children) quickly build up a tolerance to fear. Since the repercussions are rarely enforced, they usually aren't taken seriously.

Incentive motivation promises a reward for behavior. This method is often used in business as a way to increase productivity and is also frequently used by people in the process of altering habits. The problems associated with this motivation system are that the rewards have to keep escalating to merit the same impact and withholding the reward represents a punishment. Incentive motivation doesn't satisfy your desire for achievement.

The most effective motivation is self-motivation, being inspired by the pure joy of accomplishment. Approaching life from this point of view is extremely empowering to yourself and to those around you. It can be very freeing to not need outside stimulus to induce action. This can be difficult because the results of your actions are often intangible or may not be realized for a long time.

Ability is what you're capable of doing. Motivation determines what you do. Attitude determines how well you do it.
— Lou Holtz

Self-motivation is an attitude that takes time to develop and fully integrate into your life. It may take longer to master motivation in some areas of your life than in others. The clearer you are about your purposes, priorities and goals, the easier and more natural it's to become motivated by the sheer act of attaining your goals.

Your history plays a major role in attitude development. Throughout your life you have been influenced to some degree by your environment and the people around you. Your cumulative experiences and feelings impact your perception. For example, you may view a certain task as boring while someone else might find the same task exciting. One technique for altering your feelings about an activity (and thus making it easier to accomplish) is to remove any negative descriptive terms associated with it.

The principal factor in motivation is goals. Without goals, motivation has no direction. You can even create goals about motivation. Your mind is a powerful tool that is ready and waiting for you to utilize it more effectively. If your motivation is still blocked, do some clearing exercises as described on page 39 or the Dissolving Problems exercise on page 48 of this chapter.

Figure 3.13

10 Ways to Sabotage Motivation

1. Refrain from having written goals.
2. Set unattainable goals.
3. Agree to take responsibility for goals or activities that you don't believe in.
4. Set goals in such a way that they take a long time to accomplish without small successes along the way.
5. Establish important goals that conflict with your values or other aspects of your life.
6. Withhold rewards on big projects until they're fully completed.
7. Refuse to acknowledge your successes.
8. Maintain a negative attitude about yourself, your abilities, your goals and your activities.
9. Ignore your mental, physical and emotional well-being.
10. Listen to the skepticism of your friends, family and colleagues.

Boost Career Longevity

• Career Longevity Components •

According to career counselor Randall S. Hansen, Ph.D., "Recent studies indicate that the average worker will change careers—not just jobs—several times over the course of a lifetime."[1] But what if you're already in (or attending school for) your second or third career, and you want it to be your last? Or what if you're just beginning your career in this field and want to be in control of when—or if—you leave it someday?

Although there are no easy formulas that guarantee career longevity, steady efforts in the areas of professional development, positive attitude, communication skills and self-renewal are a good way to plant seeds for success—and excel in your career day to day.

The principal components of career longevity are: personality characteristics; client interactions; technical capabilities; business savvy; and self-care. Most of the suggestions for longevity are the same for those who are self-employed as they are for those who work as employees.

The additional skills critical for employees to master are interpersonal communications with staff and management, and knowing how to adapt to various management styles. Most employers look for highly skilled practitioners who are positive and professional, flexible and adaptable, and who have an ability to put clients at ease. They want mature, team players with good people skills, and an ability to take initiative. They are also looking for employees with the wisdom to seek self-renewal, which enables a practitioner to function at his or her best and avoid burnout.

If you ask me what is the single most important key to longevity, I would have to say it is avoiding worry, stress and tension. And if you didn't ask me, I'd still have to say it.
— George Burns

Personality Characteristics ✳

Successful practitioners are confident in their abilities, possess a positive mental attitude, maintain healthy boundaries, enjoy working with people, and are willing to take risk, such as speaking in public. They are willing to press through challenges and be uncomfortable for a while. They are determined and focused. They do what is necessary to ensure quality and success.

If you think you can, you can. And if you think you can't, you're right.
— Mary Kay Ash

Along with this determination is flexibility. Flexibility is crucial in the hands-on aspect of the work, as well as in business operations. For instance, there may be times when practitioners find themselves needing to change the type of work or treatment plan right in the middle of a session: perhaps a client isn't responding well to a particular technique; doesn't like what's being done; or it becomes apparent that the treatment needs to go in a different direction.

Flexibility is also needed to sail through the changes that occur in one's career. This includes adding modalities to one's repertoire and branching into other areas, such as teaching. Employees in particular need to be flexible, as they rarely have much control over their work.

The most important personality characteristic is loving your work and appreciating people for who they are regardless of their physical condition. The work you do is not limited to your technical abilities. Clients need to feel comfortable with you and know that you truly care for them.

Client Interactions ✳

Practitioners who have been in the industry for a long time have a reverence for the inherent magnificence of the human body and spirit. They respect their clients regardless of their physical conditions or the particular reasons that they seek care. A highly judgmental person rarely lasts long in private practice, as clients sense subtle messages. Successful practitioners say that a client-centered approach is important, that it's crucial to stay present with clients and to listen to what they're really saying. They customize each session to address clients' long-term goals *and* immediate concerns.

You can improve client relations by taking courses to enhance communication skills, learning effective intake interviewing skills, and creating treatment plans that encourage clients to take an active role in their own wellness.

Technical Capabilities

Practitioners with staying power possess a high level of expertise and excel in what they do. They consider their initial schooling to be just the starting point, and they invest in regular continuing education. They stay current with the trends, read the new literature, attend seminars and learn new techniques. While some long-time practitioners do well as generalists, most specialize in a particular technique, condition or aspect of wellness care.

Note to students and new graduates: The first step to career longevity to is to gain a solid base of experience to integrate what you've learned in school with hands-on practice in the field. Recognize that in the first few years of practice, it's vital to continue your education to expand your portfolio of skills and techniques. In fact, it's common to find successful wellness practitioners with several years' experience who have taken hundreds of hours of additional training. Continuing your professional education throughout your career opens many doors—to both personal fulfillment and professional growth. A commitment to lifelong learning provides a strong foundation for ongoing success.

Business Savvy *

The majority of people enter this field with limited business knowledge and many bear a negative attitude about business. Plenty of books, classes, marketing products and online resources abound to assist practitioners in expanding their business knowledge. The savvy practitioner takes advantage of these tools.

The more you make business a natural expression of who you are, the more successful you will be.

Take every opportunity to learn all you can about effective communication. Successful professionals are those who have learned to communicate clearly and openly and who have a knack for creating win-win solutions to everyday problems. They avoid defensive communication and focus on mature two-way communication grounded in respect for others. They make it a practice to listen with empathy and full attention. When others slip into gossip or criticizing a co-worker, boss or competitor, they often bring up the bright side or positive qualities of the person.

Learning to work smarter, not harder, is a chief tenet of success. Take the time to stay organized and keep excellent records. Look to the long term and consult with experts.

Self-Care *

Helping others is difficult if you neglect your own wellness. Developing a habit of self-renewal helps you stay energized and ensures you're at your professional best. Carve out time for daily walking, yoga, meditation or your favorite exercise. Enjoy time in nature and take a little time to laugh and play each day. Enjoy your friends and family. Schedule fun outings. Participate in sports that relax and energize you. Make time for a weekly touch therapy session.

Trade wellness sessions with other practitioners weekly. Not only do you benefit from the work, it's also a great way to build your knowledge of different techniques so you can make informed referrals for your clients. Even if you have a favorite practitioner, try out others. You may discover a technique or body of knowledge that is absolutely wonderful; you can then take the necessary steps to learn it and incorporate it into your practice. In addition, receiving these sessions on a regular basis can assist you in being more attuned to your clients' needs. How can you resist this wonderful opportunity to take care of yourself and grow professionally at the same time?

Grow a Strong Client Base ✸

Keep in mind that the number one key to career longevity is a solid base of clients. After all, without them you don't have a practice. Exceptions do exist, such as when you work in a destination spa or resort where there's a continuous flow of new guests, or your work is of a particular approach or philosophy that advocates working with a client only once or twice.

Doing what you love doesn't mean sitting in your office waiting for the phone to ring; it's about taking action to attract new clients and actually *doing* your work. If you don't have a full client load, either invest that free time in educating people about your work or donate your services (*do* what you love)—then the money will come.

Chapter 16
for marketing tips.

Effective marketing in this field includes a mixture of promotion, advertising, community relations and publicity—with the emphasis on promotion. The core of client retention is a solid customer-service plan. The best plans are founded upon making clients feel safe and welcome, finding effective ways to support clients' wellness and stress management efforts, and addressing any wellness needs.

✸ Prevent Burnout ✸

In today's fast-paced world avoiding professional burnout can be challenging. As a wellness practitioner, your personal well-being and balance is a major influence on your everyday effectiveness. Some common pitfalls that contribute to burnout are: scarcity consciousness, sloppy time management, poor boundaries, stress and boredom syndrome. We explore each of these pitfalls and ways you can prevent burnout and thrive every day in your work.

Scarcity Consciousness ✸

I attended a party where a woman mentioned that although her three-year-old practice was okay, she was considering getting a part-time job to help out. It wasn't as though she was just starting out and needed to transition into her career. If you figure that it takes approximately three hours of marketing to get a new client—why settle for an $8 an hour temporary job when you can spend these three hours to earn at least $50 instead of $24 (and that's if the client only comes in once). Her shortsightedness was staggering. This is a classic example of poverty thinking and scarcity consciousness at work. Keeping a realistic frame of reference is crucial. Many people operate with a "go with the flow" philosophy in most areas of their lives, but when it comes to their business their perspective often changes to one of scarcity. Poverty thinking burns you out faster than anything else. Overcome this negative thinking by utilizing the tools covered in this chapter and reminding yourself of the value of your work and. Do the math!

Sloppy Time Management *

Not paying enough attention to time management can also contribute significantly to burnout and imbalance. Practitioners who don't set appointments at accurate intervals, don't pace themselves well to accommodate breaks for clearing and centering, don't allow sufficient preparation time for clients, or don't schedule time just for themselves, are inviting burnout. A sloppy approach to time management prevents you from giving your best to your clients and creates a more stressful environment for yourself. In short, it makes sense to work smarter—not harder.

Also, be sure to set aside time for planning and thinking—whether it's about your business agreements, goals, marketing, client relations or evaluating what is working and what isn't. Think before you leap. Life is much more enjoyable and successful when one is coming from a proactive position than one of reaction.

Boundaries *

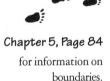

Chapter 5, Page 84
for information on boundaries.

Alongside physical injury, the inability to effectively maintain and manage boundaries with clients, co-workers and management is the leading cause of burnout for wellness practitioners. Boundaries help to protect the respect and dignity of each person. Resentment builds if you frequently allow your boundaries to be crossed. For instance, a client may repeatedly fail to respect your time by forgetting to cancel an appointment and refusing to pay for a missed session. Or you may encounter situations where others are prone to take advantage of your good nature or generosity. Learn to set strong boundaries for yourself. Practice saying "No." Create policies and adhere to them. Work with a clinical supervisor or meet regularly with colleagues for peer supervision.

Stress *

The signs of chronic stress include high blood pressure, digestive problems, sleep disorders, mood shifts, depression, anxiety and decrease in mental acuity. It is so easy to forget about ourselves, yet as caregivers we must make certain we're also care-receivers.

Body Mechanics ● ●

The number one cause of physical burnout and injuries is poor body mechanics. Take the time to find out what works best for your body. For those of you who do hands-on work, invest in a high-quality table. Additionally, for those who do outcalls, be sure to purchase and use the accessories specially designed to help tote tables. If your work involves sitting with clients (e.g., nutritional consulting), then purchase an ergonomic chair. Set up your office in a manner that supports your posture and optimizes the physical demands of your work.

Emotional Burnout ● ●

There's only one corner of the universe you can be certain of improving, and that's you own self.
— Aldous Huxley

Emotional burnout is a bit trickier. Attitude plays a critical role. You can avoid burnout by making time to meet with colleagues on a regular basis, attending conferences, varying the way you work, maintaining a strong personal support system, and enrolling in new classes to expand your knowledge and stay inspired. Set boundaries by learning to express your needs clearly and honestly so others know you expect to be treated with respect and dignity. The inability to effectively maintain boundaries with clients, co-workers and management is a leading cause of burnout for massage practitioners.

Stress Management ● ●

Take the time for your self-care: do stretches, take breaks, do breathing exercises, make adjustments in your body mechanics, use proper equipment, exercise, eat properly, meditate or do martial arts, and get some type of touch therapy weekly. Walk your talk: if you're a massage therapist, get weekly massages; if you're a nutritional consultant, eat healthy foods and take proper supplements; if you're an esthetician, get weekly facials; if you're a dentist, make sure your teeth are in great condition. How can you realistically expect clients to be convinced to regularly incorporate your services into their lives if you aren't practicing what you preach?

Regular exercise is essential for health and a feeling of well-being. If you are not already exercising, make this a habit by committing to at least three, 20-minute exercise sessions each week. In about six weeks, you will feel much healthier and best of all your body becomes more efficient at processing oxygen—the magic key to enjoying more energy. Choosing types of exercise that you enjoy or joining with others who have similar goals boosts your success in this area of self-care.

Keeping balance in mind is the key to stress management. You need to keep things in perspective. Don't react to things that aren't your responsibility. Learn to deal with interruptions: internal and external. Learn how to say "No."

Boredom Syndrome ✺

Practitioners who have been in business many years may find themselves falling prey to ennui. Sometimes a great rhythm turns into a deep rut. Here are some ideas to prevent this burnout:

- Diversify your practice.
- Alter your work environment.
- Join forces with other wellness providers.
- Start a whole new business.
- Take a sabbatical.
- Learn new skills.
- Volunteer your services.
- Revamp your business plan.

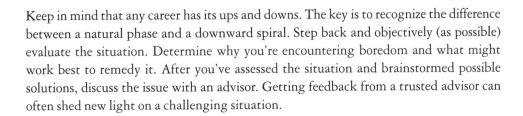

Keep in mind that any career has its ups and downs. The key is to recognize the difference between a natural phase and a downward spiral. Step back and objectively (as possible) evaluate the situation. Determine why you're encountering boredom and what might work best to remedy it. After you've assessed the situation and brainstormed possible solutions, discuss the issue with an advisor. Getting feedback from a trusted advisor can often shed new light on a challenging situation.

✺ Professional Development ✺

Learning is a lifelong process. Those who refrain from engaging their brains tend to lose their creative edge. While some people naturally gravitate toward continuous learning, others gravitate toward a comfort zone of familiar experiences. Some prefer informal to formal learning scenarios. Professional growth can take many shapes, such as workshops, to classroom settings, to participating in professional associations. It may also involve activities such as public speaking, publishing articles in trade journals or participating in research projects. Taking the time to develop a support system of like-minded professionals, as explored in the next section, can also be a powerful catalyst to professional growth.

While it's easy to say that professional development is a worthwhile endeavor, making it happen is not always so easy. Scheduling time off from work or attending weekend courses can be challenging from a logistics standpoint. It can also be cost-prohibitive at times for those on an already stretched budget. However, career experts agree that if you want to reach your full career potential, carving out time and a budget for continued professional development is a must.

If you learn only methods you'll be forever tied to those methods. However, if you learn the principles behind those methods, you'll be free to devise your own methods.
— Ralph Waldo Emerson

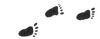

Chapter 5, Page 91
for information on professional associations.

Continuing Education ✳

Although most everyone would agree that continuing education is valuable, performance anxiety or unpleasant childhood memories of academic pressures can act as big detractors. Even with the best of intentions to grow professionally, continuing education classes can easily slip to the bottom of one's to-do list. To help you overcome these hurdles, we explore various options for continuing education.

Identifying Best Options for Continuing Education ●●

The good news is that the manner in which you continue your learning is not limited to a traditional school environment: you can read books; take distance-learning courses (e.g., correspondence, home-study, online); attend workshops; participate in self-exploration classes which benefit you directly and assist you in working with clients (e.g., movement, breathwork, communication skills); and go to conferences. Even continuing education courses offered by schools are usually administered quite differently than those in diploma programs.

Continuing education courses range from one hour to hundreds of hours. You learn the basics in school: the true integration and honing of your skills comes with practice and years of working with clients. You keep the learning process active (and thus your professional and personal growth) by taking continuing education courses—either a series of short, specific classes or a long-term, advanced training program.

Choose courses for the right reasons. Practitioners often save their pennies so they can take some new modality or product information workshop, desperate in the hope that this will bring them more clients or more security in their business. They take classes believing that "this will be the magic formula to make me successful." If they don't market themselves well now, it's unlikely that additional training is the panacea. Unless a training workshop includes a segment on how to market your new skills, it isn't likely to support your goal of creating more business.

Furthering your knowledge base is important, but don't confuse your ability to be good at your one-on-one work with the ability to market yourself well. They are different skills. If you need to learn more about marketing, take a marketing course. If you want to expand your technical repertoire, attend a modality or product knowledge training. Do each for the right reason.

Requirements ●●

Many people are required to take continuing education to keep their certification or licensure current. Check with your certifying or licensing bodies to find out their parameters: the number of hours required anually; whether all (or a certain percentage) of the classes must be given by approved providers; the scope of topics that can be taken and which topics aren't allowed; the minimum or maximum number of hours that can be allotted to certain

If you fill your mind with coins from your purse, your mind will fill your purse with coins.
— Benjamin Franklin

I am convinced that it's of primordial importance to learn more every year than the year before. After all, what is education but a process by which a person begins to learn how to learn?
— Peter Ustinov

subjects (e.g., half of the hours must be hands-on, only up to one-third of the hours can be practice management); the method of learning allowed (some certifying bodies allow a limited number of hours for reading books or writing articles, others disallow distance learning courses for certain types of courses); and specific course requirements (e.g., six hours of ethics every four years, CPR recertification every five years).

Continuing Education Sources ••

Many individuals, companies and organizations provide continuing education courses on a wide range of topics. Check out advertisements in trade journals, magazines, newspapers and newsletters; contact your professional association for a list of providers; request catalogs from schools as well as local community colleges, universities and adult education programs; peruse local specialty publications; and surf the Internet (start your search with key terms such as training, continuing education, home-study, correspondence, schools, seminars, workshops, or the specific topic you're interested in exploring).

Learning Environments ••

The best type of continuing education course to take depends on your preferred learning style. Many theories on learning abound. The two most popular for educational environments are Neuro Linguistic Programming developed by Richard Bandler; and Multiple Intelligences formulated by Howard Gardner and extended to the classroom by David Lazear. Your learning experience will be significantly more enjoyable and effective when you take a course that is best suited to your learning style. If the environment isn't suited to your learning style, you can still do it, but it will most likely be more difficult, take longer and the results won't be as clear.

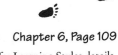

Chapter 6, Page 109
for Learning Styles details.

Some people learn best by reading or viewing a DVD and then processing the information on their own at their own pace. Distance-learning courses can be highly effective for people with this learning style. Keep in mind that these courses also vary widely: some provide reading materials while others include audio or video components. Assessments vary by course and can include multiple choice exams, written essays and documented case studies.

Others learn better in a classroom or workshop environment. Teaching styles vary greatly vary when continuing education is done "live" (e.g., workshops, classes, conferences) and the leader's style might not be best for you. Some people prefer highly structured classes; others like a loose format. Some people want to just hear what the "expert" has to say and resent class discussions. Some people enjoy group activities; others would rather work on their own. Some people do just fine in a class with hundreds of people; others withdraw. Some people want a hands-on approach, others would rather watch a video.

Once you've identified your preferred learning styles, you can assemble a list of questions to ask potential CE providers to get the best course for *you*.

Figure 4.1

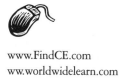

www.FindCE.com
ww.worldwidelearn.com

Questions for Colleagues about a CE Provider

- How easy was it to contact the provider about the course?
- What did you like the most about the course?
- What did you like the least about the course?
- What was the instructor's teaching style?
- Were the course materials beneficial and of high quality?
- On a scale of 1-10, how would you rate the overall value of this course?
- Did you learn what you expected to learn?
- Were agreements kept?
- Were you given a certificate upon completion?
- Do you think this was the best way to learn this subject? Why? Why not?
- What is the likelihood of you taking another course from this company?

Evaluating Continuing Education Providers ● ●

The depth, breadth and overall quality of continuing education courses vary greatly. Do proper research before enrolling in any course. The key aspect is the credibility of the company and the individual facilitating the course. The following steps guide you in ascertaining credibility:

Figure 4.2

Review Marketing Materials	Do the materials project a professional image?
	Are the courses clearly defined with specific objectives?
	Are the testimonials believable and are they from real people (not a vague reference such as "J.R. from Dallas")?
	Does the company offer a satisfaction guarantee or quality assurance?
Investigate Business History	How long has the company (or individual) been in business?
	How many classes have been given?
	How many people have taken courses?
	What are the qualifications of the person leading the classes (or the developer of a distance-learning course)?
	What are the professional affiliations held?
	Has the company or individual received any awards?
	Does the company or individual have credentialing status (e.g., an approved NCBTMB provider)?
Obtain References	Get feedback from others who have taken courses by this provider. The CE provider should give you names and contact information from past participants, but keep in mind that the referrals will most likely be slightly biased (those lists are usually comprised of happy customers).
	Talk with your colleagues and members of online newsgroups.

Research

The various disciplines that comprise the wellness professions have fascinating and diverse origins, and the unique public face of each discipline often depends heavily on these histories. Consumers vary in how they perceive these histories, and often it's these perceptions that lead them to choose one type of wellness care over another. There exists today, however, a method that levels the playing field and provides every technique an equal opportunity to prove its worth to today's savvy consumers. That method is research.

> The following information is adapted with permission from the forthcoming *A Guide to Reading the Research Literature*, by Ravensara Siobhan Travillian, Ph.D. Contact her at: www.helarctospress.com

In recent years, a growing body of research in the holistic wellness field has paved the way for wider acceptance of modalities such as acupuncture, yoga, and massage therapy by both the mainstream medical community and by the general public. By providing practitioners with access to high-relevance information, research provides solid science to document the efficacy and cost-effectiveness of treatment.

In addition to what we know through our experience and clinical judgment, and through what our clients teach us about their experience, research can promote the well-being of our clients, our profession and ourselves. It does so by facilitating the development of evidence-based practice, by providing more democratic access to high-quality information, and by giving us a common language we can use to communicate with other wellness practitioners. Finally, it can inspire us to think outside of the box, and to ask more and better questions of our profession and ourselves.

Continued research that is rigorous, focused, and of high quality will inform training programs, direct treatments, and—most importantly—guide the choices of consumers who want to know what issues a technique is good for, what it does, and why it's worth paying for. The bottom line is clear: research is essential to the long-term commercial success of the wellness professions. If you're serious about maintaining a stable and long-term career in the wellness field, study the current research, integrate research findings into your practice and marketing, and determine what role you can play in the conduct of research.

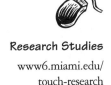

Research Studies
www6.miami.edu/
touch-research

The Scientific Method ••

In essence, the scientific method consists of observing a sequence of actions and making a testable prediction about that sequence. Research is based on the scientific method—a method that requires results to be repeatable and observable.

As an example of the scientific method used in research, a study by Ferrell-Torry and Glick focused on massage therapy treatments for patients with cancer pain. Results showed that massage lowered blood pressure in that patient group.[2] Another study by Olney applied the same treatment plan in a different group of patients with high blood pressure (hypertension).[3] This study found the same result: massage lowered high blood pressure.

In its simplest form, the scientific method consists of the following steps:

- Observe something that occurs (in our example above, in a group of cancer patients, blood pressure was lowered [indicating relaxation])
- Create a hypothesis about what you observed. Ferrell-Torry and Glick hypothesize that massage lowers blood pressure in cancer patients.
- Use that hypothesis to make a prediction about what will occur. Olney predicted that since massage has been observed to lower blood pressure in other groups of patients, it would also lower blood pressure in people living with hypertension.
- Set up an experiment to see if that prediction is accurate. Olney tested the effects of 10 back massages, (lasting 10 minutes apiece, carried out three times a week), on the blood pressure of patients diagnosed with hypertension.
- Decide whether the experiment confirmed the hypothesis or contradicted it. Olney concluded that there was a significant reduction in the blood pressure of the people who received the massages; therefore there was evidence that massage is a treatment that should be considered for hypertension patients.

Research Literacy ● ●

Research literacy refers to an ability to evaluate and apply research that may be useful in your wellness practice. At first, the idea of reading research articles may be intimidating, but remember that you don't need to analyze every detail of the article in tremendous depth. Read as carefully as you can and look for the high points: what was the research question the author tested and did that research question hold up when it was tested? That is the heart of the article; the rest is details.

Knowing how to sift gems of information and insight from research is a learned ability that comes with practice. You may want to organize a group that meets monthly to discuss research articles and information useful in day-to-day practice. It's a great way to ensure you keep up with latest developments, as well as to network with like-minded professionals. Plus it can significantly enhance your skills as a practitioner.

www.businessmastery.us/
research-structure.php
for research article structure.

You can find various kinds of articles, such as reviews, essays and research summaries in scientific journals, trade magazines and online. The structure of most research papers and articles mirrors the scientific method.

Research Capacity ● ●

Research capacity refers to the ability to carry out research. The best way to become involved in research is to become part of a multidisciplinary team that studies a particular research question. If you live near a university, you can check whether it's carrying out research in your field. If not, you can develop a research idea and approach potential funders in your community to carry it out. The funders will look closely at whether you have the skills and experience to carry out what you propose to do. Building a strong team of professionals who have solid experience in research design and implementation plays a key role in the success of such a proposal.

• Cultivate Your Support System •

A strong support system can greatly impact your career. Get advice and coaching from people who have essentially traveled the path you're on, as well as others who have greater expertise than you in specific areas concerning career growth and business development.

The four major support system categories are mentors, advisors, supervision and Mastermind groups. It is ideal to have all four in place, although finding a mentor may be the most difficult. Your support system may be comprised mainly of people you know who care about you and want to see you succeed. Then again, some, if not all, may be paid advisors. The nice aspect of paid advisors is that terminating the relationship is easy.

Experience is a good teacher, but her fees are very high.
— W.R. Inge

Find the Right Mentor •

A business or professional mentor is an individual, usually older, always more experienced, who helps and guides another individual's career development. The benefits of finding the right mentor are many. A good mentor can be an invaluable career asset and greatly enhance your potential for success. One of the most valuable things a mentor can do is to help you take an honest look at yourself and identify areas where work is needed to achieve your goals. This guidance is not done for financial gain yet can be personally rewarding for both parties. Most often people choose mentors who are in the same or related field. This person serves as a trusted confidante and the mentoring relationship usually lasts a long time—throughout a phase or throughout life.

People become mentors as a way of giving back to their community and to society at large. They may also do it to develop their skills as a teacher, manager or consultant. An effective mentoring relationship also works in both directions. A critical aspect of mentoring is to make certain that both parties are getting something out of the deal. It cannot just be a one-sided relationship; there must be give and take. Both parties must understand the benefits and demands that are going to be experienced in this process.

Chapter 5, Pages 96-99 for Social Responsibility.

Sometimes a mentor can be found through a professional or trade organization. Also contact your alma mater to find out if it has a mentoring program in place. Another option that is similar to mentoring and can ultimately lead into a true mentoring relationship is to intern or apprentice with a highly regarded practitioner.

In most instances, the best place to look for a mentor is right in front of you—perhaps someone from work or in your professional circle who you admire and respect. You might also know someone who doesn't do the same type of work as you but is an expert in the field. These are the types of individuals to approach first to ask if they would consider being your mentor.

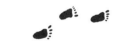

Mentor: Someone whose hindsight can become your foresight.
— Unknown

Figure 4.3

> ## Tips for a Successful Business Mentorship
>
> - The mentor must possess a high level of expertise in the area(s) in which she offers advice or training.
> - The mentee must be open to receiving feedback.
> - Both parties must have the time to commit to this process.
> - Determine the goals of the relationship and set a timeline for meeting them.
> - Create an agreement about what is expected from each party during the mentoring process.
> - Regularly check in with each other to see if the goals are being met and the relationship is still mutually beneficial.

How to Choose Advisors •

Every business has management, marketing, legal and accounting aspects. It is important to know trustworthy people for advice, particularly in areas where you lack knowledge, interest or skill. Selecting the most appropriate advisors directly affects the success of your business. Before making any major decisions, discuss them with at least one other person—regardless of your expertise in the area. All too often, the tendency is to do it all on your own and it's almost impossible to be truly objective, especially with something as significant as your business or career. Your primary advisors are your lawyer, accountant, banker and business consultant or coach.

Reliable, affordable and trustworthy counsel is crucial to your business health. Pick the members of your advisory team before you NEED them. Don't wait for an emergency when you may not have ample time to find an appropriate advisor to assist with the situation at hand. Begin to build your relationships now (particularly with a banker) so you can establish your credibility and develop rapport.

The process for selecting advisors begins by getting personal recommendations from friends and colleagues. In addition to the names get specific information about them. Find out why they recommend these advisors and what types of dealings they have had with them. Whatever you do, don't stop at this point. You must also make your own assessments. The first thing is to trust your intuition. If you don't feel comfortable with a particular advisor—keep looking. Even if you feel good about the person, do further research. She may be an excellent advisor yet not appropriate for you.

Check into the potential advisor's credentials and competency. If she has the required expertise and experience, the next phase is to discover if you're compatible. Find out the type of clientele she advises, particularly if she has clients in your profession.

Interview potential advisors (make certain this initial consultation is free of charge). See if your personalities and styles mesh. This is someone you're going to work with for a long time. You must share a similar philosophy and manner in which you like to get things done.

Government organizations that match people with mentors

www.score.org
www.sba.gov/sbdc

Assess your level of confidence and trust in this person—professionally and personally. How well you communicate with each other is one of the most critical factors in choosing an advisor. For example, this person may be totally qualified, works with many others in your profession, has an impeccable character and shares many of the same beliefs as you, but it seems as though whenever you talk, you're speaking in two different languages. You have to decide if it's worth the time (and money) it takes to work through the communication barriers to have this person be your advisor.

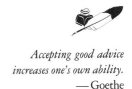

Accepting good advice increases one's own ability.
— Goethe

Finally, determine if this person desires to have you as a client. A good advisor demonstrates a sense of commitment to you and your business and is readily available to answer questions.

Create a Safe Harbor with Supervision ✳

Supervision has long been the primary professional training model for mental health clinicians. More recently, other wellness professionals have begun to recognize and use this forum to teach students. It consists of the practitioner meeting regularly with another professional (or several) to discuss client treatments and professional issues in a structured way.

Les Kertay, Ph.D., states, "If you're interested in doing work that has emotional and spiritual impact on your clients, then the most powerful way of dealing with the questions involved is to utilize ongoing professional supervision. Supervision isn't about being told how to do your job, rather it's a place to process your clients' work and your experiences of being with them."[4]

Supervision creates a shame-free setting for self-care, support and nurturance. It is the right place to receive appreciation for the good and useful work a practitioner is doing. Participating in supervision helps you to maintain an ethical practice and avoid burnout by assisting you with the following:

- Diffuse intense feelings that arise in the therapeutic relationship.
- Resolve complex interpersonal dilemmas.
- Recognize and manage transference and countertransference.
- Learn from your experiences.
- Progress in expertise.
- Ensure excellent client care.
- Enhance communication skills.
- Create balance.

Professional Supervision ✳✳

Professional (also referred to as clinical) supervision provides an opportunity to discuss with a more experienced, psychologically savvy practitioner (usually one with mental health training) how to best help a client while promoting increased self-observation and awareness.

Supervision can take place on a one-on-one basis or in a group. It is often useful to have supervision in a small group of practitioners who are doing the same kind of work. This broadens the base of learning and creates an additional support system for each member.

If the practitioner is in a group situation where she can learn from others' experiences, it's possible to master the fundamentals of practice through witnessing others' learning and not relying exclusively upon her own professional trial and error. Hearing the fears and doubts of other practitioners who are feeling challenged by unusual client situations can help practitioners feel less isolated and alone.

Rather than offering advice and telling the practitioner what to do, a good supervisor helps the practitioner to explore what's happening internally, define where the appropriate boundary is for the practitioner and the client and determine what action might correct the situation. In general, these techniques, which draw on and validate the practitioner's problem-solving skills, lead to a more effective and empowering resolution. In a group setting, the supervisor often invites other members to help navigate a colleague toward the core issue underlying the problem.

Peer Group Supervision ● ●

Peer group supervision is a valuable model of supervision for practitioners at any phase of professional life. Beginning practitioners may find it beneficial to engage in both individual and peer group supervision. Mid- and late-career practitioners often participate regularly in peer group supervision and seek individual consultations as required. Each practitioner designs a network of supervision that suits the demands and needs of his practice, phase of professional development and his personality.

Peer group supervision has easily identifiable advantages and some potential disadvantages. The strengths, limitations and success of peer groups rest with the composition of the individual members and the clarity of the peer group contract. Peer group supervision decreases professional isolation, increases professional support and networking, normalizes the stress and strain of professional life and offers multiple perspectives on any concern or problem. Peer supervision has the added benefit of being free of charge, intellectually stimulating and fun.

A brief, start-up consultation with a clinical supervisor or group specialist is helpful to define and establish the contract and framework for successful peer group supervision. When successful, peer group supervision far exceeds other forms of supervision and continuing education for individualized learning, intimacy, support, pleasure and a sense of belonging that anchors professional work. Many peer groups opt to have a clinical supervisor moderate meetings on a regular basis, such as quarterly or twice a year. It may also be appropriate to meet with this supervisor individually when additional support is requested.

How to Find a Supervisor ● ●

Psychotherapy disciplines have the longest tradition of providing clinical supervision and, thus psychotherapists are fruitful sources. Psychiatrists, nurses, social workers, psychologists and counselors are likely to be experienced supervisors. Personal recommendations by a colleague or a valued teacher are also fine ways to secure names of potential supervisors. If a referral by a colleague or instructor is difficult to obtain, it's possible to contact state or national professional organizations to obtain names of professionals in good standing.

A skillful supervisor is like a guide in unfamiliar territory, enhancing understanding and helping direct the practitioner toward constructive solutions. A supervisor often helps by asking a variety of questions about what is needed and what the practitioner was thinking and feeling when she encountered the problematic situation. In appropriate situations, advice can be offered about how to best assist a client. The most important aspect of supervision, however, is the opportunity to explore and work through a problem.

Mastermind Groups *

Joining a Mastermind group is a good way to strengthen your support system and widen your circle of professional acquaintances. Being involved in a Mastermind group is akin to having a volunteer board of directors that gives you guidance, support and shares their proven success strategies. And the only cost to you is that you give back the same. The concept of Mastermind groups was coined by Napoleon Hill in his book *Think & Grow Rich*. Hill defines Mastermind groups as the coordination of knowledge and effort in a spirit of harmony between two or more people for the attainment of a definite purpose.[5] Members of Mastermind groups serve as a confidential sounding board—they listen to business concerns and ideas are shared, analyzed and honed. The strength of this type of group is that the members are committed to supporting each other. This synergy fosters amazing creativity and results.

How They Work * *

Mastermind groups usually consist of six to eight people, but no more than ten. The members are professionals with varied backgrounds, experience and areas of expertise. They meet on a regular basis (weekly, monthly or quarterly) to brainstorm with each other, give and receive feedback, bestow their secrets for success, set goals and share their successes, as well as challenges. As an added benefit, members often provide business leads and client referrals.

Responsibilities are shared by all members. Each person takes a turn at hosting a meeting. The host sets the agenda, coordinates schedules, handles the logistics (e.g., room setup, refreshments) and facilitates the meeting.

If you cannot find an opening in an existing group, start your own Mastermind group.

Self-Assessment

You already have been doing a lot of business skill building, soul-searching and clearing throughout the process of "working" this book. Now it's time to evaluate yourself to determine the skills you need to learn or enhance. Be honest.

- What are your strengths?
- What are your challenges?
- How do you intend to alleviate those challenges?

This poster is a summation of the principles and techniques covered in this book. Post it in strategic places, such as your bathroom mirror or bulletin board. Refer to it often.

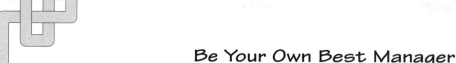

Be Your Own Best Manager

Believe in yourself!

Identify your values and operate from them.

Clarify your purpose, priorities and goals.

Design and implement an effective business plan.

Create strategic plans of action.

Learn to work smarter—not harder.

Track important components.

Eliminate time wasters.

Plan your days.

Set a schedule and keep it.

Utilize proper body mechanics.

Respect your mind's and body's cycles.

Take a stretch break every 20 minutes.

Strengthen your business savvy.

Become proficient with your computer skills.

Be dressed for "work."

Get feedback from colleagues and experts.

Collect information: quotes, articles, statistics.

Keep your work space organized.

Enhance your telephone skills.

Work from a client-centered approach.

Follow through with clients.

Market your business consistently.

Join at least one professional association.

Develop powerful networking abilities.

Keep accurate records.

Maintain healthy boundaries with clients and co-workers.

Keep up on the latest research findings.

Be a calculated risk-taker.

Be flexible.

Be willing to move on.

Make sure your needs are being met.

Exercise regularly.

Eat healthy foods.

Receive regular wellness treatments.

Create a support system.

Engage in group or peer supervision.

Take continuing education courses.

Enhance your communication skills.

Get out of the house/office EVERY DAY!!!

Have a life outside of work.

Schedule fun time that has nothing to do with your work.

Take responsibility for yourself.

Choose appropriate advisors.

Keep things in perspective.

For tasks you hate—delegate (or subcontract).

Balance your personal and professional life.

Maintain a good sense of humor.

Remember, we're all human, and we make mistakes.

Acknowledge your accomplishments every day.

Possess a positive mental attitude.

Do what you love, love what you do.

Part II

Intentional Excellence

In Part II of *Business Mastery*, the theme of intentional excellence takes center stage. Intentional excellence requires unflinching honesty and courage, and it results from making your integrity central to whatever you do. It is the result of consistent and conscious effort made visible in the behaviors, interactions and relationships you establish within your practice.

Chapter 5 focuses on measures of excellence that are different from markers of success like client numbers and bank balances. We start with a look at professional ethics, which exist not to catch people in wrongdoing but to guide practitioners toward greatness, and present guidelines for recognizing ethical dilemmas and resolving them. This discussion flows naturally into the key role that a professional image plays in building a successful practice. The last two sections consider how goodwill and social responsibility bring excellence into your practice—as you share your talents, time and resources to support causes closest to your heart.

Chapter 6 discusses why good communication skills are essential in business and highlights ways to fine-tune key skills, such as active listening and reflective feedback. It includes useful tips on how to handle the inevitable conflicts and difficult situations that are part of professional life. This chapter also offers practical insights into how communication styles differ among people of various personality types, and how to conduct effective client interviews. Excellent record-keeping is another aspect of good communication, so we discuss SOAP and CARE formats for documenting client sessions and charting progress.

Conscious Practice

❋ Ethics ❋

Ethics have been debated by philosophers great and small for millennia. While there are several aspects of human behavior that are clearly good or bad, it's extremely difficult to agree upon what is good and bad—so much depends on the situation. Ethics can be defined as: a system or code of morals and conduct of a person or group; the discipline dealing with what is good and bad or right and wrong. The book, *The Power of Ethical Management*, by Norman Vincent Peale and Kenneth Blanchard, relates ethical behavior to self-esteem: people who feel good about themselves withstand outside pressure and do what is right rather than what is expedient, popular or lucrative.

Ethics are different from morals and laws. Morals relate to character. Laws are codified rules of conduct that are based on ethical or moral principles. Laws often set the minimum standard necessary to protect the public's welfare, while ethics epitomize the ideal standards embraced by a profession.

Ethical behavior involves striving to bring the highest values into one's work and aspiring to do one's best in all interactions. It means doing the right thing for the right reason with the right attitude. The cornerstone of ethics is self-accountability. When you have a well-developed sense of self-accountability, you're honest with yourself and fully responsible for what you say and do at all times. You have the ability to look beyond the immediate moment to consider all the consequences and know if you're willing to accept them. In general, typical business ethics cover adhering to prevailing laws, upholding the dignity of the profession, being service-oriented, staying committed to quality and demonstrating loyalty to staff.

Tom Peters offers a practical definition of ethics:

> *High ethical standards—business or otherwise—are, above all, about treating people decently. To me (as a person, business person and business owner) that means respect for a person's privacy, dignity, opinions and natural desire to grow; and people's respect for (and by) co-workers.*[1]

If you help others, you will be helped, perhaps not tomorrow, perhaps in one hundred years, but you will be helped. Nature must pay off the debt... It is a mathematical law and all life is mathematics.
— G.I. Gurdjieff

For further information on ethics, refer to the book, *The Ethics of Touch* by Ben Benjamin, Ph.D., and Cherie Sohnen-Moe

We are continually faced with ethical concerns. Most of them are easily reconciled, though occasionally we encounter a major conflict. Examples of common ethical dilemmas in the wellness professions are:

- Practicing beyond your scope
- Breaking confidentiality
- Sexual misconduct
- Misrepresentation of educational status
- Financial impropriety
- Exploiting the power differential
- Misleading claims of curative abilities
- Dual relationships
- Bigotry or dishonesty
- Inappropriate advertising
- Violation of state/city laws or regulations.

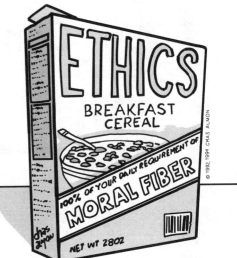

Key Interpersonal Ethics Concerns ✳

As a wellness practitioner, you may experience ethical dilemmas involving personal boundaries, power differential, confidentiality and dual relationships. Following are examples of these types of situations that may require careful consideration.

In Search of Excellence by Thomas J. Peters and Robert H. Waterman Jr.

• **Boundaries**: In relationships a boundary is a limit that separates one person from another. It protects the integrity of each person. A boundary can be as tangible as the skin that surrounds our body or as ethereal as an attitude. The primary problem in defining boundaries is that in most instances they're intangible. Understanding boundaries is crucial to creating an ethical practice and building professional relationships. By increasing your awareness of your clients' boundaries, and your own, you can improve the therapeutic relationship and avoid any inadvertent slips into unethical behavior.

The attainment of wholeness requires one to stake one's whole being. Nothing less will do; there can be no easier conditions, no substitutes, no compromises.
— C.J. Jung

• **Power Differential**: It is difficult to understand the therapeutic relationship between client and practitioner without comprehending the dynamics of power in a therapeutic relationship. There is a natural power differential in many relationships: between parent and child; between teacher and student; between employer and employee; and of course between wellness practitioner and client. A parent, teacher, employer or wellness practitioner has the more powerful position. They are the authority figures whose actions, by virtue of their role, directly affect the well-being of the other.

The power differential is inherent in any therapeutic relationship. There is an implicit acknowledgment that the practitioner has more knowledge in this area than the client. In the wellness field the power differential is amplified by the physical aspects of practice. The client takes a position—usually lying or sitting—which allows the practitioner access to his body. The practitioner positions herself within the client's physical space, often leaning over the client. Furthermore, in many professions the client is partially or fully unclothed. Finally, as the practitioner makes physical contact with the client's body, the client's physical safety is literally in the practitioner's hands.

• **Confidentiality**: Confidentiality is the cornerstone of every positive and powerful therapeutic relationship. Confidentiality can be defined as the client's guarantee that what occurs in the therapeutic setting remains private and protected. First and foremost, the issue of confidentiality concerns the client's rights to privacy and safety. These rights belong equally to every client you see regardless of age, status or relationship to you or another client. These same rights apply to both verbal and written interactions you have with anyone other than the client.

Most professionals are clear about what constitutes a major confidentiality breach such as sharing personal information about a client with a third party. However, subtle situations may occur where it can be easy to cross boundaries if one is not vigilant, such as public recognition. Clients shouldn't be acknowledged in public unless they recognize and greet the professional first. To do so puts clients in a position of having it revealed that they were seeking professional services that they may want kept private. If you work with celebrities or public figures and you think you might want to let others know (e.g., including a statement on a flier such as, "Some of my clients include [insert celebrity's name]."), it's wise to get permission—preferably in writing.

Occasions when it's appropriate to break confidentiality include: when there's a clear and imminent danger to the client or another individual; a client discloses an intention to commit a crime; suspected abuse or neglect of a child, an elderly person, or an incapacitated individual; or a court subpoena for a client's records. A confidentiality agreement that notes these situations can be an important tool for communicating to a client these exceptions to standard confidentiality practices.

• **Dual Relationships**: The term dual relationships describes the overlapping of professional and social roles and interactions between two people. Human beings naturally develop multiple relationships in various arenas—among family, friends, neighbors, employees, employers, professional peers, clients, students and teachers. People often fit into more than just one of those categories, and certain individuals play a mixture of roles. The classic depiction of a dual relationship is when two persons who interact professionally develop other roles of social interaction.

For example, you and a working colleague discover a mutual interest in tennis and begin to play together, or you and your teacher develop a longstanding friendship. Dual relationships also develop in the other direction, from the social to the professional realm: you and your sister decide to go into business together; or a social acquaintance or a friend seeks your professional services. In small towns or rural communities, dual relationships are even more common because of the limited numbers of people and choices for professional services.

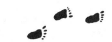

www.businessmastery.us/
forms.php#hipaa_form
for sample Privacy forms.

Chapter 12, Pages 246-249

for more information on
confidentiality and
HIPAA regulations.

Chapter 12, Pages 229-230

for more information on
Dual Relationships.

Key Business Ethics Concerns ✴

Whether you're a business owner or employee of a spa, group practice or medical clinic, you may encounter situations that require you to apply sound ethical judgment. Following are highlights of business situations involving ethical issues. The nuts and bolts of these topics are covered in depth in other chapters.

- **Finances:** In the realm of financial transactions, ethical issues can arise relating to gift certificates, fee structures and tips. There have been reported instances of practitioners deliberately setting gift certificate expiration dates or redemption policies that result in a high percentage of unredeemed certificates. On the other hand, ethical practitioners often place a reminder call to a gift certificate holder one month prior to the expiration date, or return funds to the gift certificate purchaser if a certificate is not redeemed within the allotted time. Another area of ethical concern involves scenarios in which a practitioner charges a higher fee to clients who pay by insurance versus clients who pay by cash. Lack of income tax reporting of tips from sessions is also an area of ethical concern.

Chapter 13, Pages 263-265

for more information on Product Sales.

- **Product Sales:** At times, unethical practices such as pushy sales techniques or hype can characterize product sales in wellness settings. Fortunately, this is the exception rather than the rule. Ethical product sales involve providing clients with easy access to high-quality products that enrich their well-being. As a wellness practitioner, clients depend on you to provide them with sound information and guidance in the realm of product sales. Thus, it's essential to know your products well and convey the proper use, benefits and possible side effects or contraindications of each product.

- **Client Records:** Keeping accurate records is paramount. Also, confidentiality must be maintained in a therapeutic relationship to promote an atmosphere of safety. Although confidential recordkeeping has always been a cornerstone of ethical practice, government scrutiny of this issue has added extra weight to compliance—via the Health Insurance Portability and Accountability Act (HIPAA). These regulations were enacted to ensure compliance with high ethical standards of confidentiality, and define what healthcare providers must do to protect the confidentiality of client information and recordkeeping.

State and local laws

www.smallbusiness.findlaw.com

- **Legal Issues:** A practitioner is required to comply with all legal requirements whose aspects include: complying with local, state and federal laws; maintaining appropriate insurance coverage; slander and libel; negotiating and complying with contracts; civil lawsuits; and employees. Sometimes a practitioner may feel confusion about what is legal and what seems the right thing to do. Practitioners may feel forced to find legal loopholes to justify their choices. These dilemmas require thoughtful choices.

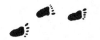

Chapter 12, Pages 256-262

for details on Insurance Reimbursement.

- **Insurance Issues:** Insurance coverage for complementary healthcare treatments is an evolving issue. Careful attention and recordkeeping can maximize the benefits for both clients and practitioners. For instance, a client's eligibility for medical insurance reimbursement may be limited to "authorized treatment." According to standard insurance definitions, treatment is warranted until a condition is corrected or maximum improvement is made. By identifying guidelines for delineating treatment versus wellness care, you can ethically apply those standards to the insurance issue: who pays for care? However, there is often a fine line between the two, especially if the condition is chronic. Ethical decision making can require careful thought and attention to treatment documentation.

• **Referrals**: Thanking people for referrals seems straightforward, yet such a simple gesture can be easily misconstrued. The key is the nature of the business relationship. It can become an ethical issue when a person in a power differential relationship makes a recommendation to a client and the practitioner receives financial remuneration for the referral. Might the concept of a referral fee come to outweigh the client's need for the best possible objective referral? Accepting payment for referrals clouds that ability and puts their ethics in a compromising position. In all cases this creates a conflict of interest.

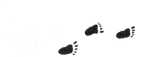

Chapter 16, Pages 361-366
for information on Building
Professional Alliances.

• **Taxes**: Taxation is a topic fraught with emotional charge. Many people resent the amount of money they pay in taxes (or how that money is spent) and use this anger to justify shady business practices. The two most common actions are concealing income (mainly cash payments and barter) and exaggerating expenses. An ethical practitioner keeps precise records, declares all income received, refrains from inflating expenses and accurately files governmental reports.

Chapter 14, Pages 301-308
for details on Taxes.

Resolving Ethical Dilemmas ☀

An ethical dilemma occurs when two or more principles are in conflict and, regardless of your choice, something of value is compromised. At such times you may find that you have several viable options, each with merit, and you aren't clear as to the most appropriate choice. You may also find yourself in a position whereby your values are in conflict. To resolve an ethical dilemma, follow this six-part process.

1. Identify the problem. This is the point at which you would gather as much relevant information as possible to determine whether it's truly an ethical problem.

2. Identify the potential issues involved. List and describe the critical issues. Evaluate the rights, responsibilities and welfare of those affected by the decision. Ascertain the potential dangers to the practitioner, client and the profession.

3. Review your profession's code of ethics and relevant laws. Determine if this issue violates either the letter or the spirit of applicable laws, regulations or professional codes. Check if your policies or procedures address this issue.

4. Evaluate potential courses of action. Brainstorm lots of ideas. Usually the first few options are based upon your personal values or an emotional response to the issue. Identify the benefits, drawbacks and outcomes of various decisions. Identify your motivations and stake in the outcome. Consider the consequences of inaction and contemplate how you will feel about yourself when all is done.

5. Obtain consultation. Engage in self-reflection and consider how society and members of your community might view these actions. Determine the impact it could have on your profession and justify a course of action based on sound reasoning which you can test in a consultation with a colleague.

6. Determine the best course of action. Map out the best way to resolve the problem. Who should be contacted first if multiple parties are involved? Do you need outside support? Do you need to talk to a supervisor? Should anyone else know about the problem?

Let's analyze a scenario using the six-step resolution model:

Figure 5.1

> ## Ethics Scenario
>
> *On Monday your session with Sally was very intense. She was experiencing significant pain in her legs and lower back. During the session she also released a lot of emotions and briefly spoke about her personal issues. Sally's partner, Terry, shows up for his weekly treatment on Tuesday afternoon. He mentions that Sally was exhausted and a bit withdrawn after her session. He jokingly makes a comment about how powerful it must have been and asks you what happened.*
>
> **1. Identify the problem:** This is a common occurrence when working with clients who know each other. They often ask how the other person is doing or how the session went. This is usually done out of genuine concern and not a need for gossip. Yet even just saying, "Oh, it was a good session" is inappropriate and may feel awkward. You determine this is an ethical problem.
>
> **2. Identify the potential issues involved.** By telling Terry about Sally's session, you would be committing a breach of confidentiality. Yet you know that it would be helpful to Sally if Terry was aware of what occurred. The potential hazards of sharing this information with Terry are: Sally may become upset with you and decide not to return; you may lose your credibility with both Terry and Sally; and you may lose potential clients due to the bad-will generated by this incident. You decide not to breach confidentiality by disclosing nothing about Sally's session.
>
> **3. Review your profession's code of ethics and relevant laws.** While you're unable to find any legal specifications, your professional Code of Ethics states that you must maintain client confidentiality.
>
> **4. Evaluate potential courses of action.** You have several options. First you need to decide what to say to Terry. You can shrug your shoulders and say, "Well, I guess it was rather intense," and then continue your session. Or you can say, "I highly value my commitment to client confidentiality. It would be best if you ask Sally directly about her session." You determine if you should pursue this any further at all (remind Terry to talk to Sally, or recommend to Sally that she talk with Terry), depending upon how Terry responded to your reply about the session and your sense of the benefits resulting from Sally sharing the information with Terry.
>
> **5. Obtain consultation.** You talk with several colleagues and get a mixed response. Some think that it isn't really a problem since the clients are partners. Other colleagues are adamant about it being a breach of confidentiality.
>
> **6. Determine the best course of action.** You choose to restate your confidentiality policy to both Terry and Sally and encourage them to share their experiences with each other.

Figure 5.2

Sample Code of Ethics

We, as wellness providers, have the responsibility to guide our actions to serve the best interests of the client. As members of this profession, we realize this responsibility can only be upheld by maintaining the highest degree of personal and professional integrity. As wellness practitioners, we make the commitment to provide personalized care and knowledgeable techniques, in a clean, comfortable atmosphere, thereby ensuring the client's safety and well-being.

Therefore, I agree to the following:

1. Maintain a professional appearance and demeanor by keeping good hygiene and wearing attire that is appropriate for the client setting.
2. Respect all clients regardless of their age, gender, race, national origin, sexual orientation, religion, socio-economic status, body type, political affiliation, state of health and personal habits.
3. Demonstrate respect by honoring a client's process, being present, listening, asking only pertinent questions, keeping my agreements, being on time, draping properly, and maintaining professionalism.
4. Maintain confidentiality of information concerning clients, and refrain from discussing client care details except under appropriate circumstances.
5. Provide a safe, comfortable, clean environment that is stocked with quality equipment and supplies.
6. Perform only those services for which I am qualified and (physically and emotionally) capable, and refer to appropriate specialists when work is not within my scope of practice or not in the client's best interest.
7. Be honest in all marketing endeavors.
8. Customize my treatments to meet the client's needs.
9. Charge a fair price for my services and offer a sliding scale when appropriate.
10. Keep accurate records and review charts before each session.
11. Educate clients by providing them with feedback and resources.
12. Make return and follow-up calls when appropriate and in a timely manner.
13. Post my credentials and policies.
14. Undergo peer review bi-annually.
15. Never engage in any sexual activity with clients.
16. Refrain from the use of any mind-altering substances before or during sessions.
17. Stay current with information and techniques by reading, receiving weekly treatments and taking at least one workshop per year.
18. Continue membership in at least one professional association.
19. Adhere to city, county, state, national and international requirements.
20. Educate the public about my services and benefits through activities such as: giving presentations, workshops and demonstrations; holding open houses and writing articles.

Codes of Ethics *

Codes of ethics are conduct guidelines. While individuals may have developed their own personal codes of ethics, codes that relate to business practices are most commonly set by professional organizations. The codes:

- Inform practitioners of appropriate ethical norms and behavior
- Supply direction for challenging situations
- Encourage practitioners to provide excellent service
- Protect clients
- Provide a means for enforcing desired professional behavior

Most codes of ethics are broad and vague, partly due to the contextual nature of "right" and "wrong." Research, consultation and self-exploration are usually required to determine what is appropriate and ethical. Among the components of a most wellness providers' codes of ethics are a statement of basic concerns: honesty, integrity, respect, compassion and making a difference; standards of service; a description of how the treatment or session is delivered (condition, place); when the treatments are given and by whom; the quality of materials used; and service guarantees.

Ideally the wellness community would develop a general code of ethics that all wellness professionals endorse with provisos for specific fields. Such a document would serve as a tool to educate the public about the basic conduct and level of professionalism they can expect from any wellness provider. Once this code of ethics is adopted we also face other exciting challenges, such as: how to implement it, determining the consequences of breaches, resolving the manner of enforcement, and educating the public. This calls for much introspection and dialogue within the industry (See Figure 5.2).

* Professionalism *

Professionalism stems from your attitudes and is manifested through the image you portray, your technical skill level, your communication abilities and your business practices. The term professionalism also relates to ethical behavior. High standards of action with clients result in both ethical and professional behavior.

No matter how many hours you work, this is your profession. There is a major distinction between part time and spare time. You may have other facets to your career besides being a wellness practitioner, but it's important to be clear about the roles each facet plays and be committed to excellence in each one. Quantity does not equate to quality. You are a wellness professional, and you're a businessperson—even if you only work three hours a week. The more you treat your practice as a business, the more professional you appear and the more successful you become. Sometimes this can be difficult, particularly if you don't have a modicum of technical business experience. Your attitudes toward yourself and your business are communicated directly and indirectly to your clients, colleagues and potential clients. You need to respect yourself and your abilities.

He who walks in truth and is devoted to his thinking, and furthermore reveres the worthy, is blessed by heaven.
— Confucius

Professionalism isn't measured by how many clients you see or how much money you earn but rather by who you are, your attitudes and how you treat others.

The basis for true professionalism lies in integrity. Someone may talk, walk and appear the part, but if that person doesn't come from a base of integrity, the facade wears thin quickly. If you don't treat your clients with the utmost respect, you won't have many clients. Integrity is often considered as a thing to have—people have integrity if they're ethical, can keep confidences and keep their word. But there is more to it than that.

Integrity can be divided into three major levels: the first level is keeping your agreements; the second is being true to your principles; and the third level is being true to yourself. Integrity is a state of being and if that's your source, you're professional. It is rare to find practitioners who put on an air of professionalism without the integrity behind it. More often they love what they do and are genuinely concerned about the well-being of their clients. Nevertheless, some neglect to develop a professional demeanor.

Webster's Dictionary defines integrity as the quality or state of being complete; unbroken condition; wholeness; honesty; and sincerity.

Professional Affiliations

Professional affiliations are an important part of the business world and the development of a professional image, in addition to the educational, social and networking benefits. Join at least two organizations: one that specifically relates to your profession and one that supports your visibility in the local community.

Numerous associations exist for wellness professions, ranging from modality-specific associations to more general health and well-being organizations. An excellent source for these groups is the *Encyclopedia of Associations* (at your library). Look under the "Health and Medical" section for thousands of listings of specialized, auxiliary and local branches of associations. You can also find online links to many associations. Membership in a professional association makes a statement of your commitment to your career field.

Involvement in business organizations also demonstrates belief in yourself as a professional. Many groups exist on a national level. Locate them by referring to the "Business" section of the *Encyclopedia of Associations*. Locally, groups such as the Chamber of Commerce and business support groups can be found by looking through the phone book, talking with other business owners, researching online, and checking the newspaper's Money and Calendar sections.

Professional Associations Directory
www.sohnen-moe.com/resourcedirectory.php

Professional Credentials

Credentials establish professionalism to the public. The three regulatory methods of credentials are known as licensure, certification and registration. Each method has its particular requirements and provisions.

• **Licensure:** requires practitioners to obtain a license to perform their services; unlicensed persons who practice break the law. Some municipalities require a business or occupational license in addition to your license to practice your trade. Legal names and professional titles cited in the law are numerous and varied. License titles are not necessarily the same as professional certification titles.

• **Certification:** from a governmental view is a voluntary option which offers the use of vocational titles to distinguish professional services from adult entertainment. Other certification documents that you can post show that you have passed specific professional tests, such as those from the National Certification for Therapeutic Massage and Bodyworkers (NCTMB) or The National Certification Commission for Acupuncture and Oriental Medicine (NCCAOM).

• **Registration:** is the means by which a government agency keeps track of practitioners by informational recordkeeping. In Canada and some states in the United States, practitioners must be registered to legally use their professional title.

Image ✳

The image you portray influences how people react to you. Your public image is determined by the way you present yourself, your office, your business practices and the manner in which you treat your clients. I'm not advocating being someone other than yourself; I am suggesting you take the time to make certain your "outward" image supports your vision of success. See Figures 5.3, 5.4 and 5.5 for guidelines to bolster your image and reputation.

Your level of integrity, professionalism and grace determine how you're perceived. Taking the time to project a professional image is always worth the investment. It isn't necessary to have a huge budget either—just creativity. Most of the above guidelines don't involve any financial outlay. The desired result is that your image is professional, and it's vital that you don't lose yourself in this process. Who you are is what makes you good at what you do. It distinguishes you from the others. Keep your style and personality intact.

Professional Characteristics

Think about someone you regard as being very professional.

- What is this person's occupation?
- What is his/her philosophy of life?
- How does s/he feel about her/his career?
- What does s/he look like?
- Where is his/her place of business?
- What does the business look like from the outside?
- Can you easily see the office from the street?
- Is parking easily accessible?
- What does the office look like?
- How does this person greet you?
- What does s/he say and do?
- How do you feel when you're with this person?

Professionalism Inventory

- Think about what professionalism really means to you.
- Describe yourself in terms of professionalism.
- Describe how you imagine others see you in terms of professionalism.
- List any of the changes you would like to make.

Figure 5.3

Exude Confidence, Competence and Compassion

- Dress stylishly yet neatly, and keep jewelry to a minimum: your attire isn't meant to be a distraction.
- Keep good personal hygiene. Don't wear heavy perfume or cologne due to chemical sensitivities.
- Keep your technical skills excellent and current: do not pretend to be an expert where you're not.
- Be punctual and prepared: make your clients feel important and respected.
- Know how to introduce yourself and others: it can be very embarrassing if you stumble over your own tongue.
- Get involved in your community: become active in civic, social and political groups.

Figure 5.4

Generate a Comfortable, Professional Ambiance

- Be aware of the noise level and make any necessary adjustments: turn off the phone bell and soundproof thin walls.
- Keep the interior clean, particularly the bathroom.
- Make sure that the building and address is visible from the street: this may mean investing in signage.
- Maintain the area outside your office: this may include landscaping.
- Keep the temperature comfortable for the client: if you don't have easy access to the temperature control, put a portable heater and fan in the room.
- Create a sense of privacy: you may have to be very inventive.
- Make certain that all equipment and furniture is comfortable and sturdy: you do not want a table to squeak and groan with every movement or to collapse under a client!
- Provide closet space or a shelf (at the very least, a hook) for your clients' belongings: most people don't like to throw their possessions in a corner.
- Keep supplies stocked and handy: you don't want your clients searching for a tissue while they're sneezing.
- Post your business license, policies, continuing education certificates and awards in a conspicuous place: these items represent the time and effort you've invested in your career.
- Have your business cards and literature available: make it easy for your clients to take what they need to help promote your business.

Figure 5.5

Your Treatment of Clients Determines
if They Become Regulars

- Be empathetic and understanding: keep in mind that not everyone shares your particular beliefs about health and well-being.
- Greet your clients appropriately: some people may not be up to a bear hug, while others may welcome it.
- Keep what happens during a session confidential: this can be tricky when your clients know each other and ask about the other's appointment. Be noncommittal and recommend they speak to the person directly. Even a casual remark can damage your trust factor.
- Remember that you're here to serve your clients: it isn't their job to counsel you during their sessions.
- Observe your clients' likes and dislikes: make the effort to do those "extra little things."
- Answer your phone professionally: you don't have to be overly formal, but remember you're a business. If you don't have a receptionist, hire a reliable appointment service. They can significantly increase your bookings.
- Return calls within 24 hours: you never know the influence and connections that a potential client may have; promptness is always appreciated.
- Answer important mail within four days and nonessential mail within two weeks: don't wait until you have the time to write a brilliant letter. Keep a supply of postcards handy. This way you can quickly acknowledge correspondence without worrying about having to fill up the page.
- Send newspaper clippings, articles and items of interest to clients and colleagues: this lets people know that you're thinking about them and are genuinely concerned.
- Acknowledge in writing any item or gift sent to you: thanking people over the phone is okay, but people usually keep cards for several days. Every time they look at your card, it reinforces their feelings of goodwill.
- Send thank-you notes for referrals: it's vital to show your appreciation. Thank-you notes are good for building goodwill and expressing sincere appreciation for your client's confidence in you.
- Set clear boundaries: don't let your personal life interfere with business.
- Return borrowed property promptly and in good condition: never borrow anything that you cannot replace should you damage or lose it.
- Never repeat a rumor that could hurt someone's reputation: it's wise to stay neutral. Gossip never reflects well on any of the parties.
- Keep accurate client files: review them before you see each client. Don't rely on your memory for all the details of your last session.

You cannot do a kindness too soon, for you will never know how soon it will be too late.
— Ralph Waldo Emerson

❋ Goodwill ❋

Goodwill is an integral component for success in any service industry and especially so in the wellness field. Goodwill is benevolence, friendly disposition, cheerful consent, willingness and readiness. In the business world, goodwill is the commercial advantage of any professional practice due to its established popularity, reputation, patronage, advertising and location, over and above its tangible assets. In other words, goodwill is an abstract impression, the "positive feelings" you inspire in others. It is based upon the supposition that you're doing the best you can and are fair and ethical in your dealings and behavior. It implies warmth, congeniality and trust.

Take a moment to think about the businesses and people that you respect. Why do you hold them in such regard? What have they done to encourage these feelings of goodwill? How have they demonstrated their concern? Your responses are the key to understanding the concept of goodwill. It is essential to cultivate alliances.

Many branches of the wellness field (particularly "alternative" ones) have substantial distances to cover before they achieve the recognition they deserve from the general public and the health industry. A major part of this guarded acceptance of touch therapies stems from a lack of standardization. The general public doesn't know what to expect. The variety of educational levels, styles, modalities, philosophies and fee structures are as diverse as those who practice them.

To gain further headway for recognition it's imperative to enhance the public image of your specific industry—that is, promote more goodwill.

The wellness field tends to rely on attraction (e.g., word-of-mouth, reputation and client referrals) rather than traditional methods of promotion. The downside is that word-of-mouth often revolves around "who" you know more than "what" you know. And even then it isn't enough to just know the "right" people. To obtain their support you need to nurture those associations. You must have good people skills. For example, you could be the most brilliant practitioner in your area, yet if you don't promote goodwill with your clients, centers of influence, colleagues and the community, you still may not do well financially. One of the most important habits to develop is prompt and gracious acknowledgment of all of the people who support you. A little recognition goes a long way!

It takes time, thought, creativity and some money to foster goodwill. Being good at what you do is only one aspect of it. Make certain that your actions reflect that you're proud of your profession and are sincerely concerned about people's well-being.

You can't buy goodwill, particularly if it's an attempt to repair a bad reputation (although corporations spend millions of dollars attempting to do just that). You can bolster the general public's opinion of you and your profession by donating your services and knowledge to charitable organizations and events—especially if you get media coverage.

You can't build a reputation on what you are going to do.
— Henry Ford

New Traditions in Business
— edited by John Renesch

Do all the good you can,
By all the means you can,
In all the ways you can,
In all the places you can,
At all the times you can,
To all the people you can,
As long as ever you can.
— John Wesley

✳ Social Responsibility ✳

Social responsibility is twofold. It holds that a business has a responsibility to refrain from unethical behavior that may bring harm to the community, its people or the environment. It also recognizes that a business has a responsibility to give back to society to help solve social problems through means such as grants, in-kind donations, community outreach and employee volunteer programs.

In short, socially responsible companies operate in environmentally friendly ways, invest in the communities they serve and focus on ways to improve working conditions for employees. A growing number of companies are recognizing that social responsibility is not just good business or a public relations gimmick—it's simply the right thing to do.

As an individual and business owner, you can make a difference socially, economically, environmentally and politically. Running your practice from a place of compassion, integrity, and personal values creates a sense of empowerment and fulfillment. Many businesses are learning how to be profitable and heed their social missions. As the concept of "quality of life" evolves, time and freedom become the dominant concerns (although financial security is clearly important). In addition, companies are becoming more ecologically aware, reducing the number of consumables, choosing "environment-friendly" products and instituting recycling programs.

As growing numbers of small and large businesses incorporate values that reflect social responsibility into their everyday practices, political pressure comes to bear upon governments to create policies and laws along the same lines. As a result of the changes in business philosophy, new operating procedures are often developed. Purchasing products and services is no longer based only on price and quality. Companies that embrace the philosophy of social responsibility often offer discounts to businesses that belong to like-minded political, professional, social or networking organizations.

Many companies demonstrate the feasibility of being financially successful while doing good in the community, treating their employees well, and providing excellent customer service. In addition, company support of volunteerism and tithing is on the rise. Many individuals and companies are donating their time, money and expertise to their favorite charities. Also, groups of individuals are joining together to form organizations expressly committed to responding to emergency conditions.

Profiles ✳

Gifts In Kind International is a wonderful example of social responsibility at work. Driven by a mission of providing an effective conduit for the donation of products and services from the private sector to the charitable sector, Gifts In Kind International is a leader in product philanthropy. It provides valuable resources to more than 200,000 nonprofits through its network of over 450 corporate partners. Large corporations, as well as small and mid-sized companies, benefit by supporting the communities where they do business, reducing inventory and warehousing expenses, and qualifying for a tax deduction. *Forbes* magazine recently recognized Gifts In Kind as one of the most cost-effective charities in the world.

A candle loses nothing of its light by lighting another candle.
— James Keller

The goodwill and heightened visibility generated by being a socially responsible business can greatly impact your success.

www.businessmastery.us/ goodwill-profiles.php for more profiles.

Ben & Jerry's premium ice cream and frozen yogurt manufacturing company believes in what they call "Caring Capitalism": a business that makes top-quality, all-natural products; is a force for social change; and is financially successful. Co-founder Ben Cohen once said, "Business has a responsibility to give back to the community." Thus the company's social mission is to improve the quality of life of a broad community—local, national and international. Ben & Jerry's product donations support the work of a wide range of nonprofit organizations across the country and it sponsors a variety of community service projects and individual volunteer efforts. In addition, some of the company's profits go directly to the Ben & Jerry's Foundation, which makes grants to grassroots organizations around the country that address social and environmental problems.

Companies of all sizes are taking action. For instance, **The Bodywork Emporium** has long maintained an active social and charitable giving philosophy. In 1996 it started The Touch Foundation, whose mission is: "It's time to touch the untouched." Dubbed "The Massage Peace Corps" by its founder, Shane Watson, the Touch Foundation reaches out to those who can't normally afford a massage or a helping hand. It coordinates a network of bodyworkers who provide healing touch to the orphaned, the needy, the elderly, the dying, the neglected, and people with disabilities. The Bodywork Emporium demonstrates commitment to volunteer therapists in the following ways: furnishing the coordinators, training, equipment and supplies; providing money to help cover therapists' basic expenses; recognizing therapists' participation; and creating a fun and rewarding environment.

You don't need to be a corporate giant to take an active stand toward social responsibility. All great movements spring from small individual actions. For example, Robert Toporek, a Rolfing practitioner in Philadelphia, had a mission to make a positive impact on the children who live in the "Badlands," one of the worst neighborhoods in Philadelphia. He founded **The Children's Project**, and every summer since 1993, he recruits volunteers go to these neighborhoods weekly to offer Rolfing structural integration, massage, music, books and computers. Since that time, he has collected, repaired and distributed more than 6,000 computers. Toporek has discovered that this is another way to relieve stress in these economically challenged families.

A unique community effort created a **Massage Emergency Response Team** in California after the Loma Prieta earthquake struck in October 1989. People at the National Holistic Institute (NHI) masterminded the logistics and got involved to help heal the community—8,000 massages were given by 300 massage therapists. It has evolved since then to become the National AMTA Massage Emergency Response Team (AMTA-MERT). There are eligibility requirements to join—although being a member of the American Massage Therapy Association is not mandatory—and members all receive standardized training in providing massage at an emergency response scene. Emergency response teams have served during the Oakland (California) Hills fire, Hurricane Andrew in Florida, the Oklahoma bombing and 9/11 at The World Trade Center.

I don't know what your destiny will be, but one thing I do know: the only ones among you who will be really happy are those who have sought and found how to serve.
— Albert Schweitzer

Gifts In Kind Int'l
www.GiftsInKind.org

Ben & Jerry's
www.benjerry.com

The Touch Foundation
www.bodywork-emporium.com/touch.htm

The Children's Project
ww.teamchildren.com

Steps You Can Take Now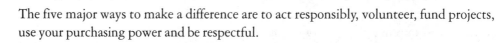

The five major ways to make a difference are to act responsibly, volunteer, fund projects, use your purchasing power and be respectful.

Act Responsibly * *

Acting responsibly requires that you be aware of your environment. In addition to embracing the slogan, "Reduce, Re-use, Recycle and buy Recycled," it's important to be knowledgeable about the world. Expand your horizons: read your industry trade journals and alternative magazines, such as *Mother Jones* or the *Utne Reader*. In your waiting room, post brochures, fliers and announcements on community events and ways your clients can make a difference.

Be an advocate: vote; write letters and place phone calls to politicians about issues that concern you; join a progressive campaigning group like Friends of the Earth, Amnesty International or an animal rights organization, such as People for the Ethical Treatment of Animals.

Volunteer * *

Donate your time and expertise to your favorite charities: join an industry group such as the AMTA-MERT or The Touch Foundation; do community service work with organizations such as Habitat for Humanity or the Literacy Foundation; donate blood; be a mentor for a child; pick a population of people who can't afford your services and "adopt" them; form a local community group; volunteer to walk a dog at your local animal shelter (there's often not enough staff to take animals for walks and you get to be a virtual pet owner—no muss, no fuss); give presentations in public schools (e.g., career day, health education week); take part in special events such as Make A Difference Day; and sponsor an activity such as "Adopt a Highway."

You aren't limited to contributing your specific vocational services. You can stuff envelopes, organize events and even build homes.

When strangers start acting like neighbors, communities are reinvigorated.
— Ralph Nader

Random Acts of Kindness by Conari Press

Make A Difference Day

This annual day of doing good was created by USA WEEKEND in partnership with the Points of Light Foundation. Held on the fourth Saturday in October, Make A Difference Day is the largest annual national day of helping others. Projects can be personal (e.g., helping an elderly relative with their chores), neighborly (e.g., organize a neighborhood beautification day), or major productions such as refurbishing a children's recreational center.

Join in with more than 1 million volunteers as they contribute to millions of others. The organizers request that if you currently volunteer regularly, make an extra effort in your volunteer activity. If you need more than one day for your project, still do a significant part of your volunteering on the fourth Saturday. If you can't participate on Saturday for religious reasons, do your project Friday or Sunday. Contact the organizers so they can include your volunteer activities as part of the DAYtaBANK.

USA Weekend   800-416-3824   www.usaweekend.com

Fund Projects ✳ ✳

In addition to donating money to worthwhile causes, you can grant scholarships and help coordinate fundraising activities. You can donate your services as prizes or raise money by sponsoring an event such as a "massage-a-thon." You can designate a charity and donate a day's revenues or run a promotion such as for every specified dollar amount (e.g., $50) that a client donates to your favorite charity, he gets a free treatment (such as a half-hour session or an adjunct service).

One of the most common ways to fund causes is through tithing. Tithing is contributing a set amount (usually 10 percent) of time or money to charitable causes. This is a convenient and effective way to give back to your community. People often associate tithing with religion, but that's only one option. Some popular forms of tithing include donating a specific amount of profits to an organization, doing pro bono work (providing services free of charge) and offering a sliding fee scale.

The greatest pleasure I know is to do a good action by stealth, and to have it found out by accident.
— Charles Lamb

Use Your Purchasing Power ✳ ✳

Let your voice be heard through your acquisitions. Purchase ecologically sound products (e.g., natural fiber linens), use environmentally friendly detergent for linens and clothes, and print your promotional materials on recycled stock. Invest wisely. Actively support businesses that are aligned with your values and boycott companies that oppose them.

Be Respectful ✳ ✳

Respect is the foundation of a socially responsible business: respecting yourself, the environment and your clients. Caregivers enter this field because they want to be of service. Clients are looking for practitioners with whom they share similar values. Be true to your beliefs, and express them in ways that respect differing viewpoints. While it isn't appropriate to foist your beliefs on your clients, you can encourage them to explore alternatives. Better yet, make sure your marketing attracts clients with similar beliefs.

Therapeutic Communications

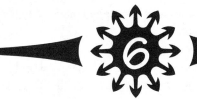

❋ Communication Fundamentals ❋

Good communication is the foundation of healthy relationships and thriving practices. In fact, one of the common threads of highly successful practitioners is effective communication skills. Advanced technical skills and business savvy are simply not enough. Without good communication skills, the growth of your business is likely to lag.

Taking the time and effort to enhance your communication skills will serve you well. Like any skill, achieving a degree of mastery takes practice—and in this case, a willingness to take a fresh look at your communication style and behaviors.

Communication skills are also known as "people skills," because, at its best, communicating involves connecting with people in positive and productive ways. As you enhance your skills in this area, you can expect to increase productivity, reduce stress and improve teamwork. You can also build stronger client relationships and minimize the potential for misunderstandings with colleagues, co-workers and clients. However, the greatest benefit manifests in clients who feel at ease and experience high levels of satisfaction with your work.

Good communication is a two-way process that involves an exchange of ideas, emotions and attitudes. The ultimate goal of communication is to elicit some type of action. The communication skills necessary in effective therapeutic relationships are the ability to establish rapport, listen to answers, effectively utilize communication technology, be patient, make astute observations, elicit information, ask open-ended questions, gain cooperation, conduct excellent interviews, ask for input, assert boundaries, use active listening techniques and show genuine concern.

To help you better understand what all great communicators know and practice, this chapter looks at the power of first impressions and rapport building, as well as several common barriers to effective communication. You will also find a wealth of practical tips and resources for developing excellent communication skills.

Seek first to understand, then to be understood.
—Steven Covey

First Impressions ✳

First impressions are powerful—and often irreversible. Your first interaction with a person sets the tone for future communication. Did you know that you have between four and 20 seconds to make that vital first impression? The elements of a first impression include characteristics such as your appearance, facial expressions, body language, what you say, what's not said, your ability to gain rapport, your energy level and the actual message. A vast amount of information is exchanged, and many judgments are formed at lightning speed in just a few moments.

Sometimes practitioners unknowingly alienate new and potential clients because they don't present themselves positively and professionally. To avoid this potential pitfall, take some time to think about how you present yourself and your work in that vital first meeting. When you're thoroughly prepared and aren't worrying about how to introduce yourself and what to say, it's easier to focus on being with your clients and listening fully to them.

Avoid prejudging yourself or your clients. This prejudice can substantially alter your first impression. Focus on building rapport and keeping an open mind. Your confidence in yourself and your abilities increases the comfort your clients experience.

Enhance Communication

www.cnvc.org
www.savicommunications.com
www.healingfromthecore.com

Building Rapport ✳

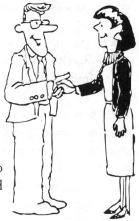

Rapport is the bond that develops between you and clients; it's based on mutual trust and accord. After you've made a good first impression, rapport can be the single most important factor in whether a client sees you once or becomes a long-term client. Rapport develops by being open and demonstrating genuine concern. Some techniques for developing rapport are to correctly pronounce clients' names, use clients' names frequently, smile, shake hands, maintain good eye contact, allow ample time for clients to talk, speak with enthusiasm and conviction, be punctual, listen, and ask a light personal question about the client's family, hobby or job.

Chapter 16, Pages 372-373

for details on developing a self-introduction.

It All Begins With You ✳ ✳

An excellent strategy for building rapport as well as enhancing understanding and impact is to begin as many sentences as possible with the word "you." This technique is also referred to as an embedded command. When you say "you," people pay attention because what you say relates to them. Incorporate expressions such as: "You are," "you have," "you will notice," "you will discover," "you will find," "you will receive," "you will experience," "you will see," "you will smell," "you will touch" and "you will feel."

Figure 6.1

Tips on How NOT to Create Rapport

- Arrive late to your appointments.
- Use language that invalidates clients' thoughts, feelings and experiences.
- Don't give the client your full attention while in person or on the phone.
- Eat or chew gum while talking to a client.
- Avoid eye contact while interviewing clients.
- Talk about yourself a lot.
- Gossip about how annoying your last client was and give lots of details, (but not the name, of course!)
- Leave intake forms and client charts strewn about your office.
- Disregard ambient noise: turn up the ringer volume on your phone, forget to turn off the stereo or television in adjacent rooms.
- Shame clients into coming back for more treatments because they don't take good enough care of themselves.
- Give unsolicited advice.
- Act like you know what's better for clients than they do.
- Be judgmental.

You can handle people more successfully by enlisting their feelings than by convincing their reason.
— Paul P. Parker

Figure 6.2

10 Keys for Excellent Communication

1. The most important thing to remember is that people act and react to fulfill needs. When you better understand their needs, you can create a better strategy for improving communication.
2. Take into consideration the person's natural tendencies and capacities. For example, if someone prefers to see things in writing, don't expect him to be very responsive to verbal communication. Also, if you're talking to someone who doesn't speak English well, avoid using polysyllabic words, rapid speech and colloquialisms.
3. Be considerate of the other person's mental, physical and emotional state, particularly if he is under a lot of stress.
4. Communicate on an equal level. Do not act superior or inferior.
5. Be honest.
6. Know the other person's opinion of you. If someone fully respects your expertise, it isn't necessary to take the time to build up your credibility. If she doesn't know you, you need to take the time to build rapport and trust.
7. Have good timing. As the saying goes, timing is everything!
8. Separate your emotions from the facts. It is difficult to have clear communication when you're coming from a reactionary position.
9. Ask questions.
10. Listen. Listen. Listen.

☀ Communication Barriers ☀

Words are imprecise vehicles of communication. The 500 most frequently used words in the English language have 12,078 separate and distinct meanings in *The Oxford English Dictionary*. On average, that's 24 meanings per word! People have to guess at what is meant by a word—usually from the context in which it's used. Often they're right; sometimes they aren't.

The biggest problem with language is that the meaning of words is in people, not in dictionaries. Each of us projects our own meanings onto the words we say and hear. The tone and accompanying body language are often more important than the actual words.

If you've ever seen someone expressing irritation or anger while smiling at the same time, you probably experienced a feeling of dissonance. Likewise, if someone apologizes to you with a smirk on his face and an arrogant tone, you'll experience a mixed message that causes you to doubt his sincerity.

Communication can also break down at the listener's end. Researchers have found that people listen four to five times faster than people speak. The listener has spare time in which to become bored and may mentally drift off to other thoughts. Also, without even realizing it, the listener may miss important elements of the message. Furthermore, we all listen through filters that screen out some messages and distort others. Our concerns, needs, moods, roles, prejudices and other factors color what we hear. The possibility for error increases when the speaker, the listener, or both experience strong feelings about the message.

The good news is that you can overcome communication barriers by applying a few basic skills and insights such as:

- Active listening
- Awareness of varied personality and communication styles
- Clarity when expressing a personal need or request
- Giving critical feedback in a positive and constructive manner
- Appropriately expressing feelings, such as anger and frustration
- Managing boundaries effectively
- Understanding how negative communications and dysfunctional patterns get in the way of good communication
- Expressing appropriate empathy

Later in the chapter, we explore how an awareness of your clients' personality and learning styles can enhance your communication.

Honor is the capacity to confer respect to another individual. We become honorable when our capacities for respect are expressed and strengthened. The term respect comes from the Latin word respicere, which means "the willingness to look again."
— Angeles Arrien

The Ethics of Touch
by Ben Benjamin, Ph.D., and Cherie Sohnen-Moe

Upset Clients and Difficult Situations

Although most of us would rather avoid upset clients and difficult situations, they're an inescapable part of professional life. In the realm of customer service, the focus isn't whether clients are right or wrong. The optimal goal is to ensure that clients feel that their concerns have been truly heard and addressed in an appropriate manner.

For instance, you may encounter a situation in which a client is having an "off" day and a simple misunderstanding can quickly gather speed. The client's emotions can start whirling, and you may find yourself in the center of a storm. It's important to realize that in some cases, no matter what you say or do, you're perceived as "wrong" by the client. Staying centered, listening carefully and responding with clarity may be the best you can do. Perhaps the least helpful thing you can say is, "There's no reason to be so upset."

Everything that irritates us about others can lead us to an understanding of ourselves.
— Carl Jung

Most of the time, you can calm an upset client by staying centered and using active listening and reflective feedback techniques. You may then need to brainstorm with the client to arrive at a solution agreeable to both parties. However, if a client is irrational, it's best to distance yourself from the client by saying that although the client may have a valid concern, you need time to think about what has been said and would prefer to respond later. You may then want to consult with a supervisor or trusted peer to explore effective ways to deal with the situation. In the worst case scenarios, you may need to involve a manager or another on-site peer to help defuse the situation.

If you as a practitioner made a mistake, did something inappropriate or inadvertently crossed a boundary, an acknowledgment and an apology would be the appropriate response in the next meeting. If a client's concerns are valid, the practitioner should take steps to correct the problem and communicate that to the client.

If a client has misinterpreted information or actions, it often works well to discuss the matter with the client at the next meeting. Sometimes a cooling off period may allow the incident to be discussed more easily. You can acknowledge how your actions could have been misunderstood and work to bring clarity to the situation.

Following are some tips on how to communicate effectively in difficult situations. As in all good communication, the first step is to carefully listen to the person's concern.

- Avoid reacting by venting back at the person with anger or frustration of your own. Though it may be difficult, do everything you can to hold your tongue. Focus on staying centered.
- Acknowledge and reflect back the person's concern and feelings. For example, "It sounds like you're really frustrated right now. If I understand correctly...."
- Don't pacify. Don't over-apologize. Upset people respond much better to a genuine apology, if appropriate, that comes from strength not weakness.
- Focus on the core issues and solutions. Don't get sidetracked by unimportant details.

Always document issues in the client's file.

Emotional Triggers ✱

If you're a wellness practitioner who specializes in hands-on bodywork, you're probably aware of how this modality can sometimes elicit emotional responses—such as crying, anxiety or anger. Your response in these emotionally charged situations can profoundly impact the positive impact of the bodywork and the long-term therapeutic relationship with your client. Thus, learning how to handle these delicate situations skillfully is essential.

If you work with clients with known trauma, it's advisable that they also see a psychotherapist.

Prior to beginning a session, many practitioners discuss with a client how bodywork can sometimes trigger strong emotions. It's also helpful to explain that emotional releases sometimes occur and are a natural part of the healing process. This type of conversation accomplishes two things. First it paves the way for a client to feel safe and at ease if an emotional release should occur. Secondly, it frames the experience in a matter-of-fact and positive way.

When working with clients who have experienced trauma, sometimes touching a particular area can trigger an emotional response associated with a past occurrence. If this occurs, the client might want to share with the practitioner. Allowing expression is usually acceptable, but encouraging it, asking questions, or interpreting it often exceeds the practitioner's scope of practice.

During an emotional release, keep the client focused on the present moment. You can suggest that the client breathe into the area, relax, and, perhaps open her eyes. If a client appears in great distress, ask the client if she would like to stop the session. If the client prefers to continue the session and asks you to work on the trigger area, you must proceed carefully. Keep in mind the significant difference between assisting a client in letting go of a memory or feeling that has surfaced, and promoting an emotional reaction or release.

Be aware of how easy it can be for a practitioner to get drawn into inappropriate responses to a client's strong emotions. Checking in with clients is appropriate, but it's best to refrain from asking questions that probe into the cause of emotional releases. Examples of some inappropriate questions are: "Do you know why you felt sad when I touched your leg?" "Were you thinking of someone in particular when you began to feel angry?" "Do I remind you of someone from your past?" Avoid playing the role of an armchair psychiatrist. Emotional release is a gray area where professional boundaries are easily crossed.

Whenever a client has an intense emotional release during a session, it's wise to call and check in the next day or so.

Unless you have specialized communication skills, knowledge and training in working with clients' strong emotions, it's best to defuse the situation and change the focus of the session with a statement such as, "This seems to be an area in your body where a strong experience is being held. Should I move to a different area?" The practitioner may then take the opportunity to explain that emotional experiences are often held in the body and mention that counseling or therapy can be beneficial in processing the emotional issues that come up in bodywork.

There is an art of knowing how to let clients have their feelings without requiring them to stop crying or express their feelings. Most times, the practitioner doesn't need to do anything except be open and available and keep working. Overreacting to an emotional release can stop the client from feeling safe.

If you encounter a situation in which you feel overwhelmed by a client's strong emotions, consider calling a time out, leaving the room, or stopping the session. All are appropriate responses that respect your professional boundaries. You can say something like, "I think it's best to give you a few minutes to let this integrate. I'm going to step right outside the door. Let me know when you would like to continue."

✳ Listening Skills ✳

Although more than half of all communication time is spent listening, very few of us have received training in the most effective ways to listen. In fact, by the time we reach adulthood, many of us have become highly skilled at tuning out messages—either from well meaning but overcritical parents or teachers, or from the constant bombardment of media advertisements.

Listening goes beyond hearing. Hearing is simply the physiological process by which the brain interprets information received through the ears. Listening involves taking the time to understand and interpret heard information. Listening means to give the speaker your full attention.

Effective listening skills affect clients in positive and powerful ways. They can help a client to feel at ease. They can also help defuse difficult or awkward situations when you may encounter an emotionally upset client. Being heard can profoundly help a client to relax and heal. After feeling truly heard, a client may breathe deeper, sleep better and feel less tension in his body—and this doesn't even have anything to do with the actual treatment.

One of the most common mistakes in both personal and professional communications is to give unsolicited advice or turn the focus back to yourself when someone expresses a concern or frustration. By jumping in with a solution or inserting your experiences into the conversation, the person you're talking with will not feel truly heard. In a professional setting you also risk traversing into territory better handled by a psychotherapist. However, with training and experience you can learn to manage the fine line between being supportive and moving into the territory of a psychotherapist.

To help enhance your listening skills, we explore how you can use the communication techniques of active listening and reflective feedback to ensure your clients feel truly heard.

Active Listening ✳

Active listening involves giving your full attention to the speaker. Oftentimes that can mean listening for the feelings behind words, facial expressions or gestures. Words convey only part of the message. To completely comprehend what a speaker is saying, a listener needs to understand what the message *means* to the speaker. That entails understanding what's said from within the speaker's *frame of reference*. It also requires a willingness to set aside wandering thoughts to stay focused on the speaker's message.

The most basic and powerful way to connect to another person is to listen. Just listen. Perhaps the most important thing we ever give each other is our attention.... A loving silence often has far more power to heal and to connect than the most well-intentioned words.
— Rachel Naomi Remen

People Skills: How to Assert Yourself, Listen to Others and Resolve Conflicts
by Robert Bolton

An active listener conveys interest with nonverbal communication, such as open body language and steady eye contact, and avoids distractions such as fiddling with a pen. The active listener also pays close attention to a client's verbal and nonverbal communication. The old saying, "Walk a mile in my shoes," captures the essence of active listening.

Figure 6.3

> ### Tips for Active Listening
>
> - Maintain steady eye contact.
> - Hold your body in an open position: face the speaker and lean slightly into the conversation.
> - Be active: nod your head, nonverbally acknowledge what is being said.
> - Use body language and tone to reflect the intent of what's being said.
> - Ask questions to clarify or get more information when necessary.
> - Pay attention to what is being said as well as what isn't being said.
> - Check in with the speaker about nonverbal cues being given.
> - Avoid distractions, turn off phone, place "Do Not Disturb" sign or "Session in Progress" sign on the door.

Listen long enough and the person will generally come up with an adequate solution.
— Mary Kay Ash

Reflective Feedback

Reflective feedback is one of the most effective techniques for enhancing communication. This involves briefly restating the feelings, concerns or content of what the speaker has said. An active listener that uses reflective feedback first allows a speaker to relate her story without interrupting, and then responds by asking further questions or rephrasing what was heard. Do not merely parrot back what someone has said. This can be counterproductive. Instead find the core of the message and reflect that succinctly and in your own words. Use tone and intention to convey what was heard and check to see if what you heard is accurate. For example, a client claims to be experiencing pain in her right shoulder. An active listener would explore that pain with the following: "Tell me a bit more about the pain." "How does this pain inhibit your activities?" "What I hear you saying is that the pain...."

Judge a person by their questions, rather than their answers.
— Voltaire

Marshall Rosenberg, founder and educational director of the Center for Nonviolent Communication, says this about reflective feedback: "If we have accurately received the party's message, our paraphrasing will confirm this for them. If, on the other hand our paraphrase is incorrect, the speaker has an opportunity to correct us. Another advantage of our choosing to reflect a message back to the other party is that it offers them time to reflect on what they've said and an opportunity to delve deeper into themselves."[1]

Rosenberg suggests practicing reflective feedback through asking questions, such as, "So what you're saying is that you've been having bad headaches since you were rear-ended last week?" Or, "So it sounds like you're feeling really frustrated that other treatments you received have not significantly decreased your pain level?" Reflecting in the form of a question gives the client the opportunity to tell you if you've heard him correctly and add any additional information he may want to convey.

Validate the speaker's feelings and experiences regardless of what you think about them. Also, refrain from expressing any judgments or personal opinions. This can be more difficult than you may think. Simple agreement or disagreement with the content of the information can be judgmental, or judgment can be more direct as in the following example: A client is very distraught because her teenage son was caught drinking last night, so you must avoid saying things like, "Wow, I hear how upset you are when your son behaves stupidly!"

Chapter 1, Page 4
for resources on
Personality Assessment.

Figure 6.4

Tips for Reflective Feedback

- Be aware that reflective feedback requires "total presence": people see, hear and feel when you're paying attention to what they say.
- Paraphrase instead of repeating what you heard word for word; only reflect back what is most important.
- Set aside your own feelings and opinions.
- Validate the speaker's feelings and experiences regardless of whether you agree with him.
- Avoid comments that express judgment.
- Use a question format to reflect back the essence of a person's concern.
- Give ample time for the speaker to complete her thoughts; don't interrupt.

Multiple Intelligences: The Theory in Practice
by Howard Gardner

✳ Communication & Learning Styles ✳

Improve your everyday interactions by leaps and bounds by developing an awareness of how different personality types view the world and the preferred communication style of each. Sometimes effective communication requires you to adjust your communication style, and it can feel a bit unnatural at first. But with basic knowledge and steady practice, you can quickly gain proficiency.

In addition, when providing client education, take into account that people learn through different channels—particularly visual, auditory and kinesthetic. Each person has their preferred learning channel. Thankfully, being an effective communicator doesn't require you to scope out each person's main channel. It simply means that the more channels you engage, the better chance a client will absorb and learn in an optimal way.

Let's look at an example of how this might work with a client. If you're demonstrating a stretching technique, it works well to discuss the stretch verbally, perform a demonstration, provide a take-away handout and inquire if there are any questions. You would then ask the client to demonstrate the stretching technique so you could observe and offer any helpful feedback.

By taking time for questions, you ensure that the client has grasped the information, and by asking the client to demonstrate the stretching technique, you provide an opportunity for body-based or kinesthetic learning. The handout serves to reinforce and support the client's at-home learning in a visual manner.

www.businessmastery.us/nlp.php
for further details on NLP.

Learning Styles

www.nlp.com

www.infed.org/thinkers/
gardner.htm

http://surfaquarium.com/MI/
inventory.htm

☀ Documenting Client Sessions ☀

The documentation of client sessions—also known as charting—is a vital activity in all wellness practices, regardless of whether the files are for recordkeeping or for insurance billing purposes. Documentation provides historical perspective, protects you in case of legal actions, demonstrates professionalism, and verifies progress. It also enables wellness practitioners to clearly communicate with each other about a client's treatment plan when needed. Note that insurance companies will not honor your malpractice coverage if you fail to keep accurate and detailed records.

Client files serve three major purposes. The first is recordkeeping, including proper documentation to support Internal Revenue Service filings. When you're in a service industry, basically the only way you can document your "work" is to create and maintain client files. The rudimentary information to include in each file is the client's name, address, phone number, session dates and amounts paid.

Second, up-to-date files document a client's needs and progress, which help you to develop the most effective treatment sessions. In group practices, client files provide continuity in treatment planning and provide the primary means for practitioners to share information about a client.

Some practitioners have clients sign contracts and waivers, and request they fill out evaluation forms after each session.

Third, client files provide documentation necessary for insurance reimbursement. Many insurance companies will not pay for maintenance care. "Reasonable and necessary" is the term used to validate a treatment modality. Thus if a wellness provider can show proof of an injury or condition (reasonable) and substantiate the success of treatment (e.g., a decrease in symptoms), the care is considered curative (necessary), not palliative.

In addition to client files, it's recommended that you have a sign-in sheet at the front desk. This form is for your protection—it verifies the client was at your office. Keep this sheet simple and don't risk breaching confidentiality by requesting personal information such as "reason for visit."

Client file and charting procedures vary depending upon the working environment. For instance, due to tight time frames at spas, charting isn't always required of practitioners. Some spas use a general intake form that a guest completes upon arrival. Due to the strict HIPAA laws, information is then passed on to the practitioner on a need-to-know basis.

Figure 6.5

Basic Charting Tips

- Review a client's file immediately before you meet with him. This helps refresh your memory and focus on the client's unique needs.
- Make concise and complete notes after each session. Include anything unexpected that may have happened during the session, techniques you want to focus on next time, client education activities and any other pertinent information.
- Be cautious of labeling or diagnosing clients in a manner way that could reflect negatively upon them. For example, if a client says, "I've been feeling low energy and moody lately," it would be appropriate to reflect the client's words as: "Client states he has been feeling…" rather than saying, "client is depressed." You never know when a client's files could be subpoenaed.
- Pay close attention to confidentiality. Although files need to contain accurate and thorough information, session records should only include information directly related to a session.
- Focus on facts; avoid analysis or judgments.
- Avoid using abbreviations or symbols not specifically defined by your employer, group practice or standard industry practices.
- In some medical and healthcare environments you may need to chart electronically. In these cases, it may be helpful to brush up on your typing skills to maintain a high level of productivity in charting.

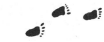

Chapter 12, Pages 246-249
for more information on
HIPAA, Confidentiality and
Informed Consent.

Client Forms

Various client file formats have been developed over the years. You may want to use "ready-made" forms, adapt them, or create customized forms.

Intake Forms

The fundamental facts to include on your client intake forms are: the client's name; address; phone numbers; medical history; chief complaints; current medication; and reason(s) for using your services.

Some practitioners also include an explanation of the range or variety of service and techniques they offer and list some of the benefits of their services on the top of their intake forms. Other practitioners incorporate a type of disclaimer. For example, many massage therapists include a statement that massage is clearly nonsexual. You must decide what purpose your client files are going to serve and choose the appropriate forms. As you and your needs change, so do the forms you use.

www.businessmastery.us/
forms.php#clirec
for printable forms.

Session Forms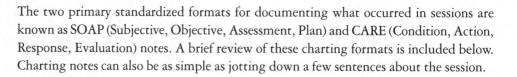

The two primary standardized formats for documenting what occurred in sessions are known as SOAP (Subjective, Objective, Assessment, Plan) and CARE (Condition, Action, Response, Evaluation) notes. A brief review of these charting formats is included below. Charting notes can also be as simple as jotting down a few sentences about the session.

Hands Heal: Communication, Documentation, and Insurance Billing for Manual Therapists by Diana Thompson

The SOAP charting format was initially used to document physical therapy sessions, and has been adapted and used widely by many wellness practitioners. Variations of this charting system have become part of the curriculum in a many schools.

However, the focus on treatment goals and the healthcare model doesn't lend itself well to many types of wellness care or spa-type settings. In recent years, the CARE charting format has been growing in popularity with many practitioners and group practices. What format you use largely depends on your work setting and your personal preferences.

Figure 6.6

Client Session Charting Formats Overview

SOAP Notes

Subjective
A description of symptoms and conditions as described by the client or the referring primary healthcare provider. Quotation marks are used to denote a client's own words. Key words are symptoms, location, intensity, duration, frequency and onset. These notes reflect a client's perception of his condition.

Objective
An account of your observations and results of the treatments you administer. This includes what the practitioner saw, felt and did.

Assessment
A record of the changes in a client's condition as a result of treatment. How the treatment worked, what changes (positive or negative) occurred.

Plan / Preferences
A list of recommended action and client preferences.

CARE Notes

Condition of Client
Provides a detailed picture of a client's condition and any relevant medical information. Includes notes about areas of discomfort, pain or tension, as well as emotional well-being or state of mind. It records a client's reasons for seeking treatment, and his goals or intentions for the session.

Action Taken
Notes the type of treatment given, the length of treatment and session details. Includes a summary of techniques used.

Response of Client
A record of physical changes noted during and after the session. It includes the verbal feedback of the client, as well as nonverbal responses. May include notes about changes in breathing, facial expressions or pain levels using a numerical pain scale.

Evaluation
Overall observations, recommendations or questions relates to a session.

☀ Client Interviews ☀

Interviews play a key role in creating lasting, healthy relationships between practitioners and clients. Information is gathered, rapport is built and ideas are shared. Ideally, they occur at regular intervals. The most extensive one is the initial intake interview. It sets the tone for your working relationship. An effective intake interview can take from 20 to 60 minutes and requires good communication skills, especially the ability to listen. An intake interview isn't simply about obtaining a client history. It is an opportunity to explain procedures, clarify boundaries, determine the course of treatment and educate clients. It is also a time to build a climate of trust by listening carefully to a client's concerns and questions.

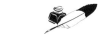

Drawing on my fine command of the English language, I said nothing.
— Robert Benchley

Timing ☀

Unless you carefully allot your time with clients, interviews can be rushed and less than effective. Conducting a thorough intake interview is time well spent. Consider that it takes approximately six times more money and three times more effort to get a new client than to keep one you already have. So, an extra half-hour is a minor investment on your part.

Allow ample time for your clients to fill out forms and ask questions. Keep in mind that your clients may not have the awareness or the vocabulary to accurately describe their conditions and goals. Your ability to ask pertinent questions and draw out useful information can make a big difference in the treatment result. A well-planned and thorough intake interview ensures the most effective experience for a client. Whether you allot three minutes or 30 minutes for an intake interview, it's important to help your client feel safe and comfortable, and for you to gather key insights about your client's condition. With time and practice, you become highly skilled at both tasks.

Figure 6.7

Tips for Keeping the Interview on Track

- Inform your clients about what they can expect to experience on their first visit. For instance, "Today we're going to go over your health history questionnaire and identify your concerns. I am gathering all of this information to get a clear picture of your specific needs. All of this is important for me to create the best possible course for you."
- Explain how you plan to allot time. For instance, "We will spend about 20 minutes talking about your concerns and health history, and the treatment on the first visit will be 45 minutes. After that sessions will usually last 50 minutes."
- If a client starts to ramble, kindly redirect him to the topic at hand and assure him you want to allow as much time as possible for his session.
- In a spa setting, it can be challenging to complete a thorough intake interview in the time allotted. Key questions to ask include: Any major health challenges or accidents in the last six months? How is your body feeling today? Any specific areas of focus? (Keep in mind that you can also can get more information on preferences as you're working.)

Artful Phrasing ✳

Of one thing I am certain, the body is not the measure of healing, peace is the measure.
— George Melton

Deftness at artful phrasing and asking clients open-ended questions is a skill that is honed over time. It involves forethought and lots of practice. Open-ended questions facilitate therapeutic communication as they encourage clients to express their thoughts and feelings. Open-ended questions usually begin with *how, what* or *could*. For example, "What would you like to achieve in today's session?" These types of questions also help the client to feel like an active partner in the treatment process. In contrast, closed-ended questions are limited in scope, as the answer is usually a simple "yes" or "no."

One of the most frequently asked questions in an intake interview is whether the client has experienced this type of treatment; for instance, "Have you ever been hypnotized before?" Two problems are inherent in this question. First of all, the scope of hypnotherapy isn't clear. A client could have listened to self-hypnosis tapes but never visited a professional hypnotherapist. Secondly, the question only calls for a one-word answer. A better series of questions would be as follows: "What is your experience with hypnotherapy?" "How often have you received hypnotherapy sessions?" "When was your last hypnotherapy session?"

Figure 6.8

Open-Ended Questions	Closed-Ended Questions
• How do you react to stress?	• Do you experience a lot of stress?
• What types of wellness activities and treatments have you done?	• Have you ever experienced this type of treatment before?
• What would you like me to focus on in this session?	• Shall we focus on your headaches today?
• How are you feeling today?	• Are you feeling better today?
• What are your concerns?	• Do you have any concerns?

Another useful practice is to incorporate phrases such as "how much?" "how long?" and "what is the level of intensity?" into your questioning routine. Let's say you're a shiatsu practitioner working with a client and you sense that the pressure may be a bit too much. If you ask, "Is this pressure okay?" the response will most likely be "yes" or "I guess so" (possibly with gritted teeth). Yet if you ask your client to rate the pressure on a pain scale (after agreeing upon what the numbers mean), you get a much more accurate response.

You can use other questions to express concern for your client's comfort and well-being. Consider the following example that frequently occurs during a session: You sense your client is getting a bit chilly. Instead of asking, "Are you cold?" or "Would you like a blanket?" ask "Would you like a blanket on your feet and legs, or would you prefer to be fully covered with a blanket?" This type of question gives the client options and shows careful forethought on your part.

Lastly, it's important to use clear and simple language when talking with clients and to avoid medical jargon and technical terms that may be unfamiliar to someone outside of your industry.

Figure 6.9

Client Interview Questions

The following interview questions help you understand your clients' needs. As each wellness modality is unique, you also need to ask questions specific to the type of work you do.

- How are you feeling today?
- Tell me about your physical or emotional condition.
- How long have you been experiencing this condition?
- When was the onset of this condition?
- What is the intensity and frequency of this condition?
- What causes you stress?
- What activities aggravate this condition?
- What actions relieve or reduce the discomfort of this condition?
- What are your long-term wellness goals?
- What do you want to achieve in today's session?
- What kind of mobility assistance might you need from me?
- Have you ever seen a {your profession here} before? If so, what were the results?
- Are you currently under medical or therapeutic treatment? If so, for what condition and what medications or supplements are you taking?
- What products have you used to address this condition?
- What questions and concerns do you have about my services?
- What are your expectations about my profession or me?
- What can I do to make this session effective and enjoyable?

I think the one lesson I have learned is that there is no substitute for paying attention.
— Diane Sawyer

Interview Stages ✳

Client interviews consist of four major stages—initiation, exploration, planning and closure.

Initiation Stage ✳ ✳

The initiation stage is the one in which you introduce yourself, establish rapport, discuss the client's general issues and expectations, describe what you can do, review your policies and explain procedures. Knowing what clients expect improves treatment results and client satisfaction.

It is what we think we know already that often prevents us from learning.
— Claude Bernard

Exploration Stage ✳ ✳

The exploration stage encompasses reviewing a client's history, performing a physical assessment and determining the treatment course of the specific session. The flow of the exploration stage varies depending upon the actual type of service you provide and your environment. Ideally, in your initial session you would review the client's intake forms, clarify any vague responses, get a sense of the client's general well-being goals and specific goals for receiving treatments, administer some type of assessment, determine the course of action and techniques to use for the current session, and then do the actual treatment.

Planning ✳ ✳

Planning is the stage that the practitioner and client create together. Long-range treatment plans are the key to having clients who receive treatments on a regular basis. Treatment plans are blueprints to follow while working with any specific client. Long-range treatment plans also serve as a reminder for the client to take responsibility for his goals.

The plan is based upon all the information gathered in the initiation and exploration stages of the interview as well as the session. It may seem awkward to break up the interview with a treatment, but it's the only way you can accurately develop a long-range treatment plan. It's usually difficult to accurately evaluate a client's condition until you've given a treatment. Also, during the session clients often discover unsuspected problems or remember previous physical or psychological trauma. This information can be crucial in designing the treatment plan.

Some items to include in the plan are: the client's short-term and long-range well-being goals; indications and contraindications; treatment frequency; specific modalities to be used; homework; and possible referrals to other wellness providers. Create a vision with your clients so they can experience themselves having attained their goals. This makes the treatment more powerful and inspires clients to take an active role in their well-being (e.g., do homework assignments and use products). This can also elicit secondary goals.

The tricky part to designing a long-range treatment plan is setting realistic goals. Many people don't know enough about themselves or your services to gauge the potential outcomes. Begin by discussing general goals and letting them know which conditions can be successfully addressed by your services. Create short-term goals (for individual sessions and the next few treatments) and long-term goals (covering periods of three, six, nine and 12 months). The difficulty here is that unless you're a primary care provider you can't prescribe—but you can describe. Make sure you're clear about the proven benefits of your work, as you can safely make those statements. It's best to let your clients determine the treatment frequency. You can provide them guidelines such as: "Other clients with similar goals obtained their desired results by coming in twice per week for two to three weeks, then once per week for three months, and tapering off to a minimum of twice monthly." or "If I had a condition like this, I would...." A statement I often used in my massage practice was, "I recommend massage as often as you can afford physically, time-wise and financially."

It can also be helpful to encourage clients to listen to their bodies to determine how often to schedule wellness treatments. Oftentimes this can vary due to life circumstances and stress levels. Clients that listen to their bodies may schedule sessions every few days or once a month depending on their comfort level and needs.

Update long-range treatment plans after each visit. Make notes for subsequent sessions, taking into account any changes in your client's lifestyle and treatment results (e.g., what worked and didn't, the areas or modalities you didn't cover, and what you want to include next time).

All too often, practitioners omit this stage, particularly with clients who have been receiving regular treatments or clients who are very educated about and involved in their own wellness. Keep in mind that most people want objective evidence that they're reaching their wellness goals. I know I appreciate it when a practitioner looks at a chart and tells me the specific changes and progress I've made since the last session and where I'm at in relation to my long-term goals.

Every person who ends up buying into your idea does so by changing it into his idea (even if it still looks a lot like your idea).
— Tom Peters

Closure * *

Closure is the final interview stage. This can be done fairly quickly with the first session since you've spent a significant amount of time designing the treatment plan. Give a very brief overview of what took place, highlight some of the client's major goals, assign homework, give the client an opportunity to ask questions, make any necessary referrals and schedule the next appointment.

Subsequent Sessions *

The first time you work with a client, the interview process is usually more extensive than in subsequent sessions. You can retain the quality of your interviews, even though the time spent is reduced, by making sure you include all four stages each time you see a client.

The initiation stage involves actions to continue building rapport, such as greeting each client appropriately and engaging in light chitchat.

The exploration stage encompasses reviewing the client's files, discussing any changes that may have occurred between sessions, documenting observations, setting treatment goals and determining the course of the specific session.

Planning is usually done by the practitioner and includes updating the long-term treatment plan and making notes for activities and modalities to incorporate into the next session.

Closure tends to take longer in subsequent sessions than with the first visit. After the treatment, review the session with your client (this doesn't need to be lengthy and can be informal). Summarize what you did, address issues that might have surfaced, and answer any questions. Briefly review the client's long-term goals and make any appropriate recommendations and homework assignments. Finally, ask when she would like to schedule the following session.

Client Compliance ✳

Many practitioners complain about a lack of client compliance (e.g., clients don't do their homework, make no lifestyle changes, don't use appropriate products or fail to return for follow-up sessions). Although you can't force someone to comply with your recommendations, your communication skills can increase the odds.

First of all, recognize the factors that prevent full compliance: lack of discipline, time restraints, insufficient funds or insurance coverage, social pressures, beliefs, and work obligations. Explain why it is in their best interest to adhere to your recommendations, clarify the instructions and discuss ways to overcome barriers. Have clients repeat instructions or perform exercises or stretches to be sure they understand them. Give them printed reference material to take home. The most important aspect is gaining your clients' concordance about their treatment plans and assignments.

www.businessmastery.us/
client-education.php
for a detailed description of
the Multiple Intelligences and
creative client education
techniques based on MI.

Client Education ✳

Everyone in the wellness field is an educator. Client education occurs in two ways: you support the body's learning how to optimally respond to states of relaxation and repair; and you increase your clients' general awareness of body function and self-care. Some practitioners offer added measures to help broaden their clients' knowledge by: describing what they're doing and why; demonstrating stretches and self-care techniques; showing videos; describing how a product works; sharing information on related wellness topics; providing educational materials; and assigning homework.

Educating clients so that they can better understand the cause of their pain or health condition, and methods to alleviate it, empowers them to take more responsibility for their wellness. They become active partners instead of passive recipients of treatments. A side benefit is that as clients learn new ways to enjoy greater wellness, they're more likely to share this information and recommend your treatment services to friends and family.

Hone Your Interviewing Skills ✳

Interviewing skills take time and practice to develop. The best way to sharpen your skills in this area is to role-play several intake interviews. Other techniques to improve communication skills are to read books, take seminars, post reminders to yourself about areas you wish to improve (e.g., ask open-ended questions, don't interrupt, suspend judgments) and ask for feedback from clients. Excellent communication skills evolve from a lifelong process of observation, study and experimentation. Have fun!

Interview Simulation

Get together with two other colleagues. Allot at least three hours for this activity. Run through an intake interview (without doing the treatment or session consultation). One person is the practitioner, one portrays a client and the third person is the observer. As you practice, focus on asking open-ended questions and listening carefully to the client to obtain useful information.

At the conclusion, the observer reports on what she noticed in terms of the overall flow, the client's apparent comfort level, types of questions asked, body language, and what did and didn't work. The client shares his reactions to the interview, and then the practitioner discusses what she experienced. Run the simulation three times so that each person gets to play every part. After all three rounds are completed, create an action plan for incorporating any desired changes.

Figure 6.10

Interview Checklist

❏ Review File
❏ Greet Client
❏ Give Client a Tour of the Premises
❏ Fill Out Intake Forms
❏ Review Policies
❏ Discuss Overall Goals
❏ Preview Session Procedure

❏ Perform Assessment
❏ Do the Session
❏ Develop a Treatment Plan
❏ Summarize Session
❏ Assign Homework
❏ Suggest Referrals
❏ Schedule Next Session

❋ Telephones:
The Client Connection ❋

Next to your technical abilities, your telephone can be the most important tool in your business—or it can be an obstacle. This section covers techniques for improving your effectiveness on the telephone and dealing with inappropriate callers.

Phone Etiquette ❋

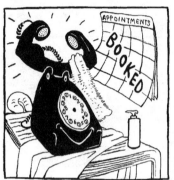

Illustration by Beth Grundvig

Every time you answer the telephone, you create an impression. The question remains what that impression will be. Within the first few seconds of a conversation you convey how you feel about yourself, your practice and the caller. Just because the caller can't see you doesn't mean that she can't sense the attitudes you convey through the tone of your voice and the words you use.

Communication is approximately 10 percent content, 35 percent voice and 55 percent nonverbal information. Given these statistics, it's easy to see why so many miscommunications occur over the telephone—more than 50 percent of the information is lost.

Without visual cues it can be quite difficult to determine the intent of someone's statement. For example, a caller might possess a sardonic sense of humor, and you could be offended by a remark that would have been humorous with visual cues. Some guidelines to keep in mind when using the telephone are:

Be prepared. You don't want to keep callers waiting while you search for supplies or information. Store needed provisions (e.g., paper, pen and appointment book) within reach and be knowledgeable about your practice.

Inspire interest. You must know how to eloquently describe in 30 seconds or less the offerings of your practice, your policies and the type of work each practitioner does. The caller may be a potential client, so you need to immediately inspire interest.

Answer promptly. Plan to answer the phone promptly: after two rings, but before five rings. By picking up right at the first ring, you may give the impression that you've nothing else to do but sit idly by the phone. Also, most people don't expect someone to pick up the phone right away, so it throws them off balance. If you wait too long to answer the phone, the effect is usually negative. The caller gets impatient or anxious that an answering system is about to pick up...then you answer in person.

Courtesy first. Greet the caller courteously. Your tone sets the stage for the whole conversation. Before you pick up the phone, be sure to smile. It sounds hokey, but smiling makes a difference in your vocal quality as well as your attitude. You never know who is on the other end of the line (unless you subscribe to Caller ID).

For instance, I was at home writing an article on telephone communications and it was late on a Saturday afternoon. I had received six or seven unsolicited sales calls in less than an hour. Lo and behold! The phone rang again and I must admit I wasn't my most "professional" self when I answered the call. After all, it was a weekend and this was my personal line. Well, it was a school owner wanting to schedule me for a seminar. He thought he was dialing my business number. I recovered the conversation (after all, I wasn't rude—just not at my best), but it took a little while to change the tone.

Identify yourself. Never assume your voice will be recognized. Also, ask to be of service. When you answer the telephone, your greeting might be like this: "Good morning. Thank you for calling The Northwest Health Center. This is Nancy. How can we assist you?"

Be clear. Speak in a clear and friendly manner. Personalize the conversation whenever possible by using the caller's name. Listen, give feedback and mirror language patterns.

Avoid distractors. One of the most important techniques for improving telephone communications is to keep down background noises. Don't drink beverages, eat food or chew gum while on the phone. Also, if you listen to music or watch television, be sure that the volume controls are close to the telephone: turn off the sound before you answer a call.

If you work out of your home and children or animals are present, you need to create a sound-proof environment around the phone. Your credibility as a professional can be adversely affected if your dog barks or children holler while you're talking with a potential client.

Avoid the hold option. Most people dislike being put on hold, so avoid it whenever possible. If you must put someone on hold, follow these guidelines:

1. Get the caller's name before asking to "please hold." When you return to the caller, address the caller by name.
2. Be specific about how long you expect to be on the other line. If it goes longer, check back in to let the caller know she is not forgotten. Even 30 seconds can seem like a lifetime when you're in telephone limbo.
3. Always ask if the person would prefer to be called back.
4. Give the first caller preference.

Follow through. Keep any promises you make to your callers. This is why it's imperative to take notes. Return all calls within 24 hours unless other arrangements have been made.

Focus on services. An effective response to a potential client who asks for prices immediately is, "Before I can answer that, please tell me what you're needing." You must understand clients' needs so that you can clearly guide them.

If your files are computerized, you can create a new client account and directly input the information.

New Client Checklist
www.businessmastery.us/
forms.php#clirec

6

Screening Clients ✴

During an initial conversation with a potential client, you've an opportunity to gather essential information that can save a lot of time and trouble down the road. By efficiently answering questions and sharing information about your services, you can quickly build rapport and inspire interest in making an appointment. After a client makes an appointment, ask for his home or business telephone number as you may need to reschedule an appointment unexpectedly. You can also effectively screen inappropriate calls by developing a set script for how you handle these inquiries, thus avoiding any misunderstandings or unwanted clients appearing at your doorstep.

Some people are naturally at ease talking on the telephone while others feel less comfortable. Consider developing scripts so that everyone who answers your phone knows how you want callers to be treated, the information you want to obtain and give, the image you desire to portray and policies for handling specific issues. Topics to cover include: prospective clients; cancellations; rescheduling; follow-up visits; disgruntled clients; fees; setting an appointment for a minor; scope of services; clients with special needs (e.g., people with disabilities); insurance reimbursement; and clients who want to speak directly with you. Rehearse the scripts and role-play scenarios.

Conduct preliminary interviews with all potential clients when they call to schedule an appointment (either by you or trained staff). Find out the reason for calling and the expectations. This assists you in determining if you're the appropriate provider for the caller (sometimes ending relationships with clients you don't want can be harder than obtaining new clients). If you're unable to talk with the potential client initially (e.g., you have a client in the next few minutes or someone else took the call), place a personal confirmation call as soon as possible.

Telephone Scripts

Design a questionnaire to ensure you obtain the information desired, disseminate your client requirements (e.g., prices, scope of services and cancellation policy) and determine if a client has special needs (e.g., assistance getting in and out of a wheelchair).

Inappropriate Calls ✴ ✴

Receiving inappropriate calls can be a source of immense discomfort. Unfortunately, many practitioners—particularly massage therapists—still get calls from people who are ill-informed about the nature and scope of wellness services. Sometimes people are indirect about wanting sexual services. You can often determine inappropriate callers by their tone of voice, awkward periods of silence, calls placed late at night and if they request late-night appointments. A common tip-off for massage therapists is when a caller requests "full-body massage."

When someone calls requesting sexual services, you have two choices: you can get upset and hang up the phone, or you can use it as an opportunity to educate the caller. Too many practitioners take these calls as a personal affront.

If you receive this type of call, it works well to stay centered in your professionalism. If people want sexual services, that's their prerogative, but they don't have the right to expect it from you or any other wellness provider. Tell them that isn't what you do, give a brief description of the services you do provide, and let them know that a legitimate practitioner does not perform that kind of work. You might also say something along these lines: "Because prostitution is not legal in most states, and prostitutes need some way to let others know how to reach them, they tend to put advertisements under massage or touch therapy. This is changing as the general public becomes more aware of the therapeutic practice of massage. If you would like further information about the therapeutic benefits of massage, I'd be happy to speak with you about it or send you a brochure."

This gives the caller the opportunity to learn more about massage or gracefully remove themselves from the conversation. Remember, these callers are human beings. Just because they want something you don't offer doesn't mean they might not want a legitimate massage in the future or don't have friends who want a professional massage. Besides, these are the people we really need to educate. They are the ones perpetuating the myths about massage and the entire healing arts field. You can transform a potentially negative experience into a positive one by responding professionally and keeping perspective.

Machines vs. Humans ☀

Since many practitioners are in sole practice and don't have a receptionist, they rely on an answering machine to take messages. These machines serve a good purpose but are generally not well suited for this field. Most people prefer talking to another human being. They may have questions, particularly if they aren't current clients, and a machine can't handle that.

Another significant drawback relates to scheduling. For example, imagine that you're working with a client and the phone rings. Someone wants to schedule an appointment right away. You have the next hour open, but by the time you're finished with the current client and listen to your messages, it's too late for the other person to come into the office. A prospective client may have called the next available practitioner while you were busy. If you had an appointment service, that person could have scheduled an appointment and been in your office by the time you were done with your current client. An appointment service is similar to an answering service, plus they book clients.

Chapter 12, Pages 236-238

for more details on telephone systems and Internet scheduling.

Appointment services are usually well worth the money! All it takes is one to three sessions to pay for this service, which could easily be done by attracting just one new regular client. Of course, you're best off researching the different services. After you've chosen one, explain the work you do to the receptionists, furnish them with brochures and then give them a complimentary session. The receptionists can help turn an inquiry into a client.

**Wellness Practitioners
Answering Service**
www.myreceptionist.com

You may also want to explore setting up an online scheduling system through the Internet. These systems are affordable, easy to work with and clients often appreciate the added flexibility that comes with scheduling appointments at their convenience. Everyone benefits from less time spent in "phone tag."

Improving Communication Effectiveness ☀

In addition to allotting financial resources for appropriate equipment, be sure to invest the time to improve your telephone effectiveness: Dress as if the caller could see you, get feedback from others, notice how others handle themselves on the phone, practice and role-play, vary your "script" and follow the telephone guidelines established previously in this chapter. Utilize the telephone wisely to build your practice. Keep in mind that every time you answer the phone you've the opportunity to gain or lose a client. Your emotional state gets conveyed and possibly misconstrued, so don't answer the phone if you're busy, distracted or upset.

We can't eliminate the inherent communication problems associated with telephones, but we can reduce distractors and increase rapport by incorporating these techniques:

Figure 6.11

Telephone Tips

- Be prepared
- Greet courteously
- Ask to be of service
- Avoid putting people on hold
- Smile while talking

- Answer promptly
- Identify yourself
- Speak clearly
- Take notes
- Follow through

Part III

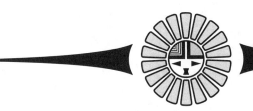

Navigate Your Way to the Perfect Job

Part III of *Business Mastery* provides an insider's look into various employment opportunities in the wellness field. You'll find valuable insights into different work environments so you can approach your job search with credibility and confidence—and tailor an educational program to your career interest.

Chapter 7 explores employment opportunities in spas. It highlights what you can expect to find in these environments, such as the corporate culture, training and scheduling concerns, and seniority issues. It also includes success tips for each of the most common types of spas: day spas, destination spas, resort spas, cruise ship spas, and dental and medical spas.

Next, this chapter turns the spotlight onto employment in the medical, wellness, and specialty fields. Medical clinics and hospitals now offer a variety of complementary and alternative services on both an inpatient and outpatient basis—which translates into a growing number of job opportunities. You'll learn what features distinguish these medical settings from other practice locations and find tips for working successfully in these environments.

Since you never know when your job situation may shift, it's wise to develop the job search skills detailed in Chapter 8. You'll find useful tips about how to research potential employers, hone your interview skills and write a top-notch resume. The chapter also reviews how to effectively navigate employment contracts, and, when the time is right, to negotiate a raise. The chapter concludes by revealing some of the secrets of successful employees.

An Insider's Look at Work Settings

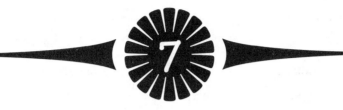

• Working in Spa Settings •

In an era in which consumers are looking for ways to slow down, rejuvenate and connect with like-minded individuals, spa visits are likely to become a desirable lifestyle experience. According to recently released data from the International Spa Association (ISPA), more than 13,000 spas were operating in the United States as of August 2006. A hefty 80 percent of them are dedicated to day spas—representing the lion's share of the industry. In spa settings, massage is generally the top-selling service.

Diamonds are only lumps of coal that stuck to their jobs.
— B.C. Forbes

Spas range in image from holistic wellness centers to posh pampering resorts. It is commonplace to find wellness practitioners—such as acupuncturists, massage therapists, nutritional consultants, estheticians, energy workers and other somatic practitioners—in all of these settings.

Today the wide world of spas includes day spas, resort and hotel spas, destination spas, cruise ship spas, medical spas and dental spas. Although the majority of spas hire practitioners as employees, some day spas and dental spas prefer to establish independent contractor relationships with practitioners, where the practitioners run their own businesses underneath the umbrella of the spa.

As the spa market continues to flourish, so do employment opportunities for wellness practitioners. New practitioners can gain valuable experience by working in a spa. In addition to building expertise through client feedback, you have the opportunity to learn proper etiquette, interact with clients in a professional manner and, in many cases, expand your skills through in-house trainings and tuition reimbursement programs.

In this chapter we examine the issues that are common to working in the spa industry in general and then cover the specifics pertinent to the sub-categories of spas.

Figure 7.1

Wide World Of Spas

Type of Spa:	Clientele:
Day Spa	Clients seek beautifying, relaxing or pampering experiences that last for several hours or the entire day.
Resort or Luxury Hotel Spa	Vacation or business travelers seek beautifying, relaxing, stress-reducing or pampering experiences.
Destination Spa	Clients seek to make healthy lifestyle changes, enhance their well-being or rejuvenate from the stresses of a high pressure career. Destination spa settings often offer the widest variety of wellness services under one roof.
Cruise Ship Spa	Passengers seek beautifying, relaxing or pampering experiences for several hours or an entire day.
Dental Spa	Clients who enjoy the convenience of spa-like services as an adjunct to their dental visits. Services may include massage, craniosacral therapy, acupuncture, reflexology, professional skin care, manicures or pedicures.
Medical Spa	Clients undergoing cosmetic surgery procedures that seek therapeutic spa services to enhance the healing process, promote relaxation and support skin beautification.

What to Expect in Spas ●

All spas share common characteristics, and the overall working environment can be similar. After you get acquainted with the big picture view of spas, we provide insights into the different types of spas. Here are some aspects of employment you may find in any type of spa: corporate culture and image; training and scheduling; ethics; defining expanded responsibilities; scope of practice issues; confidentiality; contraindications for client treatment; compensation; boundaries and sexual misconduct.

Corporate Culture and Image ● ●

Many practitioners enjoy the team environment of a spa—that is, if the corporate culture of the spa promotes a positive attitude, discourages gossip, and expects a high degree of professionalism and respect for co-workers and clients. The most enlightened spa owners aspire to build businesses in which both clients and employees thrive. The best spa managers recognize that clients perceive subtle undercurrents of disharmony, and thus aim to create a sense of community among spa team members and good working relationships with employees or independent contractors.

When it comes to image, you can expect to encounter a clear list of do's and don'ts. Ambience and image are often key elements of a spa's brand and corporate identity. Thus, spa employment requires conforming to policies about image and personal appearance. For instance, some spas may require employees not to have visible tattoos or excessive piercings. Some require practitioners to conform to a dress code or wear a designated garment.

Training and Scheduling ● ●

While some spas provide comprehensive training programs, others provide minimal or no training, (also known as "sink or swim"). When interviewing for a spa job, ask about orientation and training programs. If you ascertain in advance that the training program is skimpy and you still decide to take the job, you can adjust your expectations accordingly so you will better weather the first weeks of your new job.

Training issues are not limited to orientation. Problematic situations can arise when a spa expects a practitioner to teach proprietary treatment modalities to other practitioners, even though this may break the professional agreement between the treatment owner and the practitioner. In contrast, highly ethical spas hire professional trainers to facilitate workshops on products, treatments and other types of continuing education, which may include topics such as sexual harassment and nonviolent communication.

The most challenging aspect of spa or salon work often relates to scheduling. Before accepting employment, determine if the scheduling policies allow you to work at a comfortable pace that accommodates your special modalities and style of working. Some spas may require five to seven client sessions per shift. Others may require a hectic pace of 10 to 12 sessions per shift, sometimes without breaks between 50-minute sessions. Clarify scheduling practices prior to accepting employment so you can clearly understand what's expected. Many spas require weekend and evening shifts, while others require working on holidays.

Ethics ● ●

While most of the major ethical concerns of working in a spa are similar to those in any type of practice, the spa environment contributes additional twists. The areas of greatest concern are: establishing appropriate boundaries; addressing sexual misconduct; working outside the scope of practice; not having a detailed intake form to identify a client's health issues; compensation inequities; and breaches of confidentiality.

Chapter 5, Pages 84-90
for more information
on Ethics.

Expanded Responsibilities ● ●

Some spas ask employee practitioners to expand their skills and perform other spa treatments, such as hydrotherapy, seaweed body wraps, and paraffin treatments, when not providing their primary service. In addition, some facilities expect practitioners to assist wherever they're needed, from greeting clients to cleaning. These expectations may be present even when practitioners are not paid for nonclient interactions. Ask questions in the interview about such spa policies so you can know what to expect if you're hired.

Confidentiality • •

Confidentiality issues can sometimes occur in a spa setting—either due to the physical environment (a lack of private space) or less than professional behavior on the part of staff. Management's role is to clearly communicate and oversee professional standards and behavior. According to standard confidentiality guidelines applicable to wellness practitioners, any information shared between client and practitioner during a session or related to a session remains private (e.g., client names, details of treatment, and information shared by clients during a session are not discussed by the practitioner with anyone else). If you work at a high-end spa or wellness center, management expects strict adherence to confidentiality policies. Many celebrities or other high-profile individuals count on a spa and its employees to "go the extra mile" to protect their privacy.

Contraindications • •

You may sometimes encounter situations in which you've a concern about working with certain clients when contraindications are present such as: clients who take certain medications; those with suspicious skin conditions; clients with high blood pressure; those who request work the practitioner feels is inappropriate; and clients arriving under the influence of drugs or alcohol.

Because it's essential to accommodate clients with medical conditions, industry best practices dictate that a spa provide an intake form that includes health history and allot proper time for any needed discussion between practitioner and client. If you find that an intake form is missing in your work environment, design an appropriate intake form and diplomatically raise the issue to management with the solution in hand. An intake form protects you, the client, and the long-term reputation of the spa where you work.

Scope of Practice • •

Sometimes a client asks for a service that is outside of your skill set. For instance, a receptionist may book a specific service even if it isn't clear that the practitioner on duty is proficient in that technique.

Compensation • •

Spas often base salaries and preferential scheduling on seniority. It is important to take this into account when you're new. As in most careers, it may take some time for your income to grow to its full potential. Compensation varies greatly among spas: some pay on a commission basis, others offer a combination of base salary with a commission. The average wage is $25-$40 per hour for time when the practitioner is actually giving treatments. Employee benefits can include health insurance, paid vacations, paid sick days, pension plans, profit sharing, reimbursement for continuing education and use of facilities.

Seniority ● ●

Seniority works a bit differently at every spa, and it can affect both your salary and volume of client bookings. Like many other aspects of employment, it's a good idea to learn about seniority policies before you accept a job—rather than be surprised after you join the spa.

This can mean that during every hour that calls are accepted for appointments, the person with the most seniority gets booked first, then the next person and so on. The next hour, the process starts all over again. Thus, practitioners with high seniority may be fully booked for the day and you may have no clients for that day. Obviously, this system is less than desirable for a new practitioner. Nonetheless, if you decide to work at such a spa in spite of this initial drawback, factor this in and budget accordingly until you can move up in seniority.

Fortunately, many spas use a more balanced seniority system, such as a rotation system that favors seniority yet makes an effort to even out the bookings.

Although the seniority system can be frustrating to new practitioners, you can increase your chances of getting more client bookings by being trained in as many modalities as possible that the spa offers. The wider range of skills you offer, the better chance you will be needed in any given time slot. Many spas also have a tiered pay system that takes into account your years of experience plus the modalities you offer. Also, spas may pay you a different rate for different treatments, such as a higher rate for more physically demanding or labor-intensive treatment.

Boundaries ● ●

Understanding boundaries is crucial to creating an ethical practice, building professional relationships, and succeeding in a spa environment. By increasing awareness of client boundaries (as well as our own), we can improve the therapeutic relationship and avoid inadvertent slips into unethical behavior. Unfortunately, boundaries are often blurred in a spa environment, particularly given that people often play a variety of roles. Some spas have strict rules about boundaries and dual relationships, particularly regarding guests and practitioners.

Sexual Misconduct ● ●

In most cases when you work in a spa, you don't have to worry about sexual misconduct from clients—it rarely happens, and, if it does, assistance is nearby. More common are reports of subtle inappropriate behaviors, such as suggestive comments, offensive jokes or inappropriate touching. In these cases, terminating a session may be the appropriate response. Simply state you're uncomfortable with continuing the session, or excuse yourself from the session by saying you don't feel well.

In short, be aware of the potential for problems in this area and use your best judgment and diplomacy to deal effectively with difficult or awkward situations. Don't hesitate to end a session immediately if a client's behavior is inappropriate, and report problems or concerns to management as soon as possible. Professional ethics dictate that you refrain from talking about a client's inappropriate behavior with anyone other than management.

Figure 7.2

Success Tips for
Working in All Spa Environments

- As in any business, there are rules, expectations and guidelines to ensure profitability. By appreciating the business side of spa work, you pave the way to success.

- Prior to your interview, collect brochures or website information about the spa and its mission. Learn about its history, its clients, its spa treatments, and its unique qualities compared to competitors.

- When interviewing, ask the right questions to find out if this particular spa is a good fit for you, such as: What is the spa's vision? How long is a shift? What kind of turnover do you have? Is there a strong team environment? Does the spa value open communication and employee feedback? Is there an orientation and training program? How are practitioners compensated? How does seniority affect booking and compensation?

- When you start your new job, take the time to review policy and procedure manuals. Clarify any ambiguous policies. Clarify what's expected of you when you're not directly working with clients (e.g., paperwork, clerical duties, assisting the other practitioners, marketing, cleaning chores, providing treatments for staff).

- Recognize what the spa does for you, such as providing equipment, handling scheduling and payment logistics, paying for supplies, and laundry.

- As in many business environments, politics can sometimes get in the way of fairly resolving scheduling issues or work conditions. Make an effort to express your views in a balanced way, and then release your expectations. Accept that some things are beyond your control.

- Urban markets tend to have a higher compensation level than many resort markets.

- It helps to learn and practice conscious detachment. For example, make an effort not to take anything personally, especially when a client is difficult.

- Spa policies on tipping vary. Some spas do not allow tips to simplify logistics for clients. Others allow tips but have moved to a cashless system that enables a guest to note a tip on a credit card receipt or hotel folio.

- Spas often offer a wide variety of services. Be aware of how your service is currently marketed. Keep track of your bookings. Communicate regularly with the staff to learn about marketing plans and ask how you may assist (possibly unpaid) in promoting your service.

- Boost your chances of getting hired and increase your compensation rate by obtaining certification or advanced training in spa specialty therapies such as aromatherapy, reflexology, body wraps or energy work. A benefit of working in spas is that they often pay to train you in these modalities. This also helps prevent burnout and reduce repetitive stress injuries.

- Take advantage of opportunities to expand your knowledge base and skill portfolio by attending in-house training programs.

- Appreciate the benefits that come with spa employment, such as health insurance coverage, paid holidays and vacation, discounted services, and tuition reimbursement for continuing education.

- Overcome any phobia you have for selling products and other spa services. Most spas expect practitioners to generate from five-20 percent of their total sales in home-care products or supplies (and up to 50 percent for estheticians).

- Be a team player. Help with clients' needs that might not technically be "your job" and take courses to enhance your communication skills with co-workers.

- In most cases, the room you work in constantly changes. This can be from day to day or even session to session. It can be a challenge to focus when the room isn't yours (e.g., it lacks your personality, layout may not be what you prefer). Additionally, the treatment room may not be adequately sized or insulated, and the equipment may vary from room to room. It can require some adaptability to adjust to these working conditions.

- Learn how to do a session in the allotted time (usually 50 minutes for the treatment and 10 minutes turnaround time) without appearing rushed.

- Be prepared to work long shifts with few breaks.

- Practice good body mechanics and stretch regularly to avoid injuries.

- Follow the spa's hands-on protocols regarding how clients are to be treated (e.g., greeting, draping, the session's sequence). Consistency is paramount to spas. They want to make sure that the clients receive the same service from all practitioners.

- Develop good recordkeeping habits to ensure client files are complete and up-to-date. This helps you track client progress, any contraindications and provides a useful reference point for each session. Clients appreciate this type of thorough and professional attention to their unique needs.

- Be aware that most spa visitors are called guests, not clients.

- Expect and plan for slow seasons or open times between client appointments. If you aren't expected to perform other spa-related job duties during these times, bring reading materials, catch up on correspondence, listen to relaxation CDs, or enjoy some simple yoga stretches.

- Most spas, particularly destination spas, are team environments. Learn which spa treatments complement what you do to create the most effective and integrated experience for the guest.

Day Spas ●

Spa Finder, a spa travel company, defines a day spa as: "an establishment that provides beautifying, relaxing or pampering experiences that can last an hour or may take a whole day." A day spa can be a stand-alone business venue or connected to a luxury hotel, resort, health retreat, cruise ship or department store.

The ambiance in day spas can range from spare and simple to elegant and opulent. Whatever the means, whatever the style, all day spas aim to create a haven of tranquility and rejuvenation for clients. Working in these surroundings is pleasant. Spa clients are usually easygoing and generous in expressing their appreciation. Staff is usually available to handle marketing, scheduling, confirmation calls and financial transactions. A potential downside of this environment is that you might be responsible for generating most of your client base.

Chapter 9, Page 171

for information about being
self-employed in a salon.

Best Spa Jobs
www.bestspajobs.com

Day Spa Association
www.dayspaassociation.com

Spa Finder
www.spafinder.com

Some day spas promote themselves to the masses, while others target niche markets, such as upscale clients, aging baby boomers, moms and babies, or young professionals. In recent years, a new breed of discount spas and spa chains have emerged that offer high-quality services at affordable prices. Another growing market niche is "men-only" spas. Men now compose more than 30 percent of all U.S. spa-goers. As the day spa market continues to flourish, so do employment opportunities for wellness practitioners.

Figure 7.3

Additional Success Tips for Working in Day Spas

- Working at a day spa enables you to build long-term client relationships. It can be very rewarding to track a client's progress over time and tailor ongoing sessions to support a client's health and wellness goals.
- If you haven't seen a client for awhile, place a follow-up call to ask how she is, and invite her to visit the spa again.
- Keep detailed client files. Be sure to indicate which clients are locals. Review locals' files monthly and follow up as appropriate.
- Although most day spas hire practitioners as employees, some hire only independent contractors.

Cruise Ship Spas •

If you love the idea of traveling to faraway ports, a tour of duty on a cruise ship may satisfy your adventurous spirit. It is a great way to see the world, gain valuable experience and earn money at the same time. Five to 10 new luxury liners are built every year, which means that employment in this field is booming. Working on a cruise ship spa can be exciting. However, it's wise to gain some realistic perspectives before committing to this line of work.

A cruise ship spa can be very different from working at a land-based spa. A 12-hour workday is standard aboard ship. Wellness practitioners often administer a variety of spa treatments outside their specialty and are expected to comfortably and successfully sell spa beauty and wellness products.

Positive aspects of working in this setting are: the opportunity to get lots of experience under your belt (especially attractive to new practitioners); a major change of pace from wherever you are now; the opportunity to meet and make friends with crew members from all over the world; the ability to save some money if you budget wisely; and plenty of travel to exotic destinations.

The potential downside is that life on a cruise ship can be trying at times. If you don't mind the quirks that come with an onboard lifestyle, and being at sea for four to eight months at a time, you may enjoy working on a cruise ship spa. It can require patience and determination to ride out rough seas and cramped living quarters. In many cases you may share quarters with one to three strangers. It is common to encounter little personal privacy. In some cases you may find a lack of healthy food in the crew cafeteria. Lastly, time off is very limited.

Although training programs vary depending on the cruise line, often many luxury cruise lines offer corporate training and orientation programs that span from two to eight weeks. Recruits learn about the essential of customer services, the realities of working on cruises and how to become skilled in specialized treatment offerings.

The employment process typically begins with wellness practitioners signing an employment contract for anywhere from four to eight months, and living on a ship with room and board and laundry services provided. Compensation varies widely depending on season and ship, and can range from $200 to $1,000 per week, including tips. Benefits may include free medical insurance and reduced-price vacations for family and friends.

Figure 7.4

Additional Success Tips for Working in Cruise Ship Spas

- Working conditions are demanding. The number of sessions you're expected to give per day is higher than other working environments. You could easily do 10 or more treatments per day. Generally, you get one and a half days off per week. During off-time, you're free to do anything you like, just like a passenger, which includes going into port when the ship lands.
- Prior experience working on a cruise ship is not necessary. An upbeat attitude, high energy, flexibility and the ability to sell wellness products are a plus. A good portion of your of income may be dependent on product sales.
- You must be in excellent physical and emotional condition.
- Treatment rooms can be small and cramped.
- The actual paycheck can be very low but income is also made from a percentage of sale for spa products and client tips. Expenses for items such as accommodations, meals and laundry are usually paid by the cruise ship.
- As an employee on a cruise ship, you must be "on" nearly 24 hours a day. For all that time, you're expected to represent your company to the public, which means that you must always show a sunny personality.
- Good boundaries, an open heart and an open mind may be essential to survival.
- Beware of fictitious companies on the Internet and in newspaper advertisements that pretend to be legitimate agencies for employment on cruise ships. You should not pay a fee for a list of current job openings or to submit your resume to a cruise ship company. Also, do not fall for a "no-risk guarantee" of employment from a website that requires you to pay a fee. There is no such thing as a guarantee of employment.

About Cruises
www.cruises.about.com/
od/cruisejobs

Steiner Training
www.str.co.uk/home.asp

Destination, Resort and Luxury Hotel Spas ●

Destination spas, resort spas and luxury hotel spas share commonalities. These establishments cater to an affluent clientele with high expectations of customer service from both management and practitioners. Surroundings are elegant, the ambiance tranquil. The equipment tends to be first-rate and products are high quality. Unfortunately, little opportunity exists to build repeat business on a long-term basis, although guests often develop an appreciation for a highly skilled practitioner and schedule several visits during their stay. Practitioners are usually fully booked unless their service is uncommon or it's a slow season.

Resort and Luxury Hotel Spas ● ●

Resort and luxury hotel spas are very similar. Working at a resort spa in the Bahamas, Hawaii or the Caribbean is a great way to meet new friends and enjoy an island lifestyle. Whether you prefer ocean resorts, mountain resorts or desert resorts, a variety of spa jobs are located in these settings. You may also like some perks of the job—employees often get discounts on spa services so they can rest and rejuvenate at their leisure.

Working at a luxury hotel spa in an urban area can be very similar to working at a day spa. The pace is usually brisk and the surroundings pleasant. Most clients are vacationers or business travelers in town for a short visit. At some luxury hotel spas, people from the local community enjoy visiting the spa and partaking of its services. These clients often forge long-term customer relationships with favorite practitioners.

In these spa environments, there can be some advantages for massage therapists. Because they're often expected to perform a variety of spa treatments, this reduces the likelihood of repetitive stress syndrome, as these types of treatments are less taxing on the body than massage. For instance, a day can be divided into 70 percent full-body massage sessions and 25 percent treatments like salt glows and body wraps. The rest of time is spent in escorting clients to treatment rooms and completing paperwork.

Spa work at resort and luxury hotel spas can be demanding for all types of practitioners, but especially for massage therapists. Some industry studies report that the average massage therapist lasts about six months. However, this is not always the case, as some practitioners have found an enjoyable career niche working at resort and luxury hotel spas on a long-term basis. A lot depends on finding the right scheduling situation, with the right team and the right compensation.

Champions keep playing until they get it right.
— Billie Jean King

Destination Spas • •

A destination spa is an upscale health retreat dedicated solely to guests who come for weeklong or weekend spa programs. These types of spas are often located in the mountains or near the ocean where guests can enjoy the peace and beauty of nature while experiencing every amenity imaginable. Guests usually visit these spas to enhance their health, make lifestyle changes or rejuvenate from the stresses of a high-pressure career. Price tags range from $3,000 to $5,000 or more per week. Clients include executives, celebrities, professional athletes, health-conscious families, aging baby boomers, and just about anyone interested in enhanced well-being.

If you work at a destination spa, developing a client base becomes more a matter of retaining a "guest" and that guest's friends. As some long-time practitioners working in these settings have observed, guests often tell their friends if they find an exceptionally good practitioner. Word-of-mouth is a powerful force in building clientele, particularly when a client experiences a deeply relaxing session, gets relief from a troubling pain syndrome, or learns from a nutritionist how simple modification can make a profound change in her life.

Figure 7.5

Additional Success Tips for Working in Destination, Resort or Luxury Hotel Spas

- The pace can be demanding, especially during the busy season at resorts. One advantage is that work hours are often flexible in the off-season.
- Polish your customer service skills. Clients expect to be catered to and demand exceptional customer service.
- Practitioners may perform from eight to 10 one-hour sessions each day. Some practitioners find that the repetitive nature of this work can get tiresome.
- To find work at these spas, apply through the human resources department. By timing your application to coincide with the beginning of the busy season, you may have a better chance of getting hired.
- Practitioners with advanced training, solid experience and a wide portfolio of skills are in the best position to get hired.

Dental Spas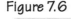

Don't be surprised if you arrive at your dentist's office one day and find a trickling waterfall or soothing candles in your treatment room. According to a recent American Dental Association survey,[1] a growing number of dentists say spa-like amenities and services persuade patients to make and keep appointments and help them stay relaxed during dental procedures.

While the idea of a dental spa may seem like an odd one, it's gaining popularity with dentists and dental patrons alike. From a 10-minute chair massage to paraffin wax treatments for hands, spa services such as massage, facials, manicures, pedicures, reflexology, acupuncture and craniosacral therapy are welcome amenities to time-pressed dental customers—or to customers that dread visits to the dentist.

Spa services offered by dentists vary widely depending on the demographics and preferences of customers. Some dentists offer full-service massage therapy within their office setting, while others find that 10-minute chair massages, facials and manicures are more popular. Although some dentists do not refer to their offices as dental spas, they pamper loyal customers and attract new ones by offering practical and relaxing spa-style comforts. A busy dental spa might hire a practitioner as an employee, while others hire them as independent contractors.

Figure 7.6

Hospitals and medical centers highlighted in the next section on Wellness Settings, serve clients with injuries or health conditions that require medical intervention.

Additional Success Tips for Working in Dental Spas

- Schedule informational interviews with practitioners who work in a dentist's office or medical spa to gain more insights into the pros and cons of these working environments.
- With the right dentist, it's possible to gain many referrals and build a loyal following fairly quickly. Most dentists who offer wellness services do so because they believe in them. This element of support boosts your chance of success. A few dentists may be experimenting with these services because they've heard it's a good way for them to increase their revenue.

Medical Spas •

The phenomenon of medical spas started in the mid-1990s and promises to keep thriving as a more holistic approach to health and beauty gains in popularity. Most medical spas are owned and managed by dermatologists or board-certified plastic surgeons. Medical spas cater to the luxury market, offering a menu of cosmetic surgery procedures, holistic health services and skin rejuvenation treatments. The services may range from massage therapy, acupuncture, aromatherapy and facials to modern laser therapies, injections and plastic surgery procedures such as facelifts. It is generally acknowledged that medical patients who schedule holistic health treatments often heal faster, feel less pain and have a decreased medication dependency after surgery. Most medical spas have high professional standards and seek practitioners who are highly educated and skilled in using appropriate medical terminology.

Figure 7.7

Additional Success Tips for Working in a Medical Spas

- Schedule informational interviews with several wellness practitioners who work in a medical spa to gain insights into this type of working environment.
- Search the Internet for information about medical spas throughout the country for insights into medical spa operations and how spas market themselves.
- When interviewing, questions might include: Is there a strong team environment? Does the medical spa value open communication, teamwork and employee feedback? Is there an orientation and training program? How are practitioners compensated?
- Gain credibility by becoming familiar with medical terminology and recordkeeping specific to plastic surgery procedures.
- Medical settings often require adaptability and flexibility due to unexpected scheduling twists or changes to client conditions.

In recent years, massage therapy has solidified its presence in traditional healthcare due to validated outcome measures (i.e., proven results). Massage is generally recognized as one of the key therapeutic interventions that support effective pain management.

• Working in Medical Settings •

In response to the public's growing interest in Complementary and Alternative Medicine (CAM) therapies, an increasing number of hospitals are establishing adjunct clinics for services such as chiropractic, massage therapy and acupuncture. Others hospitals integrate CAM programs directly into their operating environments.

Medical settings may include hospitals or clinics, such as a rehabilitation center, medical center, sports medicine clinic or orthopedic physician's office. In all cases, working in a medical setting requires the integration of the CAM therapy into a multidisciplinary team as a key member. In a hospital setting you may become a part of the medical team treating trauma patients, amputees, cancer survivors or burn survivors. You may be treating a client prior to surgery to enhance relaxation and reduce stress. Treatments may be on an inpatient or outpatient basis.

A high degree of knowledge and skill is vital to effectively and safely treat clients with medical conditions. You need to have excellent clinical skills, such as assessment, clear identification of short- and long-term treatment plans, and techniques appropriate to specific conditions. In addition, specific protocols, procedures, documentation and medical language are used by clinicians and physicians in hospital and clinic settings. Fluency in these practices and terminology is required to participate as an inclusive member of the healthcare team.

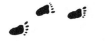

Chapter 9, Page 168

for details on working as an independent contractor.

One of the advantages of working in a medical setting is the opportunity to develop ongoing relationships with clients and observe outcomes of care over time. It can be very rewarding to see a client endure and triumph during a difficult healing journey. However, in some cases, you may see a client for only a limited number of treatments.

Working in a clinic environment requires an awareness of and adherence to policies and procedures. For instance, it's common to encounter dress codes. Many clinics approach dress formally (e.g., uniforms or lab coats), while others are more casual and allow you to choose a flexible blend of attire (e.g., black pants, white shirt). Some have stringent hygiene policies, such as long hair pulled back, no facial hair and no perfume. The personalities, styles and philosophies of the various wellness professionals must blend or conflict can arise over working conditions and what's best for the client.

Specialties •

Determine what type of medical practice or specialty attracts you. Learn about it and the types of clients it helps. Ascertain the specific skill set needed to be successful in this environment. For example, somatic practitioners are much more employable if they also are trained in lymphatic drainage, myofascial release, aquatic massage and scar massage. Most practitioners discover that they need to alter their treatments or scope of practice in a clinic setting. The time you spend with clients and the actual work you do may be determined by the lead primary care provider. You may be directed very specifically on what to do, how to do it and the time allotted.

Administration

Practitioners who work in a medical setting or clinic are expected to participate in various activities in addition to direct client treatment, such as completing various medical reports, participating in team meetings, and documenting daily workload. Working agreements may be negotiated as an employee or independent contractor, usually either by on-site appointments or contracted hours. If you're a private practitioner, allot ample time to market your services to attract new clients and obtain referrals from physicians.

Measuring Therapeutic Outcomes

To ensure the ongoing success of CAM programs, most hospitals and clinics develop practices that incorporate standard outcome measures, such as the McGill Pain Rating, Vancouver Burn Scar Index, Goniometry (for measuring range of motion) or the Arizona Integrative Outcomes Scale. These measuring tools enable practitioners to identify the therapeutic outcomes and benefits to clients in a language shared by all healthcare professionals. Evidence documenting a program's effectiveness is a key in the long-term viability of CAM programs. As wellness research continues to evolve, you may have the opportunity to contribute to research studies or be asked to share periodic research findings with physicians and administrators.

Figure 7.8

Success Tips for Working in a Medical Setting

- Schedule informational interviews with several wellness practitioners who work in a hospital or clinic to gain insights into these environments.
- Broaden your employment possibilities by learning a variety of techniques for assorted medical conditions. Seek to understand the benefits of treatment for each medical condition, as well as conditions for which a CAM is contraindicated. For instance, a client touched by cancer requires a different approach than a client that is scheduling a session for relaxation prior to surgery.
- If you work within a hospital or clinic environment, it's important to develop an awareness of the organization structures and chains of command typical in these medical settings.
- Medical settings often require adaptability and flexibility due to unexpected scheduling twists or changes to client conditions.
- Working with seriously ill or dying patients can be emotionally taxing. Many practitioners prefer part-time work of this nature.
- Gain credibility by being well versed in medical terminology and recordkeeping specific to different types of medical practices.
- After you gain some solid experience working in medical settings, consider volunteering. Many cities have formed organizations that offer free wellness care to hospital patients, especially those touched by AIDS and people in hospice care.
- Know how to conduct research and how to measure therapeutic outcomes. Medical settings often rely on funding from agencies that require this type of documentation.

• Working in Wellness Centers •

In wellness settings, clients are primarily interested in preventive care, stress management, relief from everyday aches and pains, or support for various health challenges. Practitioners are drawn to this type of work for various reasons—either as a way to find an enjoyable career niche, to supplement income while building a private practice, or to gain valuable experience working in collaboration with other professionals. Most wellness centers offer a wide range of wellness services under one roof (e.g., chiropractic, massage therapy, acupuncture, nutritional counseling, aromatherapy, yoga), while some group practices offer a single specialty.

A key advantage to working in a wellness center is peer support and supervision. You may enjoy the camaraderie and connection to other professionals (private practice tends to be more isolated). From the opportunity to ask another practitioner's opinion about a treatment scenario to discussing integrated care plans for clients whom you share in common a clinic setting easily supports a team approach to client wellness.

Your schedule may be more standardized than in a spa environment, as most clinics aren't open late evenings or Sundays.

Many wellness practitioners enjoy being part of a clinic with clear and established professional boundaries. This setting also offers many opportunities for professional development through mentoring or tuition reimbursement programs. It is also usually easier to get insurance reimbursement if you aren't already a recognized primary care provider.

When exploring job openings, evaluate the advantages and disadvantages of joining a wellness center as an independent contractor versus an employee. Sometimes you may work first as a contractor of the clinic, then negotiate a change to employee status. Or you may be offered a position as an employee after the manager has had a chance to observe your skills and success in building a solid base of clients.

As with medical settings, wellness centers also provide opportunities for case management. When a team of highly skilled wellness practitioners works together to create optimal support for a client, positive results can be greatly amplified. This requires open communication, consistent cooperation and shared values among practitioners—and carving out time throughout the day or week for informal or formal team meetings.

An ethical dilemma that can occur relates to working part time in a wellness center while maintaining a small home-based practice. Following is an example:

The old cliché is true: "An ounce of prevention is worth a pound of cure."

> A clinic client has received his total insurance-covered sessions for the current year, yet is still in need of further treatment. The rate for your services at the clinic is substantially higher than your home-based practice. The client has somehow discovered this and has requested private sessions. What do you do?

If you had previously set up guidelines, this issue could be avoided or at least resolved with minimal conflict. When you negotiate your employment contract or independent contractor relationship with a clinic, it's important to clarify how this type of situation would be handled.

Figure 7.9

Success Tips for
Working in a Wellness Center

- Schedule several informational interviews with practitioners who work in clinic or group practice to gain insights into this type of work. (If you're a student, do this while you're in school.)
- Before your interview, obtain a copy of the clinic's promotional material, mission statement and policies.
- Research industry trade journals to get insights into salary structures.
- During the interview, ask about the types of clients who are seen in the clinic. Gain a clear understanding of target markets, conditions addressed and health philosophies of the clinic.
- Ask to meet other team members prior to accepting employment. A brief team meeting or one-on-one meetings gives valuable insight into whether the clinic setting and team is a fit for you. Do you share similar philosophies and views? Do you sense that team members are dedicated to excellent client service?
- If you work in a chiropractic or acupuncture clinic, you need a firm grasp of clinical terminology and protocol, and skill at insurance charting.
- Define parameters for working with clients outside of the clinic.
- Clarify what is expected of you when you're not directly working with clients (e.g., paperwork, janitorial chores, clerical duties, assisting the other practitioners, providing treatments for staff, marketing). Whether you get paid for these activities depends upon your employment status.
- Working at a wellness center even part time can help a practitioner feel a sense of community and support often lacking in private practice.
- Be prepared to do cash flow forecasting to budget, particularly if you receive deferred insurance payments.

*Make sure to have questions prepared if you are going to meet with potential employers.

• Working in Specialty Centers •

Specialty centers are businesses that specialize in one type of wellness service, such as acupuncture, massage or chiropractic care, and often at a discount. They range from a group of like-minded practitioners joining forces to nationwide franchises that encourage clients to become members and get discounted treatments. The average price for a treatment even for nonmembers is usually slightly less than the going rate in the area.

There are many advantages to working in this type of setting. It is a great way for new practitioners to gain valuable experience and often receive free continuing education as an employment benefit. Practitioners who are in transition or who have recently relocated can kick-start their practice by working in this setting. There is also the advantage of walking into a situation in which everything is provided: you just show up to do the work. The disadvantages are that often the pay is low as the fees being charged are low, and clients tend to be more loyal to the business than the individual practitioners.

Figure 7.10

Success Tips for Working in a Specialty Center

- This work environment is very similar to that of a wellness center, so also refer to those tips in the previous section.
- Enjoy what is provided for you, such as scheduling services, laundry and marketing.
- There can be a lot of competition between practitioners when you all do the same thing. Go the extra mile with clients so your work stands out.
- Improve bookings by incorporating small touches such as aromatherapy or hot towels during the session.
- Increase commissions by using retail products in your sessions. If a client enjoys the product, you can tell him how to purchase it for home use.

Employment Fundamentals

• Research Potential Employers •

After you have determined what type of setting is the best fit for your skills and personality, the next step is to research potential employers. Look through the Help Wanted sections in newspapers, trade journals and online job posting sites. Check with the local schools to find out if they have any job postings. Contact school alumni to see if they have any openings in their practices. If you're unable to get a list, then perhaps there's an alumni newsletter in which you can place a classified ad for "Position Wanted." Check your professional association's website for job postings, and if none exist, you can often find contact information for practitioners in the area where you wish to practice. Also, consider posting your resume on professional online bulletin boards.

If you're still in school, you can jump-start your career by having a job lined up before you graduate. Most students are so overwhelmed with all the tasks necessary to complete their education that they don't start their job search until after graduation. Take advantage of this to get your name higher on the "potential employee" list. One of the personality traits employers highly value is initiative. Contacting potential employers while you're still in school demonstrates foresight and strong initiative.

Create a list of potential employers. Note the addresses, phone numbers and the names and titles of the people who have hiring authority. Meanwhile network, network, network. Talk to people, let them know you're available. Ask for leads. Remember, quite often it's who you know that gets you the job.

There is no security on the earth, only opportunity.
— General Douglas MacArthur

Figure 8.1

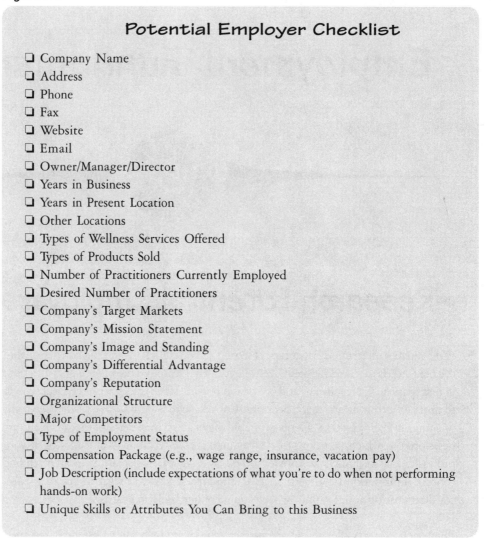

Potential Employer Checklist

- ❏ Company Name
- ❏ Address
- ❏ Phone
- ❏ Fax
- ❏ Website
- ❏ Email
- ❏ Owner/Manager/Director
- ❏ Years in Business
- ❏ Years in Present Location
- ❏ Other Locations
- ❏ Types of Wellness Services Offered
- ❏ Types of Products Sold
- ❏ Number of Practitioners Currently Employed
- ❏ Desired Number of Practitioners
- ❏ Company's Target Markets
- ❏ Company's Mission Statement
- ❏ Company's Image and Standing
- ❏ Company's Differential Advantage
- ❏ Company's Reputation
- ❏ Organizational Structure
- ❏ Major Competitors
- ❏ Type of Employment Status
- ❏ Compensation Package (e.g., wage range, insurance, vacation pay)
- ❏ Job Description (include expectations of what you're to do when not performing hands-on work)
- ❏ Unique Skills or Attributes You Can Bring to this Business

www.businessmastery.us/
forms.php#busman
for a printable copy of this
checklist.

Informational Interviews ●

Informational interviews are a good way to gain valuable insights into different work environments and the people who work in each. They are also a way to make valuable contacts; people may remember you when there is a job opening down the road. Before you start the formal interview process with employers, meet with several practitioners and managers who work in the type of settings you're targeting in your job search. Most people are willing to schedule a half hour to share insights and guide you in your research. The following are sample questions to ask during an informational interview.

Figure 8.2

Informational Interview Questions

- What are some attributes of practitioners who have been most successful in this environment?
- Is there a strong team environment?
- What do you think is the most challenging part of this work environment?
- What do you like best about working here?
- How would you describe communication between management and staff? Are there regular staff meetings?
- Because so much depends on seniority, how did you endure the slow days in the beginning when you were not scheduled for many treatment sessions?
- What advice do you have for doing the best job possible and developing a career in this type of setting?
- What advice do you have for adjusting to this environment and management (e.g., rules, personalities)?
- How does the hiring process work (e.g., are there several rounds of interviews or just one)?
- If you're a student: What do you suggest I do while in school to increase my odds of getting hired by this spa/wellness center/medical center?

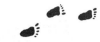

Chapter 16, Pages 357-360

for more specifics on networking.

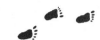

Chapter 15, Page 337

for information on the Differential Advantage.

• Contact Potential Employers •

Sometimes it's possible to make an initial contact by phone. In other cases, you may need to send your resume and cover letter by mail. When calling about a job opportunity, ask to talk to the manager that makes hiring decisions. If you're fortunate enough to connect directly to that person, be prepared to express your interest in employment opportunities and ask how the interview process works. Answer any questions concisely and completely. If you gauge that you've established rapport and there is mutual interest, ask about scheduling an interview.

If the hiring manager is unavailable when you call, make a note of the person's name, title and confirm the correct spelling. Then send a resume with a cover letter to the attention of the manager. Although some job openings are filled through online applications or resumes, it's a good idea to send a paper resume and letter. It shows you're willing to take some extra time and effort in your employment search.

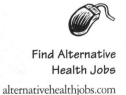

Find Alternative Health Jobs
alternativehealthjobs.com

If you haven't received a response within five days of the potential manager having received your letter, call to follow up. Continue to place follow-up calls weekly. Sometimes endurance pays off. If you keep yourself so visible that a manager is aware that you really want to work for her company, you may get the job out of sheer persistence.

• Polish Your Interviewing Skills •

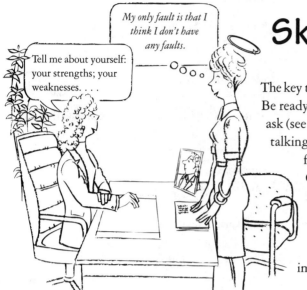

Tell me about yourself: your strengths; your weaknesses. . . .

My only fault is that I think I don't have any faults.

The key to a successful interview is preparation. Review your research. Be ready with answers to questions that an interviewer is likely to ask (see Figure 8.5 for sample questions). To get comfortable with talking about your skills and experience, and what you're looking for in a job, practice role-playing an interview with a friend. Get feedback. Work on polishing your answers to possible interview questions and asking meaningful questions about the job. Focus on concise phrasing and conveying a positive attitude. Keep in mind that the best communicators are also the best listeners. You must be confident, and most important of all, you must be prepared.

Figure 8.3

Interview Tips

- Dress appropriately and be well groomed.
- Be enthusiastic, confident and polite.
- Bring an appointment book or a PDA (personal digital assistant).
- Bring extra copies of your resume.
- Bring a printed sheet with at least three references.
- Be on time.
- Be prepared. Have all necessary documentation available.
- Be well poised, centered and relaxed.
- Maintain good eye contact.
- Use positive wording and listen carefully.
- Control the interview yet don't monopolize the conversation.
- Know what sets you apart from the other candidates.
- Have a list of unique skills, education or attributes you can bring to this business.
- Know your strengths and weaknesses and how you plan to compensate for those weaknesses.
- Be prepared to discuss each item on your resume or job application.
- Have at least three questions that you can ask the interviewer.
- Prepare a response to the inevitable interview question, "Tell me about yourself."
- Look for closing signals.
- Avoid discussing salary and benefits in the first interview.
- Thank the interviewer when done.
- Send a thank-you letter to everyone with whom you've spoken.

Tough Questions

During the interview you're talking up your strengths and experience and how you're a good fit for the job. You can also expect an interviewer to ask you some tough questions. For example: "What are your weaknesses?" Think carefully about your response. Whatever weakness you choose, it shouldn't be a true liability. Turn a weakness into a strength. A good example: "I have a tendency to be hyper-responsible, but I also work to keep a sense of balance about this." This conveys that you're conscientious and interested in self-improvement.

Another tough question an interviewer may throw at you is: "Why should I hire you?" This is often asked toward the end of the meeting. This is a point when taking interview notes can come in handy. Refer to your notes, and say: "Based on our meeting, I believe you're looking for . . . based on my experience and training [elaborate], I know that this would be a good fit for my skills and abilities." Another sample answer: "Based on our meeting, it sounds like you're looking for a highly skilled, flexible person with initiative and an ability to put clients at ease—someone who is dedicated to doing their professional best each day. My experience tells me that I'm a good fit for the job . . . [elaborate]. Also, I like the company and admire its success. It seems there is a good team environment here and I value that." In short, communicate why you're a good match for the position. (See Figure 8.5 for common interview questions.)

www.businessmastery.us/
test-massage.php
for tips on giving a test
massage.

Take Charge of the Interview ● ●

Instill confidence in your potential employer by asking several thoughtful questions. At some point in the beginning of the interview, ask the interviewer to describe the skill set that he or she is looking for in the position. This information helps you determine what education and experience you'll highlight in the interview.

Usually toward the end of the interview, you will be asked, "Do you have any questions for me?" This is your chance to shine. Here are some sample questions you can pose:

Figure 8.4

Interview Questions You Pose

- What was it about this company that made you want to work here?
- What does this company value the most?
- What is the most important thing I can do to help within the first two months of my employment?
- When senior practitioners leave the company, why do they leave and where do they usually go?
- What do you see as my strongest assets and possible weaknesses?
- Do you have any concerns about me fulfilling the responsibilities of this position?

Figure 8.5

Common Questions Employers Ask

Work History

Of all your jobs, which one was the most rewarding, and why?

Of all your jobs, which one was the least helpful to you and why?

What would your references say about you?

What accomplishments bring you the most pride?

What do you like best and least about your profession?

School History

Why did you choose this field?

How did you pick the school you attended?

What were your favorite courses? Why?

Ability & Personality

What would make you successful in this job?

How do you cope when work is very demanding?

What experience have you had dealing with the public?

How would you describe your personality using 10 words or less?

How do you motivate yourself?

What was the most difficult situation you've ever been in?

Has there ever been a time when you changed your schedule to accommodate work? What was the situation? How did you respond when asked?

What are the situations when you will not bend or give in?

Do you have a goal-setting system to determine priorities and get them completed?

Manageability

How do managers get you to do your best work?

What would the perfect relationship between a manager and employee look like?

Describe the best and worst managers you ever had.

How can a manager reward you for doing a good job?

Communication

What was the most difficult communication situation you've dealt with?

How do you deal with people when there is a disagreement?

Have you ever had a time when you turned an unhappy customer into a happy one?

What type of people do you get along with best?

How do you work with people you do not like?

Describe a time when you had to make an immediate decision that you may not have had the authority to make. Why and how did you make the decision?

What kinds of decisions do you not like to make?

Team Building

What is your strategy in working with a group to accomplish a goal?

What are some of the things co-workers do that irritate you?

Job Suitability

What is the most important thing you do in your job?

What do you think a typical day would be like here?

Describe your perfect job.

What does success mean to you?

What types of clients do you like to work with?

In what area could you expect to make the biggest impact?

Why should I consider you for the job?

Future

How will this job help you reach your personal and professional goals?

How long do you plan on staying with this company?

What are your plans for future education?

Polish Your Answers to Interview Questions

Schedule an hour or so to review the above questions and jot down your answers. Then spend some time with a friend who will give you tips on how to polish your answers. You need to articulate your strengths. Use concrete examples and stories to emphasize how your skills and abilities are a fit for the job. Know the company's mission and explain why you want to work for the company. Be yourself, remember to relax, and prepare clear and concise answers to potential interview questions.

• Resume Writing Made Easy •

A resume is a tool with one specific goal: to inspire a potential employer to interview you. A resume that clearly highlights your professional training and experience, and that conveys an understanding of an employer's mission, is the one most likely to lead to an interview. To create an effective resume you need to learn about the company's history, its mission, needs, and problems. Determine the ways in which your skills and experience can contribute to the company's success and emphasize these points. Finally, find the name and title of the person in charge of hiring (which isn't always the personnel administrator).

The two major types of resumes are chronological and functional. The chronological resume is used when you want to emphasize a good work history that's directly related to your desired job. The functional resume is used when you want to emphasize your talents, abilities and potential—not your work history. In most instances, practitioners use more of a functional resume or sometimes even just a targeted inquiry letter. A resume is a useful tool for promotion, even if you own your own business. If nothing else, the process of developing your resume clarifies your strengths and reinforces your self-esteem.

Resume Magic: Trade Secrets of a Professional Resume Writer by Susan B. Whitcomb

Figure 8.6

Resume Checklist

❑ Does the resume focus on why the employer should hire you over your competitors?
❑ Is the resume targeted to the employer rather than a one-size-fits-all document?
❑ Have you included a concisely stated career objective?
❑ Does the resume clearly describe your training, experience and accomplishments?
❑ Does the resume have a visually pleasing, polished presentation?
❑ Are margins even on all sides?
❑ Are design elements like spacing and font size consistent throughout the document?
❑ Is the resume free of spelling errors and grammatical errors?
❑ Is there a good balance of white space and words? Does the resume look overcrowded with words, or is it too skimpy and vague?
❑ Have you asked friends or colleagues to proof it for accuracy and to share feedback?

Resume Resources
www.rockportinstitute.com/
resumes/html

www.office.microsoft.com/
en-us/templates/
CT101043371033.aspx

www.creatingprints.com

Resume Formats •

The following chart highlights the elements of chronological and functional resumes. Also included are sample resumes for wellness practitioners. (See Figures 8.8 and 8.9.)

Figure 8.7

Chronological Resume Format	Functional Resume Format
Highlights Work History & Experience	**Highlights Talents, Abilities & Potential**

Chronological Resume Format

Highlights Work History & Experience

Heading

Name, address and contact information. Centered at top of the page.

Objective

This is optional, particularly if you address it in your cover letter. If you do use an objective, make it very specific and concise. State what you can contribute to the organization. Objectives can help focus resumes when you have an eclectic background or you're embarking on a new career. This can also be a place to state your healing or therapeutic intentions: a sentence, statement or paragraph which communicates your desired goals and effects of treatments.

Work Experience

Start with your present or most recent job. It isn't necessary to give the month and day, just the year. List your employer, job title and a brief description of your duties. Emphasize your major accomplishments and abilities. You don't have to list each position change within a company.

Education

Include the name of the school, year graduated (optional), degree(s), certification(s) and any awards or honors. If your education is within the past few years, it should be the first thing listed after the heading, otherwise put it at the bottom.

Personal

This is optional. Only include information you feel is valuable toward getting you the job.

Functional Resume Format

Highlights Talents, Abilities & Potential

Heading

Name, address and contact information. Centered at top of the page.

Objective or Professional Profile

This is optional, particularly if you address it in your cover letter. If you do use an objective, make it very specific and concise. State what you can contribute to the organization. Objectives can help focus resumes when you have an eclectic background or you're embarking on a new career. This can also be a place to state your healing or therapeutic intentions: a sentence, statement or paragraph which communicates your desired goals and effects of treatments.

Function

List your strongest abilities or accomplishments in four or five separate paragraphs—put them in order of relevance to desired job. Have a major headline for each paragraph. If you have a strong work history, it can be by position (e.g., Staff Management). If you have limited work history and are relying on your education, list by modality (e.g., Sports Massage, Hydrotherapy) or related skills such as Organizational Skills.

Education

Put at bottom unless it was within three years.

Work Experience

(Optional.) List a brief summary at the bottom of the page. Include dates, employers and titles.

Personal

This is optional.

Figure 8.8 Sample Chronological Resume

Nikki Mountain, LMT

4141 Winding Way

Tucson, AZ 85750

520-555-5555

nikkimountain@example.com

Professional Profile

Highly skilled massage therapist with more than 10 years' experience in a wide range of healing modalities. I am seeking to join a wellness center as a partner or associate. The ideal setting would include practitioners who value open communication, high ethical standards and dedication to providing high-quality client care. My goal is to provide bodywork that honors the body, mind and heart of each client, combining my skills in Swedish massage, deep tissue massage, aquatic massage, energy work, Asian style belly work and nonviolent communication.

Work Experience

Moving Spirit Massage Therapy, Tucson, AZ

Sole Proprietor. 1997 - Present.

- Highly skilled in combining various healing modalities, such as Swedish massage, craniosacral therapy, deep tissue massage, energy work and Chi Nei Tsang.
- Responsible for managing business tasks, including scheduling, bookkeeping, marketing and publishing monthly newsletter for clients.
- Maintained a diverse practice, including many long-term clients of five years or more.

Wellness Institute, Tucson, AZ

Massage School Coordinator. 2002 - 2005

- Coordinated and managed multiple aspects of massage therapy education program, including curriculum development, course planning, scheduling and faculty relations.
- Maintained Filemaker Pro database of all student records.
- Developed and presented study skills training for students.
- Coordinated professional development programs for faculty.

Healing Arts Spa, Tucson, AZ

Assistant Manager. 2000 - 2001

- Responsible for working with marketing consultant to develop new logo, promotional brochures and business cards.
- Maintained appointment books and confirmed client appointments.
- Responsible for tracking product inventory and ordering products for resale.
- Coordinated laundry service to ensure smooth operation.
- Developed weekly schedules for spa practitioners; helped to troubleshoot last-minute schedule conflicts.

Education

Mountain Institute Holistic Health, Tucson, AZ

- Completed 750-hour Therapeutic Massage Program, 1997
- Arizona Licensed Massage Therapist, 1997
- Reiki I and II with Susan Wright, 1997-1998
- Chi Nei Tsang I with John Sterling, 2001
- Introduction to Craniosacral Therapy with Mary Suntree, 1998 and 2000

Figure 8.9 Sample Functional Resume

David Waters

2001 N. Pine Road

San Francisco, CA 94995

415-555-5555

dwaters@example.com

Objective

To establish an acupuncture practice working with clients who seek a safe and natural way to get well and enjoy vibrant health. My goal is to join or create a group practice at a holistic health center with other practitioners, such as physical therapists, chiropractors, bodyworkers, naturopathic physicians and medical doctors.

Specialty Focus

Areas of special interest include pediatrics, pre- and post-surgery support, and eye diseases. Received letter of commendation from faculty for demonstrating highly effective diagnostic assessment and acupuncture treatment skills during my senior internship.

Education

California College of Traditional Chinese Medicine, Master of Science in Health Science, Oriental Medicine Program (O.M.D.), San Francisco, CA. 2006.

Curriculum and training focused on history and philosophy of Chinese medicine, diagnostic assessment, acupuncture needling techniques, Chinese herbology, tongue and pulse diagnosis, adjunct treatments such as moxibustion, case studies, ethics and business management.

California Licensed Acupuncturist, 2007

Clinic Practice and Internship

The California College of Traditional Chinese Medicine curriculum and internship practice focuses on blending the holistic approach of ancient Chinese acupuncture and herbology with modern healthcare.

The program closely aligned with current O.M.D. training in China. Clincal practice and internship included:

- **Assistantship** (60 hours). Assisted acupuncturists in treatment procedures such as moxibustion and cupping, and withdrew needles from the patient.
- **Junior Internship** (240 hours). Provided acupuncture treatments to patients under close supervision and performed diagnoses with guidance from a clinical instructor.
- **Senior Internship** (270 hours). Diagnosed and treated acupuncture clinic clients with minimal supervision.

As an adjunct to the clinical training component of the program, I annually attended two grand rounds conducted by California College of Traditional Chinese Medicine faculty. During these sessions, faculty presented interesting or difficult cases and demonstrated appropriate treatment.

Acupuncture Work Experience

San Rafael College of Acupuncture, San Rafael, CA. Business Manager, 2001-2002.

Managed student acupuncture clinic. Responsible for patient scheduling, bookkeeping, ordering clinic supplies, coordinating laundry services and maintaining student practitioner attendance records.

Cover Letters ●

Your cover letter is an integral part of your resume packet; it complements your resume and inspires the recipient to read further. A cover letter is where you build rapport. Keep your tone friendly and use terminology that's appropriate to your field. The best cover letters clearly communicate your understanding of an employer's needs, and convey your professionalism and personality.

Writing a good letter can be a challenge. Experienced writers often write, rewrite, edit, and edit some more. Plan to do the same. Do not expect to complete your letter in one sitting. Write the first draft, and come back to it later to edit. Find the hot topics, concerns, trends and buzzwords by researching trade journals, newsletters and consumer publications targeted for your particular industry.

Cover letters typically consist of three sections: an opening, body and close. The opening establishes rapport and communicates your interest. The body conveys how your skills and experience will meet the needs of your employer, and highlights unique aspects of your professional experience. The closing thanks the reader and suggests the next step, such as a telephone call or interview. Type your cover letter on stationery that matches your resume, and keep the letter length to one page. Some career experts suggest sending your letter and resume in a 9 x 12 inch envelope so the presentation of your letter is a bit crisper.

The closest most people come to perfection is when they fill out a job application.
— Don L. Griffith

Figure 8.10

Resume Cover Letter Tips

- Employers hire humans not robots. Beyond your professional experience, they like to get a sense of your personality and interpersonal skills.
- Use conversational language in your cover letter, and avoid copying sample letters word for word. Find your own voice. Include brief insights into your career experiences or why you chose your career path.
- Sample phrases:
    Some of my most rewarding work has centered on….
    I am passionate about….
    I love my profession—the satisfaction that comes from….
- Avoid overly formal language and refrain from starting the cover letter with a sentence such as, "Enclosed please find a copy of my resume…." Instead use: "I am writing to express interest…."
- Briefly highlight relevant experience; avoid repeating information verbatim from your resume.
- If you've recently graduated from an educational program, reference your intern experience or include testimonials from those who have experienced your work in a student clinic or other apprentice program.
- If applicable, mention a referral source. For example, "Jane Doe mentioned you were looking for an experienced nutritional consultant to join your clinic."
- The best cover letters focus on how you can meet an employer's needs, and convey unique aspects of your personality, training and professional experience.

Figure 8.11 Sample Cover Letter

Nikki Mountain, LMT
4141 Winding Way, Tucson, AZ 85750
520-555-5555
nikkimountain@example.com

July 10, 2020

Ms. Susan Sample, Center Manager
Desert Wellness Center
1234 East First Street
Tucson, AZ 85750

Dear Ms. Sample:

You recently advertised an opening for a highly skilled, licensed massage therapist at the Desert Wellness Center. My cousin and several of her friends are clients at your center. They speak highly of the quality care they receive and how comfortable they feel.

Given my 10 years' experience in this field, unique skill set and dedication to high-quality client care, I would make a great addition to your team.

During my years in private practice, I greatly enjoyed seeing how regular massage sessions helped long-term clients weather stress and navigate through health challenges and surgery with greater ease than they thought possible.

I enjoy working with a diverse clientele. I am in excellent health and can easily work with a large number of clients each week.

I would appreciate the opportunity to personally convey what I might contribute as a member of your center.

Thank you for your time and consideration.

Sincerely,

Nikki Mountain

Enclosure

Targeted Inquiry Letters •

Another type of job search tool is a targeted inquiry letter. This type of letter is appropriate when you've a identified a company that fits your profile of a place where you would like to work. It is particularly valuable when you want to focus on your abilities—regardless of whether you've had much experience or training. In this case you aren't targeting a job opening. You are introducing yourself and your unique talents, and proclaiming your interest in a future job opening. You must determine the type of job you want and specify it up front with a title and possibly include a short description if the title doesn't fully convey the job description.

As with a cover letter, the first thing to do is develop rapport. Then identify the type of job you want (e.g., spa coordinator, massage therapist, esthetician, yoga instructor, staff counselor), and give a concise, dynamic summary of your experience, capabilities and achievements that relate to the targeted job.

Include specific work history and education, but keep the focus on what you have to offer, including any unique training or internship experiences. Close the letter by suggesting a time to get together. Type your letter on stationery that matches your resume (in case you send one in the future), and keep the letter length to one page.

www.businessmastery.us/
resumes.php
for more sample resumes.

www.businessmastery.us/
scannable-resume.php
for scannable resume tips.

www.businessmastery.us/
targeted-letter.php
for a sample Targeted
Inquiry Letter.

Assemble Your Resume Kit

Create templates that can be easily customized to a specific employer. Keep this information in one folder. Include the following documents:

- Resume
- Cover Letter
- Targeted Inquiry Letter
- Reference List

• Employment Contracts •

The old saying, "The devil is in the details," certainly applies to contracts. Although it may seem a cumbersome task at first glance, the time you take to carefully review a proposed employment contract can save many headaches down the road. Many practitioners have a legal or business advisor review a contract prior to signing it. Before meeting with an advisor, make a list of points that you would like to clarify, or where you would like to add new information to the contract. In some cases, you may want to negotiate terms that you perceive are more equitable. Often you can clarify any questions in a brief conversation with your potential employer. A careful and thorough review of your contract is smart business.

The following sample contract (Figure 8.12) is for illustrative purposes only and not intended for use as a legal document. Most employers don't create written employment agreements (although it isn't a bad idea).

Figure 8.12

Sample Massage Therapy Employment Agreement

This agreement, dated July 4, 2020, is by and between Holistic Health Clinic ("Employer"), with principal offices located at 1776 Independence Way, Washington, D.C., and Frank Benjamin ("Employee").

Services to Be Provided by Employee

Employee agrees to provide massage therapy services within the scope of licensure. Employee is responsible for maintaining appropriate certification and licensure (including all costs thereof). Employee agrees to dress in a style consistent with the Employer's image, including uniforms. Employee shall maintain client records in the manner prescribed by employer.

When Employee isn't engaged in treatments, Employee shall assist with other office duties as directed, including but not limited to:
a. Assisting other practitioners with clients.
b. Performing clerical duties.
c. Cleaning and organizing the clinic.

Services to Be Provided by Employer

Employer shall provide the following: a safe, clean environment; a room furnished with a chair, stool, hydraulic table, settee, hydrotherapy equipment and storage area; receptionist services; appointment scheduling; insurance billing; marketing; and all necessary supplies and materials used in the performance of services (e.g., oils, lotions, linens and music).

Other Provisions

a. Employee has the right to perform services for others during the term of this Agreement, however such services are not to be performed on Employer's premises.
b. Employee shall not solicit or provide services to Employer's clients for private practice while employed or for six months after termination of employment, except as noted in "c."
c. Upon termination of employment Employer and Employee shall discuss which clients, under what conditions and with what compensation Employee may maintain continuity of service.
d. All client records shall remain the property of the Employer.
e. All Employee's nonclinic marketing materials that include any information about Employer, must be approved in advance.

Fees, Terms of Payment and Fringe Benefits

Employee shall be compensated at the base rate of $10 per hour, with an additional $5 per half-hour massage and $10 per hour massage, not to exceed 30 hours per week. Employee shall be paid biweekly. Employee shall receive payment on all services performed regardless of the collection time. Employee is eligible to participate in any of the following fringe benefits: health insurance, vacation time and employee pension plan (see policy manual).

Local, State and Federal Taxes

Employer is responsible for paying all required local, state and federal withholding, Social Security and Medicare taxes.

Workers' Compensation and Unemployment Insurance

Employer will provide Workers' Compensation and Unemployment Insurance.

Insurance

During the term of this agreement, Employee shall maintain a malpractice insurance policy of at least $2,000,000 aggregate annual and $1,000,000 per incident. Employer shall maintain insurance coverage for liability, fire and theft.

Term of Agreement

Either party may terminate this agreement, given reasonable cause, as provided below, or by giving 30 days written notice to the other party of the intention to terminate this Agreement:

a. Material violation of the provisions of this Agreement.

b. Action by either party exposing the other to liability for property damage or personal injury.

c. Violation of ethical standards as defined by local, state and/or national associations and governing bodies.

d. Loss of licensure for services provided.

e. Employee fails to maintain the standard of service deemed appropriate by Employer.

f. Employee engages in any pattern or course of conduct on a continuing basis which adversely affects Employee's ability to perform services.

g. Employee engages in any pattern or course of conduct on a continuing basis which adversely affects Employer's or other employees' ability to perform services.

h. It is agreed that any unresolved disputes will be settled by arbitration, including costs thereof.

This constitutes the entire agreement between Employee and Employer and supersedes any and all prior written or verbal agreements. Should any part of this agreement be deemed unenforceable, the remainder of the agreement continues in effect. This agreement is governed by the laws of the District of Columbia.

Signatures

Employee: _____Frank Benjamin_____ Date: ___July 4, 2020___

Employer: __Marshall Taylor_____ Date: ___July 4, 2020___

Witness: __Joy Cronkite_____ Date: ___July 4, 2020___

• Negotiating a Raise •

Meeting with your manager to discuss a raise can be an excruciatingly painful process—or may flow as smoothly as a river running downstream. Your comfort level in talking or thinking about money hinges a great deal on two factors: your attitude toward money and feelings about your self-worth. Money is simply a medium of exchange for products, services and ideas. What is your attitude toward money? Do you view money skills like any other skill—requiring education and practice to achieve optimal results? Do you manage money matters by default and let this part of your life operate on autopilot? Do you set financial goals?

Chapter 14, Pages 285-286

to further explore the concept of money.

Developing a healthy attitude toward money can take time and effort, and this doesn't happen overnight. It requires developing basic knowledge about money matters and then practicing what you've learned. There are plenty of good books and magazines that can help you build your money skills and confidence.

A strong sense of self-esteem is vital to discuss or evaluate your compensation package with ease and confidence. Self-esteem is a feeling—how you feel about yourself. It isn't based on what you look like, how much money you have or your position in the business world. If all your accomplishments, looks and material goods were taken away—how would you feel about yourself? Do you believe in yourself and your ability to be your best and overcome obstacles? Who you are goes beyond the externals. Simply stated, self-esteem is how you feel about who you are.

Rate Your Performance •

When exploring a raise, keep in mind that who you are as a person doesn't necessarily correlate with your value to an employer or client. You may be dedicated, outgoing and honest, yet you still may not live up to external performance standards. The better you can distinguish "you" from your actions, the easier it becomes for you to analyze your strengths and create a powerful negotiating base.

My father taught me always to do more than you get paid for as an investment in your future.
— Jim Rohn

First of all, you must be sure that your services are worth more than you now receive. Your financial desires and needs have nothing to do with your worth as an employee. Your skills may not be as valuable in the eyes of your company as you would like them to be. When you've finished answering these questions and you aren't certain about being qualified to ask for more money, don't worry. Think about the areas you want to improve and set goals to improve your performance. Strengthen the areas that are weak. Take a seminar or read a book. Identify and follow through on whatever is necessary for you to grow and improve your skills. Keep track of your accomplishments. Regularly review your accomplishments and goals. Then when you feel more confident about your results, schedule a meeting with your manager to discuss a performance review.

Assess the Worth of Your Services

In analyzing your worth to an employer or client consider these self-analysis questions:

- Am I achieving my goals?
- Am I performing at my peak level in quality and quantity?
- How have I improved my business skills?
- How have I improved my technical skills and knowledge?
- Am I reliable and consistent?
- Do I get my work done on or before deadline?
- Are my clients achieving their desired treatment goals?
- In what ways have I taken initiative?
- How have I contributed to the success of the company?
- Are my relationships with co-workers pleasant and productive?
- How have I improved my leadership abilities?
- In what ways have I given better/more service than I was paid to give?
- If I was my employer, would I be satisfied with my performance?

The Performance Review Meeting •

One of the first steps to prepare for your performance review meeting is to look at the big picture. How long has it been since you received a raise? Is your income comparable to your peers? Research industry salary surveys and economic indicators; look for articles in trade publications that provide facts and charts about salary trends. If data are available, research your company's history: how often has it given raises? What is the average percentage increase? What are some of the available perks?

Review Your Performance Record ● ●

Review your performance records. Many practitioners like to create a file to track accomplishments and training achieved during each year along with thank-you notes from happy clients. Note the times that you've exceeded expectations or achieved outstanding results under difficult circumstances. Compile a list of your accomplishments. Refer to the self-analysis questions. Write a summary of your accomplishments. Whenever possible, include numbers. Be specific. Some examples are: "Clients are completing their treatment courses on or before projected date," "The number of clients on maintenance programs has increased by 40 percent," "My department's productivity increased 20 percent," "My promotion idea garnered us a $15,000 corporate contract," "Turnover rate has decreased by 50 percent," "Product sales increased by 42 percent," and "We were $5,000 under budget this year."

Also include some of the less tangible results. For example, "Morale has improved," "Case management is more effective," and "I am more organized." Actually, you could figure out how much money you were saving the company even with the intangible results by analyzing the amount of time saved and multiplying that by the average salary per minute. Unfortunately, many people either overlook or underestimate the financial value of time.

Carefully evaluate if your desire for more money is based upon your needs or your performance. Assess your company's, supervisor's and clients' standards for excellence and compare them with your standards. Make certain your perceived priorities are the same as theirs.

Mental Preparation ● ●

The next step in preparing for your raise is to imagine asking for an increase in compensation. Brainstorm the possible objections you might encounter and have responses to each one. Include "why" questions: Why don't you feel this job is worth $40,000 per year? Why don't you think I deserve $35 per hour? What do you think I need to do differently in the next six months to earn a performance increase? We would all hope the discussion wouldn't get to this point, but it's best to be fully prepared. This may seem like a lot of work, but, asking for more money is like selling—you're communicating the benefits of what you have to offer and asking for appropriate compensation for your talents and abilities.

Factor in Benefits ● ●

After evaluating yourself and following the suggested steps to prepare for a performance review, take stock of the employee benefits you already have. Sometimes employers may not be willing or able to give you more money, but they may increase benefits. Alternatives to cash include: an expense account; a company car; stock options; profit sharing; pension and retirement plans; insurance; paid travel; vacations; use of corporate lodge or resort; professional association dues; educational expenses; memberships to health clubs; tickets to sporting events and theatrical productions; company discount on products or services, nursery and day care centers; and flexible working hours.

The Negotiation Presentation ● ●

Chapter 12, Pages 252-253
for more information on
negotiation skills.

This is when the fine art of negotiation comes in. Tailor your presentation to the manager's communication style and personality. Be grounded in your capabilities and accomplishments. Remember, timing is very critical. What is a good time for you may not be the right time for the other person. Although substance is important, style can play a big role in successful communication. Your attitude tremendously impacts negotiations. Before you ask for an increase in compensation, role-play your presentation with a friend. Listen to feedback. Visualize a win-win experience in your mind's eye. Imagine everyone getting what he or she wants. Have a positive mental attitude. You know you and your services are worthy of earning more, and you've prepared an excellent presentation. You are now ready to ask for that raise!

• Career Success Secrets •

How do you make sure your talent and hard work get noticed, appreciated and rewarded by your employer? How do you create the best chance of a promising career path?

First, follow the success tips of highly successful people. You can find a list of these career building secrets in Figure 8.13.

Next, make it your aim to land a job with an employer—either a company or an individual—that values happy employees and a positive work environment. Besides making it more enjoyable to go to work each day, it's simply good business.

I have found enthusiasm for work to be the most priceless ingredient in any recipe for success.
— Samuel Goldwyn

A recent international study showed that companies with positive employee attitudes are more profitable.[1] As a result, these employers are also more likely to recognize and reward talented and dedicated employees accordingly.

Oftentimes, gauging whether an employer offers a positive work atmosphere starts with first impressions. How are you greeted when you arrive for an interview? How were you treated on the phone when you were contacted about scheduling an interview? Were the people you talked with engaged with their job, or were they in zombie mode, barely there?

When you arrived for the interview, did you sense positive and upbeat energy and a sincere interest in providing the best customer experience, or ho-hum energy and a focus on quantity versus quality? Did you observe professionalism versus an overly informal approach to business? Did you sense a strong team environment?

Although there are times when first impressions are not always representative of a company or individual's business persona, more often than not they're a good indicator of what's to come.

Of course, you will have already done your best to research the company and its mission, and what you can expect in terms of hours, clients and salary range. These are the measurable and tangible elements of your job search. Just as important are the "vibes" you get when you interact with people in the company. Observe carefully, consult your research and talk with trusted advisors—then follow your instincts.

Keep in mind that sometimes when you're first starting out, finding the ideal employer may not happen right away. However, in time, the right door will open for you as you build your skills and expertise, and keep a clear focus on finding your ideal employer.

Figure 8.13

What Highly Successful Employees Know

Highly successful employees share these common traits and career success secrets.

Respect. Respect for others means honoring clients, co-workers and managers as unique individuals. Although others may have different outlooks or ideas, it means treating others as you would like to be treated.

Respect can manifest in social courtesies such as greeting co-workers pleasantly each morning. Or it can mean holding back an angry or unkind remark during a difficult conversation. It can also mean coming in to work on time or even a little early. Respect also includes going out of your way to pitch in when others need help, and, if you share a room, making sure you leave that room clean and appropriately stocked for the next practitioner.

Whatever shape it takes, respect requires a conscious effort to honor both the terms of your employment and your team members' need to be treated in a positive and kind manner.

Appreciation. To appreciate is to acknowledge the positive effort, unique talent or personality characteristics of co-workers and employers. It creates a sense of teamwork and inspires people to be their best.

Solution-oriented. An employee who can identify creative solutions to problems, or find new ways at looking at old problems, stands out from the crowd. If you see difficult situations and difficult people as opportunities to put your creativity to work and learn new skills, you're sure to shine. Most companies highly value and reward these type of employees.

Communication skills. Great communicators are good listeners. They know how to communicate with clarity and genuine respect for others. They take every opportunity to hone their skills through practice, continuing education and study.

Positive attitude. Simply put, attitude is everything. A positive attitude is like a magnet. It attracts good people and fortunate circumstances. It ensures that you excel in your career. Keeping a positive mind-set isn't always easy, but always worth it. When challenges loom large, a good sense of humor can work wonders to help revive a positive attitude.

Approximately 70 percent of all people who are fired are fired because they cannot get along with other people.[2]

Part IV

Business Beginnings

The phase known as business start-up is crucial to your future success. It provides the necessary groundwork for a business to grow and prosper. Studies show that most business failures are due to improper management or undercapitalization, not because the owners were underskilled in the performance of their profession. Part IV of *Business Mastery* encourages you to take the time to master the basics of business start-up, so that you can maximize your chance of success and avoid common pitfalls—such as financial woes and poor planning—that befall many small business owners.

To help you launch your ideal business, Chapter 9 takes an in-depth look at private practice options, such as working in a home office, a business setting or on an outcall basis. It also explores group practice settings, where one or more wellness practitioners share office space and expenses such as rent, maintenance and office staff. In addition, this chapter offers insights into building a business as an independent contractor in either a group practice, other wellness settings (e.g., salons, fitness clubs, corporate wellness programs) or working at special events.

Chapter 10 looks at the nuts and bolts of a business start-up. It covers how to assess the feasibility of your business idea, find start-up financing and determine client fee structures. You'll also find tips on how to select a good location, enhance the positive effects of your practice with the ancient art of feng shui, navigate zoning and licensing regulations, and procure appropriate insurance coverage. Also included is valuable information about marketplace research, various legal structures, and what to look for when buying a practice. The information in this chapter is useful to know even if you plan to be an employee. It helps you to understand what's involved in establishing a business and the costs of running it, thus giving you a better appreciation of what an employer offers. This knowledge is crucial if you plan on moving into management.

Finally, Chapter 11 provides detailed instructions for creating your business plan—an indispensable tool for mastering both short- and long-term success. The chapter details the major components of a business plan, including how to create a financial forecast to realistically assess the finances required to launch and maintain your business. We also include a guide of additional useful resources to help you create a solid business plan.

An Insider's Look at Practice Settings

• Your Ideal Practice •

As a small business owner you need to develop a solid base of business knowledge and understand the advantages and disadvantages of various practice settings. To help you establish your ideal business, this chapter looks at career options such as private practice in a home office, business setting or on an outcall basis. It also explores a group practice where practitioners share office space and expenses such as rent, maintenance and office staff. In addition, there are insights into building a business as an independent contractor in either a group practice, other wellness settings, or to work at special events. This chapter provides the insights you need to make a wise choice on whether private practice or group practice is best suited to your personality, skills and interests.

Your profession is not what brings home your paycheck. Your profession is what you were put on earth to do with such passion and such intensity that it becomes spiritual in calling.
— Vincent Van Gogh

Figure 9.1

Private Practice, Group Practice & Independent Contractor Working Environments

Private Practice
Home Office
Stand-alone Office in a Professional Building
Room in Another's Practice (e.g., chiropractor's office)
On-site or Outcall Settings
Corporate Wellness Program
Salon, Day Spa or Dental Spa
Fitness Center, Gym or Health Club
Hospice
Personal Practitioner for a Celebrity or Professional Athlete

Group Practice
Holistic Healthcare Clinic or Wellness Center
Specialty Clinic or Center (e.g., only acupuncturists)
Medical Clinic

• Private Practice •

At some point in their careers, most wellness practitioners choose to be self-employed. These sole proprietors work in private practice settings, either out of home offices or business offices. These businesses may also include outcall services. Practitioners often work in multiple environments. For example, a practitioner might see clients three days a week from a home office, go to several clients' homes each week, and work as at a corporation one day per week.

Independent Contractors •

Chapter 10, Page 195
for Sole Proprietorship regulations.

Oftentimes private practitioners pursue short-term or long-term independent contractor arrangements as an effective way to supplement their income. In these settings, you're technically a separate business operating within another business: you generally rent office space on a flat rate or percentage basis of the income you generate. Some practitioners even work as independent contractors for several companies and rarely see clients in their own offices. These opportunities provide a degree of variety that appeal to many.

If you're thinking about working as an independent contractor for one or more companies, keep in mind that while it means you operate as a business owner (sole proprietor), you may be treated more like an employee without the employee benefits. In these settings, your start-up business tasks are fewer in number and complexity than practitioners who establish a private or group practice.

Independent Contractor = Self-Employed.

If you're an independent contractor and also operate a private practice, define parameters for working with the "company's" clients in your private practice setting. Consult with a business coach, attorney or financial advisor before finalizing and signing an independent contractor agreement. The time and money you invest in consultation more than repays you by avoiding lost time, disappointment and potential legal problems resulting from conflicts. In most cases, to qualify for independent contractor status (according to Internal Revenue Service standards), you would work part time with any given company, but most importantly, have revenue from other practice settings.

Key Aspects of Private Practice •

The main reason people start a private practice is control. They can choose when they work, how they work and with whom they work. A private practice provides freedom and flexibility (e.g., you choose the attire, clients, environment, music, lighting, ambiance, creativity, modalities, fees and scheduling). You can essentially do anything you want as long as it's legal, ethical and moral. Besides the overall start-up tasks and the general practice management activities covered later in this chapter, a sole practitioner must contend with some aspects unique to this working environment. We briefly review these aspects and offer tips on how to effectively manage them.

Autonomy • •

Although you may enjoy the freedom of private practice, a potential drawback is a sense of professional isolation. Private practice can be a stark contrast to educational programs which offer plenty of opportunities to share professional opinions and insights with colleagues. Nonetheless, some practitioners thrive in a private practice setting. Others find they must actively work to minimize isolation. Some good ways to do this are to join a networking group or attend industry conferences as your time and budget allow.

You may also experience days when the endless array of business tasks seem to take on mammoth proportions. As the appointment scheduler, bookkeeper, business manager, marketing director and wellness provider, you are responsible for making sure everything gets done—until you can afford to hire an assistant.

Safety • •

Safety is a standard concern for any business owner, but even more so for a wellness practitioner in private practice. Take a vigilant approach to personal safety. For instance, first-time clients can present potential trouble spots, as it's difficult to know much about their character or background. In most cases you can quickly and aptly sense unbalanced individuals, an unsafe neighborhood or other safety concerns and remove yourself from the situation with haste or end a session if need be. However, operating this "inner radar" at top efficiency requires that you first develop an awareness of potential personal harm and take it seriously. Fortunately, safety incidents are rare in private practices. From a safety standpoint, it's best to only work hours when someone else is in the building (or your home). In addition, lock your treatment door or main office so uninvited people can't wander in. The old saying, "An ounce of prevention is worth a pound of cure," certainly applies here.

Finances • •

When you're the only source of revenue in your business, you must carefully manage your cash flow. You need to plan for items such as tax payments, supplies and equipment purchases, insurance premiums and marketing expenses. To help launch your business on solid footing, meet with a financial advisor or work with a business self-help book to map out an effective system for estimating monthly operating expenses and revenues, and making quarterly tax payments. Learn about tax deductions and set up an easy-to-use recordkeeping system to save time and headaches at tax time.

Benefits • •

The only "employment benefits" you receive are the ones you pay for yourself (which kind of defeats the whole concept of "perks"). As a sole practitioner there are no true paid vacations, holidays or sick days. Some practitioners find it helpful to open a savings account to set aside cash resources as "self pay" for vacations and days off.

9

Figure 9.2

Success Tips for Private Practice

- Minimize professional isolation by establishing a support system of colleagues and advisors. Trade tasks with a colleague (e.g., you balance her checkbook and she helps you develop your marketing plan).
- Find mentors and trusted advisors with whom you can consult.
- Network! Attend at least one networking event each month. It is a great way to make new friends, generate leads, and find employment opportunities.
- If you are just starting out, it can help ease financial pressures if you work part time at another job until you can build a strong client base.
- Hire someone to handle time-consuming business tasks such as bookkeeping so that you can focus on working with clients. This makes good business sense and frees you up to do more of what you love. For instance, if you pay someone $10 per hour for 10 hours a week ($100) and that frees you up to do eight more sessions at $50 each ($400), you'll net $300.
- Take safety precautions by screening new clients, make sure outdoor lighting is adequate, and call a friend before and after sessions.
- Don't hesitate to end a session immediately if you encounter inappropriate comments or behavior. You may excuse yourself by saying you don't feel well, or simply state that you're uncomfortable continuing the session.
- Create a reserve account for purchasing high-ticket items.
- Keep good records in an easy-to-use system that works. Track where your time and money go so you can monitor results and change course if needed.
- Allot ample time each week to focus on marketing tasks.
- Research health and disability insurance options to find the best value and coverage. Ask colleagues for their recommendations.
- Verify that your auto insurance covers lost income if you're in an accident. Typically, this isn't a standard coverage feature.
- Develop clear policies about cancellations and no-shows. Include this policy on your client forms and review it with clients.
- Schedule efficiently. A mistake many practitioners make when they are new is to work whenever clients want. This can lead to burnout. Make a schedule that works for you, includes ample breaks and allots time to take care of yourself. Take off at least one day per week and two days in a row when possible.
- Take the time to write a business plan that includes a vision statement and maps out best-case and worst-case financial scenarios.
- If you rent a room in a medical facility such as a chiropractor's office, place your business cards and brochures on display at the reception desk. Create good signage. Offer to give free demonstrations of your services to clients waiting for chiropractic services. Offer referral incentives. Hold educational meetings for your clinic staff. Explain the benefits of your work, give demonstrations and show them tips for self-care.
- Make lifelong learning a priority.

Salon and Day Spa Environments

Salons, which many classify as a close cousin to day spas, range from bustling turnstiles to tranquil escapes from everyday stress. Although most day spas hire wellness practitioners as employees, opportunities may arise to work as an independent contractor in this type of setting. Salons customarily rent rooms to practitioners and rarely have more than three wellness providers (usually somatic practitioners and estheticians).

In some salons or day spas you're assigned a permanent treatment room, and you can personalize the decor to some extent. In most cases you share the treatment room with other practitioners. A potential drawback is that some treatment rooms are located in close proximity to other salon activities and lack room-specific temperature control units. Some aren't well-insulated from sounds and odors. Be prepared to include supplies and equipment in your operating budget. Most salons require you to purchase all supplies and equipment, particularly linens, treatment chairs or massage tables.

In this setting, you must actively and consistently market your services through a brochure, special introductory offers, gift certificate programs or other means. In general, body therapies and other wellness services are of primary interest to spa visitors. In contrast, building a successful wellness practice in a salon may require considerably more time and effort. On the plus side, demand for wellness services in salons is growing steadily.

Figure 9.3

Success Tips for Salons and Day Spas

- If you work in a salon, place your business cards and brochures on display at the reception desk. Create good signage.
- Be sure to set clear cancellation policies.
- Make sure that everyone who works at the salon experiences your services. Be visible. Give free demonstrations of your products or services to clients waiting for other services. Offer referral incentives. Hold educational meetings for your co-workers. Explain the benefits of your work, give demonstrations, and show them tips for self-care.
- Ideally, arrange the treatment room so it isn't adjacent to hair designer stations (to avoid intrusive noise of hair dryers) or where harsh chemicals are used.
- Have the front desk place your brochure in the bags when clients purchase products.
- If you haven't seen a client for a while, place a follow-up call to ask how she is and if she has any concerns or feedback she would like to share about the last session.
- Ensure client files are complete and up-to-date. This helps track client progress and provides a useful reference point for each session. Clients appreciate thorough and professional attention to their unique needs.
- Expect and plan for slow spells or open times between client appointments. If you aren't expected to perform any other spa-related job duties during these times, bring reading materials, catch up on correspondence, listen to relaxation CDs, or enjoy some simple yoga stretches.

Salons provide you with a built-in clientele of people who *need* your services—the other employees!

Salon Employment
www.salonemployment.com

www.businessmastery.us/ start-spa.php for tips on starting your own day spa.

Chapter 7, Pages 127-139
for information on being a spa employee.

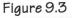

Fitness Centers and Health Clubs ●

Working at a fitness center, gym or health club requires you to tailor services to your client's health concerns and interests. Many highly motivated career professionals and aging baby boomers have taken the initiative to develop a personal wellness program at local fitness centers, and enjoy the convenience of scheduling massage therapy, bodywork, yoga classes or nutrition consulting under the same roof. This provides ample opportunities for practitioners who prefer to work in fitness settings.

Building a practice at a fitness center, gym or health club setting can be a good way to gain valuable experience if you're a new practitioner—or if you're an experienced practitioner who likes working with the type of health-conscious clientele common to these settings. You may particularly enjoy this type of work if you're interested in sports injuries or if you like working with athletes or clients who are looking for effective ways to manage chronic pain or health conditions. It can be fun and rewarding to work with regular clients and witness progress in their efforts to reduce stress, heal from injuries and enjoy good health.

Figure 9.4

Success Tips for
Fitness Centers and Health Clubs

- Place your business cards and brochures on display at the reception desk. Create good signage. Be sure and set clear cancellation policies.
- Education is the key to building a practice in this environment. Offer free demonstrations and classes.
- Offer special "welcome" marketing programs (e.g., $10 discount coupons for first visit, gift certification promotions) to help build your business.
- Network with other wellness practitioners in your area who work in similar settings.
- Utilize a comprehensive intake form, so you can become aware of and accommodate a client's medical conditions or contraindications. Practice conservative treatment.
- Take classes and exercise at the facility. This is an informal way to network and market your services plus get a good workout!
- Make sure that everyone who works at the facility experiences your services, especially the personal trainers. Educate staff on how your service helps clients meet their health and fitness goals.

Private Practitioner for a Celebrity or Athlete ✳

Sometimes working at a fitness center or health club can lead to a job as a personal practitioner for a celebrity or athlete. These clients may be patrons of the establishment, and, after getting to know your skills and abilities firsthand, they may offer you a job traveling with them on concert tours, movie sets or during the game season.

On the other hand, you may hear of these types of career opportunities through personal or professional contacts. In most cases, you work as an independent contractor, although occasionally you may be offered employment. As in any working environment, it's important to assess the advantages and disadvantages, and take a realistic look at what the job involves. Although these types of jobs can be glamorous, they're often physically demanding and require a great deal of flexibility in terms of scheduling and adapting to travel and lifestyle issues.

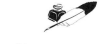

Nothing great was ever achieved without enthusiasm.
— Ralph Waldo Emerson

Figure 9.5

Success Tips for Working with a Celebrity or Athlete

- Work with a legal advisor to carefully review the terms of your employment contract or independent contractor agreement. Clarify what is reasonable in terms of scheduling (e.g., minimum and maximum number of treatment sessions per day and per week, time off, and the time limit after which you would not be available). Maybe you don't mind working at 2 a.m., but maybe you do. Will you be paid a weekly salary or compensated by the number of hours worked? Determine if there is a bonus for working beyond the standard number of hours each week.

- If you will be traveling, clarify how expenses for air travel, lodging, meals and incidentals such as laundry will be handled. Document this in your employment contract or independent contractor agreement. Will you have an allowance for these expenses? Will all charges be handled directly by your client?

- If you work for a client who is on tour, you may be on the road for six to eight months. Think about how you will handle the logistics of maintaining a home base while you travel or what storage solutions may work for you.

- Consider lifestyle issues. Are you willing to adapt to your client's preferences in terms of restaurants and hotels? Clarify expectations around the times when you will not be providing wellness services. For instance, are you expected to run errands or handle other chores?

- Good communication skills and boundaries help create a professional working relationship that balances your needs with the needs of your client.

Corporate Wellness Programs •

According to a recent report from the Wellness Councils of America[1], the return on investment in corporate wellness programs is no longer in dispute. Every one dollar that an employer spends on wellness programs saves as much as three dollars in healthcare expenses. Faced with steadily rising healthcare costs, most large employers are expanding workplace wellness initiatives. This helps to create a healthy, happy and productive workforce—and a healthier bottom line.

Corporate wellness programs may include on-site seated massage, table massage, acupressure, chiropractic care, fitness classes, smoking cessation, nutritional consulting and yoga classes, either through a company gym or sponsored program at a health club. Hospitals may offer wellness programs for staff to help reduce stress and enhance health. Recognized benefits of employee wellness programs include reduced absenteeism, reduced number of sick days and an overall reduction in healthcare costs. An article titled *Massage Is In Business*[2] reported that of the companies mentioned as the "100 Best for Working Mothers," 77 percent offered massage therapy to their employees.

The expansion in corporate wellness programs bodes well for wellness practitioners. Many companies offer flex benefits which allow employees to apply eligible dollars to wellness services and classes. You may also find opportunities working within wellness programs at upscale retirement communities. In the majority of cases, wellness practitioners work as independent contractors.

Figure 9.6

Success Tips for Corporate Wellness Programs

- Join a local chapter of the Wellness Councils of America (see welcoa.org). Get to know the wellness professionals in your area and network.
- Contact local hospitals, colleges and universities about wellness programs for employees and staff. Send the contact person a letter with articles about other companies that offer such services. Follow up with a phone call to request a meeting to introduce your service and its benefits. Offer to give a demonstration of your services during your introductory meeting.
- Many massage practitioners approach on-site chair massage as a complement to their private practice. It is a good way to grow some extra income and make contact with prospective clients.
- Gain experience in corporate wellness by working for an established on-site employer that provides services to corporate clients and at health fairs.
- Employee participation is higher if the company pays for on-site wellness care versus if the employer pays only partial costs. Negotiate this from a win-win standpoint. The more employees who participate, the healthier they become, which ultimately translates into lower employer healthcare costs. Also suggest that the company pay you by the hour rather than by the session. This takes into account the transition time between clients; otherwise you will be on-site and unpaid for this time.

Hospice

Many practitioners find working in a hospice program rewarding and fulfilling. In medieval times, the word "hospice" referred to a way station where travelers were cared for and refreshed. Today, hospice programs combine advanced medical technology with compassionate care, enabling individuals with terminal or incurable health conditions to live as fully and comfortably as possible, in familiar surroundings, in the company of family and friends.

Those who apply to hospice program are usually required to have an opinion from a medical professional that their disease is likely to lead to death in six months or less. Although some hospice programs are part of medical centers, the majority of hospice programs offer in-home care and support.

People of all ages are admitted to hospice programs. In this setting, you may very well work with patients from 3 to 93 years old. In most hospice settings, wellness practitioners work on a part-time basis as independent contractors. Practitioners are typically paid a flat-fee rate, not including travel time. Once a referral is made through the hospice program, a practitioner often continues visits on a weekly or bimonthly basis. Hospice work can be emotionally demanding and is not for everyone. Hands-on work often needs to be adapted in this environment to meet clients' needs. For instance, you may need to work with clients in their beds.

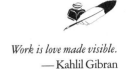

Work is love made visible.
— Kahlil Gibran

Figure 9.7

Success Tips for Hospice

- Allot ample time for recordkeeping, and document patient sessions carefully. A record of a wellness session is usually placed in a patient file for reference by other team members, such as the patient care coordinator or visiting nurse.
- A good working knowledge of contraindications for medical conditions and familiarity with medical terminology are important in this environment.
- Many practitioners prefer to work on part-time basis, as hospice work can be emotionally taxing.
- Acupressure, reflexology, polarity, energy work and gentle touch therapies are often effective in easing the pain and anxiety experienced by hospice patients.
- Be prepared to adapt to unexpected schedule changes, and be flexible in your access to clients.

9

On-Site and Outcall Settings ❋

Mobile practices have become very popular in the past few years. Many wellness practitioners prefer to go to a client's home or office. The major advantage is very low overhead for the practitioner—no rent to pay! Clients also love the convenience of receiving services at their home or work.

The disadvantages include lugging around heavy equipment and driving a lot. You may spend more time with clients when you're in their home setting up and breaking down (which doesn't happen when there is another client waiting in your office). Also there can be many distractions you cannot easily control.

Figure 9.8

Success Tips for On-Site and Outcall Settings

- As a safety practice, call a friend (while the client is nearby) and tell him that you will call him after your session.
- Keep safety concerns foremost. Avoid problematic situations with first time outcall clients by clarifying the scope of services you offer. Avoid booking appointments in unfamiliar neighborhoods at night. Be cautious with late-night appointments for new clients, unless it's through a hotel or agency you trust to carefully screen clients.
- Try to set up your session area in a peaceful space away from telephones, kids and other distractions.
- Set a price that takes into consideration drive time as well as setup and breakdown.
- Set good boundaries to avoid spending too much time at the client's premises. One idea is to schedule a business or personal appointment within an hour after the expected completion of the session.
- Schedule wisely: Whenever possible group clients who are in the area on the same day. Allow enough time to get to your next client in heavy traffic.
- Give a discount for more than one client per location.

Working in a Primary Care Provider's Office ✳

Another practice option is renting a room in the office of primary care provider (PCP), such as a chiropractor, medical doctor, naturopath, osteopath or a physical therapist. These situations range from sharing a room to having the room to yourself. The fee structure also varies. In some situations you pay a flat rate for the room or you pay per session. Payment based on sessions provides a safety net for new practitioners, since they only pay when they see clients.

As with all practice settings, this one has advantages and disadvantages. On the positive side, you may have a good source for new clientele from referrals. On the negative side, you may rarely get referrals. Some PCPs simply have other practitioners there to lower their costs and look good, while others do it because they believe in what you do and want to have alternatives available to their patients.

Other pluses can include sharing marketing expenses, a sense of community and possible shared reception or office help. As an independent contractor or renter, you usually supply all materials used in your work. Before you agree to work in the office, make sure you know how the PCP plans to interact with you and how referrals and marketing are handled.

Figure 9.9

Success Tips for Working in a Primary Care Provider's Office

- Place your business cards and brochures on display at the reception desk. Create good signage.
- Have a good marketing plan to make your services known to current patients. Make sure that everyone who works at the office experiences your services.
- Give free demonstrations of your products or services to patients waiting for other services. Offer referral incentives. Hold educational meetings for your co-workers. Explain the benefits of your work to co-workers and patients.
- If you pay a rental fee per session, negotiate a ceiling of how much you will pay per week or month.
- Have a clear agreement or contract about exactly what your role is for things such as marketing, scheduling and office staff.
- Fluency in medical terminology is a plus in this environment.
- Keep good client records for marketing purposes as well as creating team treatment plans with the PCP.
- Determine what to expect as far as referrals from the PCP. (Will you need to supply most of your own clients?)

• Group Practice •

If you're interested in joining or establishing a group practice, the primary settings are holistic healthcare clinics, wellness centers, specialty clinics or medical clinics. Typically, holistic healthcare clinics and wellness centers offer a variety of services, such as chiropractic, acupuncture, massage therapy, nutritional counseling and aromatherapy, under one roof. In contrast, specialty clinics focus on a single specialty, such as chiropractic, acupuncture or massage therapy. Medical clinics may take the shape of sports medicine clinics, physical therapy clinics or orthopedic medicine clinics, where massage therapists or acupuncturists work in tandem with medical doctors or physical therapists. Though these group practices have different objectives, they're more similar than not when it comes to what you need to know to make it work for you.

Group practices can be formed as an association or partnership. In most instances, wellness practitioners prefer to form associations rather than partnerships. The reasons for this vary, but they primarily center on ease of operation, minimal commingling of funds, liability issues and more independence for each practitioner. A typical association arrangement involves several practitioners who operate separate businesses joining together to share office space and expenses such as rent, maintenance and administrative support. Later in the chapter, we explore various types of business structures so you can determine the best option for your situation.

The benefits of a group practice are numerous. Many practitioners enjoy the camaraderie and creative synergy that happens when two or more professionals work together on case management or everyday brainstorming. In addition, group practice often provides a variety of wellness services under one roof, which can attract new clients and lead to greater income potential. Other benefits include access to a ready-made professional image and extensive office resources (e.g., staff to handle scheduling, greet clients, manage financial transactions), along with an increased sense of personal safety when dealing with problematic clients.

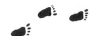

Chapter 10, Pages 195-199

for information on
legal structures.

Group practice offers added flexibility when you're ill or want to take a vacation, as you can make arrangements with other staff to provide services for your clients during these times. Group practice can also be highly cost-effective. You often encounter reduced overhead and greater buying power via discounts on quantity supplies and holistic healthcare products for resale. Lastly, it can be more fun and rewarding to share space with others in a team environment—providing the team works in harmony and shares professional values.

Some aspects of clinic or wellness center work require careful consideration if you join the group as an independent contractor. Finances tend to be complex, especially in view of the need to maintain fairness in shared expenses, client scheduling and revenues from product sales. It's vital to create clear, written agreements with other group practitioners to avoid entanglements and misunderstandings. From a cash flow standpoint, keep in mind that if you're dealing with insurance reimbursement, you may not receive payment for months after you've done the work. Track your operating expenses and continuing education events so you can confidently raise your prices periodically to account for cost factors and your growing skill level. It is also usually easier to get insurance reimbursement if you aren't already a recognized primary care provider.

Although holistic healthcare clinics, wellness centers, specialty clinics and medical clinics have unique aspects, they all share common operating and marketing challenges—and potential pitfalls. The next section explores a range of topics which can help you find a group practice setting that best matches your talents and interests.

Before we launch into the above-noted exploration, we look at a brief case study that serves as a cautionary tale. Unfortunately, many practitioners develop business alliances without creating a proper operating structure. The following scenario demonstrates the importance of planning and foresight when entering into a group practice arrangement, and emphasizes the importance of a written business agreement.

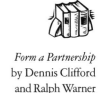

Form a Partnership
by Dennis Clifford
and Ralph Warner

Group Practice Case Study

Steve, a chiropractor, decides to share an already established office with chiropractor, Terry. The office is situated in a prime location, and Steve has been feeling rather isolated in his practice. He has known Terry for several years and respects her work. Steve asks Terry to create an association agreement, but Terry refuses and acts offended. This red flag should have immediately sent Steve running in the opposite direction. Steve decides to proceed anyway. After all, they're both caring, responsible adults, and he feels confident they could work out any problems.

Things go fairly well for several years. Terry starts getting involved in accounts that take her outside of the office, so she brings in another chiropractor, Stacy, to work with clients in her treatment room. This is done without consulting Steve. Now there are three people sharing the total space, yet Steve is still paying half of the expenses. Resentment brews. Then Steve discovers something that sends him over the edge: Several times clients had called to book sessions with him when he wasn't in the office. Stacy talked with the clients and instead of trying to figure out another time when they could schedule with Steve, she booked the appointments for herself.

He could not resolve these issues, and no guidelines had been set for how to deal with unresolved conflicts. So Steve gives notice. He wants to leave as soon as possible but agrees to stay for several months. Meanwhile, things go from bad to worse. He feels uncomfortable in his own office. He realizes that communication is difficult, so when the time nears for him to leave, he submits a written, 30-day notice. The next day, Steve goes to work only to discover that the locks to the office had been changed. Ultimately, the situation gets resolved, but not without unnecessary grief and anger (as well as the intervention of an attorney).

9

Key Aspects of Group Practice •

You can avoid the pitfalls described above and garner the benefits of working with others by paying careful attention to some nuts and bolts of business start-up, such as scheduling time for self-assessment; performing careful interviews with potential associates; clarifying roles, goals and expectations; evaluating legal status options; defining image and marketing goals; creating a game plan for product sales, setting up financial operations; defining office logistics; and establishing scheduling procedures for clients.

Self-Assessment • •

The first phase in choosing an associate or partner is clarifying your reasons for wanting to share your business (or space) with another person. For instance, are you doing this because you want to or is it mainly stemming from financial considerations? Assess your temperament to determine if it's appropriate for you to have another person involved in your business. Think about how you want to share your space and how much control you need to exert: if you're uncomfortable when things aren't done in a specific manner, it may become difficult for you to share an office, let alone be in partnership.

If you decide to go ahead with the idea, you need to be clear about the desired relationship with your potential associate or partner. Do you want this person to play an active role in your business, or would you rather just have someone to share ideas and expenses? Do you want to bring someone into your business or join an already existing practice? It might be beneficial to affiliate with someone who does something totally different from you. On the other hand, you may prefer someone who does similar work as you.

Interviews • •

Memories fade. Avert problems by referring to a partnership document.

After you've clarified your reasons for wanting an associate and have envisioned their qualities, it's time to conduct interviews. This process is helpful whether you're thinking of joining a practice or bringing someone into yours. Your closest friends or colleagues may not be the wisest choices when looking for a business partner. Invest the time required to do this well; after all, this is someone you may be seeing every day. Share with each other your dreams, goals and concerns. Some of the questions to consider are: How long do you intend to stay in this location? What kind of work schedule do you prefer to keep? What type of atmosphere do you want? Who do you want as clients? Do you ultimately want additional associates or employees? Do you plan on incorporating other services or products?

Look for the commonalities and possible areas of conflict. Do your businesses complement each other? Are your fee structures similar? Also, get to know each other's communication style and see if your personalities are compatible. Everyone has their own personality and way of doing things, and these styles don't always mesh well in a business setting. For example, if you prefer a methodical approach to business and your partner tends to work best under pressure or in chaos—you may be in for a tempestuous association.

Roles, Goals and Expectations ● ●

After you decide to become associates, the next step is to delineate—in writing—your roles and expectations. List all of the things that are important to each of you in running your business.

In addition to writing your shared vision, goals, roles and expectations, create a dissolution (or buy-out) agreement. Who knows what the future holds? People's goals change or major life-altering circumstances happen. Make sure that all parties have a realistic means to ethically and amicably part ways. If you decide to become partners (and not just associates), I highly recommend you design a full business plan before the partnership is official. The process of developing your business plan compels you to evaluate your strengths and weaknesses, clarify your financial arrangements, delineate your roles, determine legal responsibilities and refine your business vision. Also, memories aren't always accurate; you can avoid many misunderstandings by referring to a written agreement.

Be certain to agree upon the image you wish to portray. Nothing is quite as frustrating as sharing space with others who don't hold similar visions or standards.

Legal Status ● ●

Most group practices are associations, not partnerships: the practitioners get together to share resources and expenses while keeping separate business identities. A partnership is two or more people contributing assets to a jointly-owned business and sharing in the profits or losses (although not necessarily equally). To be considered a partnership, you don't need to use the term "partner" or have a written partnership agreement. The operative phrase is "jointly owned."

In many states, if you're perceived to be a partnership, you could be held liable for something your associate does. Legalese aside, your reputation could be on the line if anyone else within your group does something unprofessional. Avoid any misconceptions about association status by posting a sign in the office reception area that states that each person in the office operates her business separately.

Finances ● ●

Financial obligations can be a major source of entanglement in an association. Usually one person is required to assume responsibility for each major account (e.g., rent, utilities and telephone). If you commingle too many funds, you are in essence creating a partnership.

Avoid misunderstandings by drawing up a contract that outlines each person's financial obligations, and how profits are to be distributed. Next, agree upon an operating budget and perform financial projections. You may want to involve a financial advisor in the planning process or simply have the advisor review any financial contracts or plans before finalizing them. Be cautious when jointly making major purchases, unless you are indeed partners.

9

Product Sales • •

Product sales are a great diversification method and profits from them can defray overhead expenses. The three biggest problems are choosing the product lines, determining who is responsible for overseeing sales, and calculating who gets what profit—particularly when a client sees more than one practitioner in the group setting. If your business is a partnership, the funds can be commingled. If you're part of an association, consider one of the following models for handling the logistics of product sales:

Option 1 —Individual Profit Centers • • •
- Designate a weekly or monthly order date. Combine practitioners' product order lists and place one order. Each practitioner pays for his portion of the order.
- Each practitioner receives requested product quantities and sells products separately.
- Each individual collects payment for product sales and retains the profit.

Option 2 —Distributed Profits • • •
- The group assigns one practitioner to manage product sales. Tasks include tracking inventory, stocking products, placing orders, handling payment through the manager's individual account (this assumes an office assistant handles payment processing tasks).
- The product manager is compensated for her time in managing product sales. Remaining profit is applied to lower shared overhead expenses (e.g., rent, linen service, telephone and marketing).

Marketing • •

Many marketing activities and expenses can be shared even when group practices are associations and not partnerships. Actually, this is one of the strongest benefits to being in a group practice. The combined energy, expertise and financial resources can provide diversity and afford you the opportunity to experiment with avenues that were previously unaffordable or infeasible.

Determine what percentage of marketing is handled jointly. Next, develop a joint marketing plan that defines goals, target dates and a budget. Before placing any long-term advertising, such as a Yellow Pages ad, create a payment agreement to cover the possibility of an associate leaving.

Interaction Levels • •

Some people get involved in a group practice merely to share expenses while others desire more contact and camaraderie. Although communications and time spent together vary, it's important to clarify your desired levels of interaction. It takes time, energy and concern to maintain decent relationships. Holding weekly or biweekly office meetings can be a good way to keep everyone up to date about business matters and talk about concerns or new ideas.

Office Logistics • •

Office logistics encompass the day-to-day activities in running a business, such as preparing the office for clients, stocking supplies, cleaning and coordinating repairs. Most people in group practices develop a task list, designate who is responsible for what tasks and agree upon weekly or monthly schedules.

Although few people thrill at the thought of writing a policy and procedure manual, it's an essential tool to smoothly operate a business. It simply documents how the group has agreed to run the business—what policies apply to what situations and how office procedures work. It doesn't have to be elaborate. It just needs to state the facts simply and clearly so everyone knows what to expect. Topics can run the gamut from ethics, to how to answer the phone to, what is considered to be a clean kitchen (e.g., dirty dishes belong in the dishwasher, not the sink). It can be helpful to all parties to clearly define what consequences apply when there is a serious or repeated violation of policy or procedures. This is especially important if you hire employees because establishing grounds for termination is essential from a legal standpoint.

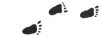

Chapter 12, Pages 225-233
for more information about developing policies and procedures.

Scheduling Clients • •

In most group practices, each individual is responsible for booking his own clients. This gets fuzzy when clients come in from shared marketing activities (particularly a Yellow Pages ad or website). You can avoid many misunderstandings and resentment by creating a new client scheduling policy. For instance, make a list of all the practitioners and place a check next to each one's name every time she gets a new client. In general, it's best to match the first caller with the first practitioner on the list and then proceed down the list. This isn't always possible when a client wants an appointment at a certain time (or desires a specific service) and the only person available is the one who received the last referral. But if you review the list, whoever answers the phone knows that practitioner B gets first choice of the next new client.

9

Figure 9.10

Success Tips for Group Practice

- Before interviewing potential business associates, clarify your reasons for entering into or developing a group practice.
- Meet with all group members before joining a group practice. This gives you valuable insight into whether the situation is a fit for you.
- If you're pursuing a partnership, make a list of the characteristics of your ideal partner. Highlight qualities that are absolutely essential.
- Develop a detailed agreement that defines roles and expectations.
- Include a section on image in your agreement. Cover items such as the way clients are greeted, practitioners' attire, physical layout of the office, funding for available beverages, music and noise level.
- Be prepared to do cash flow forecasting to budget, particularly if you will be receiving deferred insurance payments.
- Schedule time for a marketing review each week. Develop a checklist and timeline for ongoing marketing activities. Prior to your business launch, set up logistics for a gift certificate program and special introductory offer coupons.
- After you've located the best group practice situation, make plans to jointly develop a long-term business plan and a professional code of ethics. Document in writing the policies and procedures you and your associates agree upon. Distribute a policy and procedure manual to everyone who joins your business.
- Create a written telephone script for greeting callers, and find an existing educational resource that includes a guide to proper telephone etiquette.
- Make certain the types of therapy offered aren't in conflict. For example, a massage therapist who works with elderly clients and does a lot of quiet guided meditations would not co-exist well with a counselor who does Primal Scream Therapy (which can get very noisy).
- Make an effort to coordinate office decor to avoid a hodge-podge look. First impressions do count.
- Hold group meetings to discuss decorating plans for special occasions. Also, agree upon how expenses are handled for ongoing items, such as fresh flowers or other office decor.
- Schedule a group meeting to create an action plan for product sales, including goals and a budget.
- Include each practitioner's name on the office lease.
- If you work in a chiropractic or acupuncture clinic, you need a firm grasp of clinical terminology and protocol, as well as insurance charting.
- Define parameters for working with clients outside of the clinic.

Business Start-Up

10

• Where to Start •

As a new small business owner, you may be wondering where to start. You have a huge checklist of business start-up tasks and the energy, enthusiasm and inspiration to match. Because knowledge is power, it makes sense to start with knowing your market—your clients, colleagues and competition.

Many of life's failures are people who did not realize how close they were to success when they gave up.
— Thomas Edison

Scope Out the Competition •

Begin by exploring your career field. Find out the number of other businesses that are the same or similar to yours. Start by looking at listings and advertisements in the phone book, Internet and local newspapers. Spend some time browsing through industry trade journals, magazines and books related to your field. Attend professional association meetings, and subscribe to their newsletters. This gives you a good sense of the competitive landscape and an appreciation for effective and lackluster marketing.

Interview the owners of these businesses, ask them how they got started, the services they offer, what trends they see happening that will affect the success of this field, and then ask them for any advice. Most people like to talk about themselves, although some might not eagerly share this information. It helps if you can give them a name of someone who suggested that you contact them. If this isn't possible, find something about them that grabs your interest (check their website, brochure, card or phonebook listing). Start off by telling the practitioner what intrigues you about her practice and then ask her if she would be willing to share some insights with you.

Figure 10.1

> ### Questions to Ask When Interviewing Business Owners
>
> * How long have you been in practice?
> * What obstacles did you have to overcome?
> * What are some of the smartest decisions you made in terms of business success?
> * What are some poor decisions or mistakes that you made that I should avoid?
> * What are the keys to long-term success in this industry?
> * At what point in your career did you first feel successful?
> * How much has your business model changed now from when you first started?
> * What advice do you have for me about gaining the best results with a business support group?
> * If you could do it all over again, what would you do differently?
> * For those of you who are students: What would you suggest I do while in school to prepare me for being in business?

Chapter 15, Pages 327-329

for the details on analyzing your competition.

People with Insider Information •

After conducting an Information Interview, send a thank-you note to express your appreciation for that person's time and professional generosity.

Another way to gain valuable business perspectives is to meet with professionals who provide services or supplies to your segment of the wellness industry. They can often shed light on trends and potential trouble spots for a new business owner. Schedule several informational interviews with sales representatives, product suppliers, equipment manufacturers, bankers, accountants or consultants.

Research your potential markets. You may do an informal survey or hire a marketing consultant to do the research. Discuss the industry with other people who service your potential clients. Let's take athletes as a sample target market. The professions and companies that provide products and services to athletes include massage therapists, medical doctors, sports psychologists, chiropractors, trainers, sporting goods stores, nutritionists, equipment manufacturers and hypnotherapists. These people may give you a broader view than someone who does your specific type of work.

Chapter 15, Pages 339-349

for details on identifying Target Markets.

Determine the Business Feasibility •

Ascertain the economic capacity of the community to support your business. You may find you need to expand your target markets or diversify your practice to increase your business viability. This information gathering process is also crucial when expanding or revamping a current business. "It's never too late to start over" is a common saying, although one not normally associated with business. Yet you can start over, regardless of how long you've been in practice. Although it can be more difficult to make changes after you're established, it's often worth the time and energy.

Figure 10.2

Evaluate Your Business Potential

Gather Income Statistics, Client Usage and Trends

- U.S. Department of Labor
- Professional Associations
- Practitioners in Your Field
- Trade Journals
- State and Local Licensing Agencies
- Online Resources

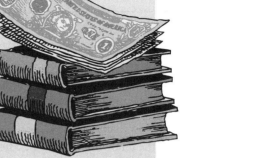

Research Potential Markets

- People most likely to utilize your services
- People or conditions you want to work with

Estimate Supply and Demand

- Calculate the numbers of potential clients
- Find out the average number of people receiving your type of work
- Determine the average number of sessions per client
- Ascertain the number of practitioners in your field in your city
- Project the average number of clients seen by current practitioners
- Divide the potential clients by the number of practitioners

2002 National Health
Interview Survey
nccam.nih.gov/news/
report.pdf

U.S. Department of Labor,
Bureau of Labor Statistics
www.bls.gov/oco

Supply and Demand ● ●

The old economics cliché states that business success is based upon supply and demand: find the demand then supply what's needed. This information is crucial for determining where you choose to practice and whom you target as clients. It is important to look at the general demand for wellness care in your city and the specific need for your particular services.

Figure 10.3

Supply and Demand Example

- Population: 100,000
- Average number of people receiving your type of work: 15%
- Average number of treatments per year that a client receives: 10
- Current practitioners in your field: 100
- 100,000 x 15% = 15,000 people receiving your type of work
- 15,000 x 10 = 150,000 sessions per year
- 150,000 ÷ 100 = 1,500 sessions per practitioner per year
- 1,500 ÷ 48 weeks per year = 31.25 sessions per week

In this example, it's likely that this city can support a few additional practitioners.

10

Assess Supply and Demand

Determine the supply and demand for your services in the city you wish to practice. Calculate how many additional practitioners the city can easily accommodate.

Self-Assessment

Now that you have a good picture of the business landscape, take a few minutes to answer the following questions. They will help you realistically assess your plans and pinpoint any actions needed to move you closer to your ideal practice.

Self-Exploration Questionnaire

- How well does your educational and career experience fit this industry?
- How soon will you need advanced training to compete effectively and grow your business?
- Have you interviewed colleagues and industry experts?
- Do you feel comfortable with the "business" aspects?
- Does this business provide sufficient opportunities?
- Are you aware of industry trends and regulations?
- Have you assessed your strengths and challenges?
- Do you have adequate financial resources to start your business?
- Is the time commitment compatible with the rest of your life?
- Are your friends and family supportive?
- Can you identify at least two target markets that will eagerly embrace your practice?
- Have you identified what makes your business unique and gives you a competitive edge?
- Do you have the personality and aptitude to market your services?
- Do you have a support system of colleagues and advisors?

Chapter 15, Page 337

for information on the Differential Advantage.

• Start-Up Financing •

The costs of starting up and running a business can be daunting, which is why many people opt to work for others. According to the Small Business Administration (SBA), the median start-up costs for a solo business owner to just open the door is $6,000. The actual start-up costs depend on the scope of the business, the location and build-out costs, and the requisite equipment. Many wellness practices are fairly easy to set up, particularly since the initial costs tend to be minimal. In many instances, you can operate out of your home, rent space by the hour or provide on-site work.

People often build their private practices slowly while working for another company. This is an acceptable route to take as long as you develop an action plan for attracting clients and actively market your practice. Otherwise you may find yourself with a permanent, part-time practice.

When determining start-up costs, include operating and personal living expenses for at least six months. Decide whether the costs are essential or optional. A realistic start-up budget should only include items that are necessary to start the business. Research similar businesses and seek advice from a realtor, accountant and lawyer. Also contact your local SBA, and SCORE office (Service Corps Of Retired Executives).

Initial Expenses: Opening a business checking account; telephone installation; equipment; first and last month's rent and security deposit; business cards, stationery, brochures, logo design; opening promotion package (e.g., ads, direct mailers); decorations; office supplies; furniture; music system and CDs.

Annual Expenses: Property insurance; business license; permits; liability insurance; professional association membership; legal and accounting fees.

Common Monthly Expenses: Rent; utilities; telephone; bank fees; supplies; networking club dues; education; promotion; Internet access; postage; repair and maintenance; business travel; inventory; business loan payments.

Financing your business (whether for start-up or expansion) can be frustrating. Even though a lot of venture capital is available, it's extremely difficult to procure investment money for a service business. Be extremely wary of any company that guarantees (for an up-front fee) to find you venture capital. There are a lot of scam operations. To find reputable sources of funding, check out the resource guides at your local SBA office.

A bank may be willing to give you a loan; the amount is usually based upon your assets. Applying for a loan (or venture investment) takes a lot of work: research, correspondence, proposals, refining your business plan—including financial statements and cash flow forecasts (they want to see numbers) and putting together an impressive presentation.

The most valuable of all capital is that invested in human beings.
— Alfred Marshall

Be creative in obtaining services and supplies. Consider bartering and buying previously owned products. Your creativity, talent and persistence are the qualities that help balance out the shortage of start-up resources.

10

Chapter 14, Page 295
for specific information on business costs.

Most small business owners finance their company with money from personal savings or through loans from friends and relatives. If you decide to borrow money from friends or family, treat them with the same consideration that you would give to a formal lending institution. Make an official presentation and submit a loan proposal and a business plan. Clearly delineate the terms of the loan and the repayment schedule. If you follow these guidlines and set your boundaries, it can be a rewarding experience—one in which everyone benefits personally and financially.

Figure 10.4

Options for Financing a Practice

Personal Savings	Be conservative in your spending so you can build a start-up nest egg.
Personal Loans	If you own your home, you could take out a second mortgage or an equity loan. Some people use their credit cards (not usually advisable due to high interest rates). Another option is to cash a retirement account.
Student Loans	If allowable, maximize the amount of your student loans and put the extra into savings.
Family & Friends Loans	Avoid potential discomfort and resentment by designing a loan contract that clearly delineates the terms and repayment schedule.
Private Investor Loans	Most private investors want to make a healthy return either in dollars or a percentage of the business. This route requires research, correspondence, proposals and a refined business plan.
Bank Loans	The amount loaned is usually based upon your assets, and banks require a complete business plan.
SBA Loans	The SBA offers several types of funding from guaranteeing up to 85 percent of a commercial bank loan to directly loaning money.
Grants	Many organizations provide grants to people who fall within the parameters of special interest groups, either as the business owner or the market you plan to serve. At a minimum, this route requires research and proposals.
Partnerships	This affiliation can vary from a "silent" partner (more of an investor) to someone who works alongside you to build your business.
Community Development Corporation (CDC) Investors	Local organizations that partner with government, business owners and community leaders to provide economic assistance (e.g., loans, grants, consulting, subsidized office spare). This is usually geared toward specific populations or the enhancement of a particular area of the city.

• Buying a Practice •

The idea of buying an existing practice may seem very appealing. After all, you avoid the process entailed in building a strong business foundation. Although it may be easier and faster to buy an established practice, you also inherit the previous owner's problems, and there is no guarantee the clients will stay on with you.

Figure 10.5

Steps to Buying a Practice

- Evaluate your reasons for buying.
- Determine the "fit."
- Conduct a preliminary evaluation.
- Analyze documentation.
- Evaluate the business premises.
- Clarify legal agreements.
- Open negotiations.
- Offer a letter of intent.
- Purchase the business.
- Begin the transition stage.

Evaluate Your Reasons For Buying •

Chapter 14, Pages 316-318

for tips on how to price a business.

There are many advantages and disadvantages to buying an existing practice. Before you jump into a purchase, do the following exercise to assess your reasons for taking this route.

Self-Assessment

Ask yourself the following questions:

- Why do I want to buy an existing business?
- What are the potential risks versus the perceived benefits?
- What liabilities will I incur (e.g., lease, unclaimed gift certificates, payroll)?
- What conditions need to be present to make it worthwhile?
- Does the business generate enough money to meet my financial goals and loan repayment?
- Are the practice's image and philosophy compatible with mine?
- Why might buying this practice be inappropriate?
- Would it be more cost-effective to set up my own practice?
- What are my other options?

10

All businesses aren't created equally. Clarify exactly what you're buying. Determine if you're purchasing one or more of the following: rights to use a well-known business name; a client list; established contracts; goodwill and reputation; an office location; equipment.

The most common instance of a wellness provider buying another practice is when that practitioner is just starting out, or moving to a new location. An established practitioner might purchase a practice if she is interested in expanding her current target markets or wants to branch into another area.

Practice Sale Scenario

A seller is asking for $15,000 for her practice. She has been in business for five years, and, during that time, her clientele has steadily increased. She sees an average of 15 clients per week and charges $50 per session. Her office is in a small professional building. Her monthly operating expenses run approximately $1,000. She is making a major life change and has decided to move to a tropical island. She is including her equipment and supplies as part of the package.

If the assets are items you want and you could retain the majority of her clients, this would be a reasonable price. You can minimize your risks by requiring that, in addition to the hard assets, the remainder of the selling price be based on the actual number of clients who stay with the business. Two examples are: making payments only if the business meets certain client retention requirements (e.g., at least 50 percent of the clients stay); or you only have to pay the seller a set percentage of the fees received from the current clientele (e.g., 40 percent of fees collected until the original loan is repaid).

Determine the Fit •

When meeting with a potential seller, attempt to discover the true reason for the sale. This could dramatically influence your decision. For instance, if the seller is moving to another state or retiring, that's one thing; but if the move is within 30 miles, you may not be buying anything, because the majority of the clients may still continue to see the practitioner at the new location.

The seller may not be versed in the protocol for selling a business. Usually, sellers view their practices in terms of the work they've invested in making it successful. It may not be set up for someone to easily take over. It is rare to just step in and retain all the clients. They may not like you and vice versa. More than anything else, assess the "fit" you would have with the business. Your chances for success are much greater if your knowledge, training, personality, modalities and style are similar to that of the seller. One way to determine this is by receiving a session from the seller. Ask to be treated as though you were a typical new client. Although the seller will most likely be on her best behavior, this experience gives you insight into her style, as well as what the current clients are accustomed to receiving. If the company's policies and procedures don't suit you, or the types of treatments offered are outside your desired scope of practice, it most likely isn't in your best interest to buy the practice.

Conduct a Preliminary Evaluation ●

Many factors come into play in judging the viability of a business. The seller should have a fact sheet that encompasses the company history, mission statement, business description (including the number of clients, the services offered, the equipment and products used, location description, fee structure, client profile, position statement, competition analysis and differential advantage), assets, financial history, reason for sale and pricing terms.

Obtain this fact sheet and samples of promotional materials, before making an offer. Ask to view the current appointment book. Check to see how many appointments are scheduled each week and how far in advance the practitioner is booked. After reviewing these materials and receiving a session, you're in a better position to decide whether to make an offer.

Analyze Documentation ● ●

When you make a written offer, be sure to state that it's contingent upon verification of the detailed documentation. This documentation should include the following: a detailed business description; a copy of the lease; names of all owners, associates, and staff members; profit and loss statements for the past three years; tax returns for the past three years; copies of current contracts; a listing of accounts payable and receivable; a list of fixtures, equipment and inventory with their replacement value noted; and a portfolio of promotional materials about the company and owner.

Evaluate the Business Premises ●

One of the most beneficial aspects of buying a practice can be obtaining a lease on a "prime" location. Sometimes this is more important than the actual number of clients the current owner has. Let's say a massage therapist has a concession in a very busy, upscale gym, but this therapist hasn't been marketing his practice very well. If you're willing to invest the time in marketing, you could probably do quite well, and it would be worth a reasonable selling price. But, do the proper research before you allow a location to inflate the selling price of a business.

First, verify the building is zoned for your particular profession. Don't assume that because someone is currently running the same type of business in that location, it's therefore legal. Zoning may have changed or the current business might have somehow slipped through without anyone noticing (yet).

Next, find out if the current lease can be subleased or assigned, or if a new lease needs to be negotiated. Be sure to verify the particulars about the lease. Determining the worth of a lease during the negotiations of a selling price is a rather subjective process. After researching the property, weigh your findings with the perceived importance of the space to the current clients.

10

Clarify Legal Agreements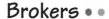

Another positive consideration is whether the business has outside contracts to provide ongoing wellness services to a business or seasonal work for conferences.

Open Negotiations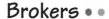

Deciding on a fair price for a practice is difficult at best. The seller sets what he feels is a realistic price. You must do the math. Calculate how much time, energy and money it would cost you to build your practice to the same point as the seller's, remembering that there is no guarantee the current clients will stay with you.

Most buyers take out loans (from friends, a bank or the seller) to finance the purchase of a business. When a service business is sold, the seller often becomes the loan holder.

International Business Brokers Association

www.ibba.org

Institute of Certified Business Counselors

www.icb-c.org

Brokers • •

Many brokers work on either an hourly consultation rate or a flat transaction fee. A qualified broker knows what questions to ask and can identify potential problems. You can locate a broker through the resources listed here or in your local telephone book. In your initial interview, ask if the broker has ever negotiated a sale for the type of practice you desire (or a similar type of sale). The most important factor is that the two of you communicate well with each other. Also have your accountant interview a potential broker. Your accountant already knows your business, has your best interests at heart and can determine if the broker is qualified. After the sales contract has been negotiated, have an attorney review it before you sign.

Final Stages •

Chapter 14, Pages 312-320

for information on how to sell a practice.

The final two stages are the completion of the purchase and the transition time after the sale. The ideal situation would be to work as an associate for several months before actually purchasing the business. This way the current clients would get to know you, and you could assess whether you like working in that environment, particularly if an office space or working with other practitioners is part of the sales agreement. In addition, this would give you an opportunity to discover little nuances of the business and become familiar with the logistics of running the business. It is also guaranteed to make the actual transition much smoother.

As a buyer, it's wise to understand the process a seller goes through, so please refer to the section on selling a practice. Buying an existing practice is very risky, yet the potential benefits can be rewarding. Keep in mind that even if the practice is a strong one, you need to continue nurturing it through marketing and an active client retention program.

• Legal Status •

The most common legal entity choices for your practice include sole proprietorship, partnership, corporation and Limited Liability Company (LLC). The majority of new businesses open as sole proprietorships, mainly because this is the simplest, fastest and least expensive structure. The decision to opt for a different structure is usually based on tax and liability considerations. Consult with an accountant or tax attorney, because each person's situation and needs are unique, tax laws frequently change, and requirements vary by locale. This section describes types of business structures and some of the advantages and disadvantages.

Consult with appropriate advisors before deciding which structure best suits your needs.

Sole Proprietorship •

If you don't incorporate, create a partnership or form an LLC, your business is automatically considered a sole proprietorship. The Internal Revenue Service (IRS) usually allows a married couple to operate as a sole proprietorship. In all other cases in which two or more people co-own, a business they must choose an entity other than sole proprietorship.

The major disadvantages of sole proprietorship are having to be responsible for all business aspects, relative difficulty in obtaining financing, and unlimited liability. All business debts and liabilities are the personal responsibility of the owner. Damages from lawsuits brought against the business can be taken from your personal assets.

Success seems to be largely a matter of hanging on after others have let go.
— William Feather

The main advantages of sole proprietorship are the ease of formation (minimal governmental regulation on how the business is operated), possession of profits, control of all decisions and relatively simple financial record keeping.

The type of business license required for a sole proprietor who is a wellness provider varies from state to state. You may even need more than one license.

From a legal standpoint, as a sole proprietor, you and your business are one entity. You can't be treated as an employee of the business. You may withdraw money from your business, but it isn't considered a wage and can't be deducted as a business expense. Although you don't pay payroll taxes on "draw," you pay self-employment taxes and income taxes. The business doesn't file income tax returns or pay income taxes. In the United States, you file a Schedule C with your 1040 form and pay personal income taxes on the profits.

10

Partnerships ✻

Having an associate or partner can be quite beneficial. It can help ease the loneliness of being self-employed, allow you to take time off, and add diversity of services and approaches. It can also infuse capital, decrease overhead expenses, enable you to share the activities involved in running a business, and provide you with another person with whom you can brainstorm. It could also be a nightmare. A written partnership agreement is crucial.

A partnership is when two or more people contribute assets to carry on a jointly-owned business and share in the profits or losses. To be considered a partnership, you do not have to use the term "partners" or have a written partnership agreement or equally share ownership. The operative phrase is "jointly-owned."

A partnership is similar to a sole proprietorship in that governmental regulation is still fairly minimal. The financial recordkeeping is a bit more involved, although it's insignificant compared to a corporation. You must obtain a federal identification number (contact the IRS and request Form SS-4). Partnerships file a Schedule K-1 (Form 1065, partnership informational tax return), but the partnership itself pays no taxes. Each partner submits a copy of the K-1 to report his share of profits or losses on his individual tax return (Form 1040).

You can be held personally responsible for debts and legal obligations incurred by the partnership, even for those made without your knowledge or consent. Incorporation, or forming a Limited Liability Company (LLC), is the best way to protect yourself against this kind of liability.

Corporations ✻

The major categories of business corporations are C Corporations, S Corporations and Professional Corporations. The type of business you operate and your tax requirements determine which structure is the best for you. Many people incorporate because they think it gives them an air of legitimacy—without considering all the legal implications.

A corporation provides a business entity that is separate from the owner as an individual. That distinction assists in creating clear boundaries between your work and the rest of your life—an important consideration—since wellness practitioners have a tendency to become so enmeshed in their work that it becomes difficult to "switch off." Owners who work in an incorporated business are considered employees and are paid as such.

My relationship to my work dramatically shifted when I incorporated my business: I became more detached (which is good); the ups and downs of business are a bit easier to take; and I pay myself regularly. Now there is Cherie, the person, and Sohnen-Moe Associates, Inc., a company which I happen to own. Of course, I always knew there was a difference between me and my company, but I hadn't really experienced the separation on an emotional level.

A corporation tends to be the most costly legal structure to form and dissolve in terms of finances and time. There are required filings with the IRS, as well as with the state in which the corporation is formed. Though there are no federal fees involved, the state may require an initial filing fee and annual report filing fees.

Contact your state Corporation Commission or Secretary of State to ascertain the specific requirements and fees for incorporation. The minimal components of the incorporation process are:

- Adopting and filing Articles of Incorporation
- Developing corporate Bylaws
- Holding the first board of directors and shareholders meeting and preparing meeting minutes
- Issuing stock certificates
- Filing for an IRS Employer Identification Number (EIN, Form SS-4)
- Filing Subchapter S status if so adopted within 75 days of incorporating or start of business (IRS Form 2553 which requires your new EIN)
- Setting up your corporate book that contains all corporate documents

There are myriad details involved in each step. The incorporation process varies from state to state according to each state's regulations, and so do the requirements for the content of your bylaws. Be sure your bylaws include the approval of telephonic meetings for shareholders and directors. This saves time and helps to minimize travel expenses.

The general minimal requirements for maintaining a corporation are conducting annual meetings and filing the minutes in your corporate book, as well as filing required documentation with the state on an annual basis. In the event your corporate status is questioned by the IRS or the state, the first thing they do is inspect your corporate book to make sure you've followed all the requirements. If you haven't, your status as a corporation can be nullified, which could result in severe tax consequences. Keeping your corporate book up to date is essential. Even though there are do-it-yourself incorporation kits, it's strongly recommended that you consult with an accountant and an attorney.

One of the primary motivations for incorporating is to limit liability. If your business is a sole proprietorship, you could lose your personal assets (e.g., your home or car) if your business is sued. Wellness practitioners in partnerships often incorporate to shield individual owners from possible losses and lawsuits stemming from actions (e.g., a malpractice suit) of the other partners. In most cases, incorporation protects your personal assets from being taken by creditors; but it doesn't shelter you from lawsuits.

Other popular reasons for incorporating include the ease in which the business can be transferred, the ability to raise capital by selling shares of stock, potential tax advantages, and fringe benefits, such as health and life insurance premiums, tuition reimbursement and tax-sheltered retirement plans, which can be deducted partially (and often fully!) as business expenses.

IRS Publication 542
www.irs.gov/publications
Incorporation Services
www.corporate.com
www.mynewcompany.com

10

C Corporations • •

C Corporations are subject to a corporate income tax on the net business profits. Although there is the potential for double taxation (the corporation as well as an individual), most small business owners use all the profits as tax-deductible salaries and fringe benefits, or they retain money to expand the business. Income can be divided between paying money to shareholders (salaries and dividends) and keeping the rest of the profits in the business. This process is called income-splitting. The retained earnings are taxed at the initial rate of 15 percent, which is usually lower than the individual income tax rates of the owners.

C Corporations must file annual returns (Form 1120) by the 15th day of the third month after the close of their fiscal year and make quarterly estimated tax payments.

S Corporations • •

S Corporations are taxed like partnerships but retain the liability protection of C Corporations. They have the same basic structure as C Corporations and file corporate tax returns, but the corporation doesn't pay federal income tax, as the profits are passed on to the owners who pay the taxes at their individual rates. Losses are treated in the same manner.

A primary tax advantage of an S Corporation is reducing the potential for double taxation. Another financial consideration is that start-up businesses often show a loss in the first year or two. Given those circumstances, an S Corporation might be the most appropriate choice, because it allows the owners/shareholders to directly declare business losses on their individual tax returns.

One of the prime eligibility requirements for S Corporations is that the number of stockholders be 75 or less. To form an S Corporation, fill out IRS Form 2553 (Election by a Small Business Corporation) within 75 days after incorporating. S Corporations must file annual returns (Form 1120-S).

Personal Service Corporations (PSCs) • •

Wellness providers, as well as other service professionals (e.g., accountants, attorneys, engineers, business consultants and performance artists), often opt for this status. In some states, these types of service providers are required to choose this incorporation designation. The benefits include the separation of the owners from the business entity (which also makes it easier to carry on the business should one shareholder withdraw), fringe benefits similar to those under C Corporations, and limited liability protection. If you're a sole business owner, a PSC might not be advantageous. This designation is more common with group practices, particularly given that most states require all owners of a PSC to be licensed to render the same type of service.

Professional corporations lost their popularity in the late 1980s when tax laws changed. Now they're taxed at a higher rate than other corporations, and income-splitting is not allowed. Limited Liability Companies are preferred.

Limited Liability Companies ● ●

A Limited Liability Company (LLC) is a hybrid of a partnership and a corporation. Most states require a minimum of two owners (they can be spouses) and these owners are generally called members (membership title and status changes depending on the type of LLC chosen).

LLCs offer many of the benefits as S Corporations with fewer drawbacks. This designation gives the individual owners a separate entity from the actual business and provides them with a limited personal liability shield. The profits from an LLC flow through to the owners (as in a sole proprietorship or partnership).

The paperwork isn't as complicated as with other types of corporations. You must file Articles of a Limited Liability Company, develop an Organizational Agreement, and file for an IRS Employee Identification Number. There may not be any requirement for annual meetings or additional filings with the state. Since regulations vary, contact your Corporation Commission or Secretary of State. Currently, LLCs file an IRS Form 1065, and each member files a Form K-1 at the end of each year. Then, each member reports her share of the profits or losses on her individual income tax return.

● Business Name ●

Choosing an appropriate name for your business takes some contemplation. Most wellness practitioners are their business and thus need not go further. If you choose this route, I recommend that you also include a title, such as Tracy Jones, D.C.; Steve Smith, L.M.T.; or Terry Richards, Licensed Esthetician.

You may want a separate business identity, particularly if you have a group practice. If so, choose your name carefully and avoid anything gimmicky. Select a name that conveys the essence of your business in a manner that inspires people to find out more about your services. Names such as Riverside Wellness Clinic are okay, but they lack oomph. One of the best names for a massage centers is The Right Touch (located in Tucson). The Relaxation Center, Just Feet, Transformations Day Spa, and The Athletic Edge are examples of names that convey a company's mission or identify target markets.

When you've selected a potential company name, say the name out loud several times to be sure it's easy to pronounce and understand. Test the name out on your friends and potential clients. Verify that your business name doesn't mean something derogatory in another language.

Naming a business can be an arduous process. In two decades, I still haven't found a name that encompasses the many facets of my business. If I decide to change my company's name, the transition will be a bit bumpy because Sohnen-Moe Associates is well known (even though it's extremely difficult to understand over the phone).

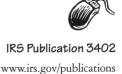

IRS Publication 3402
www.irs.gov/publications

Internet Trademark Search Companies:
www.thomson-thomson.com
www.corsearch.com

U.S. Trademark Office
www.uspto.gov/main/ trademarks.htm

10

Trademark: How to Name a Business & Product
by K. McGrath and S. Elias

Check the Trademark Electronic Search System to see if your desired name already is internationally trademarked. www.tess2.uspto.gov/

If you choose a business name other than your own, request a name search with the Corporation Commission or Secretary of State. They usually do this by phone and let you know if the name is available for use. Regulations and fees vary, as do forms. In some states, there is a difference between a "trade name" and a "trademark." Each has its own form and fees. With the trade name, you're registering the actual name of your company (e.g., Hands That Heal). A trademark is the registration of your logo and its description, which can be a design or set of words. If you plan to use a company name, specific word(s) or a logo in interstate commerce, consider obtaining a federal trademark. This is a somewhat complex process which needs to be carefully done. The fees as of 2007 are $325 per mark per classification. The fee is nonrefundable regardless of the results.

Whenever your business name is different from your personal name, most states require that you publish a DBA ("Doing Business As"), also referred to as a Fictitious Name Certificate, in the classified section of at least one newspaper in the county where you operate. Contact your county clerk for forms and procedures.

EIN Application

www.irs.gov/businesses/ small/article/ 0,,id=98350,00.html

As a sole proprietor wellness provider, you don't need an employer identification number (EIN) unless you have employees or a Keogh plan. (See IRS Publication 583 for specifics.) Otherwise, you can use your Social Security number. To get an EIN, file form SS-4 with your local IRS. You can complete the application online, mail or fax the completed and signed form. Contact the IRS at 800-829-4933, or go online to get the fax number for your region.

❋ Location, Location, Location ❋

You spend a lot of time in your office, so it's critical to choose a location that you like and that also attracts clients, fits your business image, accommodates your business needs in terms of size and layout (and potential expansion), is properly zoned and is priced within your budget.

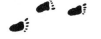

Chapter 14, Page 293

for details on home office tax deductions.

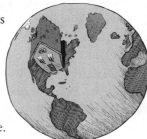

A large number of practitioners business site. Even those with see some clients at home. A advantages: it's cheaper to run you can take a tax deduction; between sessions; you can family; and there's no commute. have home offices as their main commercial office space still home office yields many than a commercial office; you can do household tasks spend more time with your

The flip side is that some people are not productive at home. They are too easily distracted and lack discipline. Other problems arise from family members not respecting their boundaries. Plus zoning restrictions often restrict or prohibit home businesses. Commercial office space conveys an image of professionalism that is rarely found in a home office, no matter how nice it is. Although this perception is changing as more people in diverse professions are working at home.

Most people want their offices close to home, yet that choice can be disadvantageous. The most important questions to ask are, "Will your clients want to come here?" and "Is there convenient parking?" The building in which your office is located impacts the atmosphere you wish to create. Your room (or office suite) doesn't exist independently of its surroundings. Your clients are affected by the totality, including the lobby, restroom facilities, the parking area and even the building itself.

Most practitioners don't generally have a large walk-in clientele—although locating a business in a high-traffic area can provide exposure. They tend to choose office buildings where the tenants are wellness practitioners or other service providers.

Office prices vary greatly depending on the actual location and the local economics. Check out the going rates on other comparable office space. "Comparable" is the key word. Read the fine print. The quoted price might not include such things as utilities, parking, leasehold improvements (lighting, decorations and structural changes to the floors and walls), maintenance and signage.

Make sure the office space is right for you before signing a lease. Research the office's historical information: find out why the space is vacant; ascertain the number of tenants who have held the space in the past 10 years; and get a listing of other current tenants, including their types of businesses, office hours and schedule of lease expiration dates. Visit the area at different times of the day and night to get a sense of the traffic flow. Ask the landlord or leasing agent for a copy of the operating rules and regulations to ensure compatibility with your practice. Determine if the building is properly zoned for your type of work.

Inspect the physical structure; make sure the roof is sound, the heating and cooling system is in good condition, and the building is secure (e.g., appropriate exterior lighting, stable stairs, lockable lobby door). Check with building and fire inspectors to see if the space has been cited.

The last step before finalizing a lease agreement is to review all legal documents with an attorney. The relatively few dollars spent with counsel can save you thousands later on should disputes arise.

Safety Note:
If you work at night, make sure other tenants keep evening office hours.

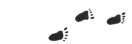

Chapter 13, Pages 280-284
for information on relocating your practice.

Zoning: Your Rights & Responsibilities

Now that you've found an excellent site, can you practice there? Zoning ordinances can be a potential source of frustration and financial cost. You must know the local zoning requirements before opening up a business, buying an existing practice or even remodeling your current office space. Wellness providers are often required to obtain several types of licenses and permits. It can be difficult to discover the requirements, because each locale has different zoning laws, and it isn't always clear which departments issue the various permits.

The two main purposes for licenses and permits are raising revenue and protecting the health and safety of the public. Zoning ordinances essentially divide an area into sections in which various activities and businesses are allowed or prohibited. The four major types of zoning are residential, commercial, industrial and agricultural. Within these categories are subsections which define the types of allowable activities. For example, a commercial area might be zoned for professional businesses only, retail, a combination of professional and retail, light industry or major manufacturing. Some residential areas allow certain types of businesses (mainly professionals) but not others. The level of enforcement varies widely. Some areas have negligible standards of operation and others are strict. Often it becomes important only if someone complains.

In some cities you're required to meet certain codes before you open your business (e.g., building, health and safety). Health practice items commonly regulated in zoning ordinances are off-street parking, signage, wheelchair accessibility, shower facilities and types of business activities. For example, hydrotherapy is an area in which many practitioners encounter restrictions. A touch therapist in the Southwest was told that unless his office had a shower he could not do light steam treatments—even though he was using professional equipment. Before investing money in adjunct equipment, make certain that the zoning regulations allow its use. If the zoning doesn't, do your best to get a variance (see below).

Keep in mind that ordinances are amended frequently, and just because a similar business is in operation, doesn't mean that yours will be allowed. The other business could have been in place before a zoning change was made, and, as such, is allowed to stay in operation. But any new business or one that changes hands would have to meet the new requirements. Consider this case in point.

Warning!

Get your information in writing. It isn't unusual for two different people in the same office to give conflicting information.

Zoning Scenario

Susan Smith, L.Ac., decides to open an office in a well-established professional building. The tenants are a mixture of accountants, attorneys, counselors and a reflexologist. The office she wants formerly belonged to a massage therapist. She assumes that she won't encounter any problems since the businesses are similar and a wellness practitioner previously rented the office. She proceeds to sign a lease and decorate the office. Within a month Susan opens the doors, only to be served with a cease-and-desist order. She wonders how this could possibly happen.

If she had researched the zoning ordinances, she would have discovered that two years ago, the regulations had changed. Since the previous therapist had already been there before the new regulations, he did not have to comply with the changes. But the moment Susan applied for an occupation license, it set off a chain of events that resulted in the zoning board discovering that she did not make the necessary changes to legally operate an acupuncture practice in that building. Any time you apply for a business permit, license or building permit, it tags your business for scrutiny.

Talk with the licensing bureau to find out which ordinances pertain to your practice. The staff should provide a list of the types of permits you need—or at least the names of appropriate contacts. Next, talk with people at city or county hall. Then meet with the planning department and the health department. If you experience any difficulties in obtaining the necessary information, go to the library, the office of economic development or the state office of industrial development.

Figure 10.6

Office Leasing Checklist

Logistics
❑ Is the building in an area that is easily accessible to your target markets?

❑ Is there adequate parking, storage and space for signs?

❑ Are the other businesses in the building compatible with your practice?

❑ Do other allied professionals work nearby?

❑ Will your clients feel comfortable transitioning from your office to the outside—or will it be culture shock?

Ambiance
❑ Does the location and the building itself fit your image?

❑ Are the other businesses in the building compatible with your practice?

❑ Is the noise level suitable? (It is difficult to mask the sounds and vibrations if an aerobics class is in the adjacent room or if a band rehearses next door.)

Comfort & Safety
❑ Is the building in a safe neighborhood?

❑ Is the building accessible to the physically challenged?

❑ Does the space provide privacy and security?

❑ Are the utilities sufficient (e.g., do the air conditioning and heating units have adequate capacity)?

❑ Do you have direct access to the temperature controls?

Remodeling & Improvements
❑ Can you alter the layout?

❑ Do the premises need major improvements or remodeling in order to be appropriate for your practice?

❑ Once you've furnished and organized the space, will it blend in with the style and decor of the rest of the building?

❑ Does the premises provide space to expand your business?

Business Terms
❑ What are the terms of the lease?

❑ Who is responsible for the repairs and maintenance of the premises?

❑ Who is responsible for upkeep or possible replacement of major items, such as the roof or air conditioning unit?

❑ What type of insurance coverage is provided?

❑ Who pays the utilities, taxes and insurance?

❑ What are the sales options or renewal provisions?

❑ By what formula are lease increases determined?

❑ Can you sublease, and, if so, are the terms the same as the original lease?

Home Office Regulations • •

Home office requirements are often more stringent than those for commercial office space. Check your deed covenants for any specific limitations. Residential offices are often restricted to the amount of vehicular traffic generated, parking, the numbers of clients allowed in the home at any one time, signage, hours of operation, the percentage of floor space devoted to business and storage facilities. Many permits require a separate office entrance with an attached bathroom. In some locations, home businesses are not allowed to have employees or sell products.

Now that more than 44 percent of American households have members who work at least part time in their homes, city officials are beginning to ease up on home office restrictions.

Still, it's risky to open a practice in a location where zoning is questionable. If possible, get the zoning changed before it's a necessity. If you operate a home business, you may opt to take a "let's wait and see attitude" and not worry about the zoning ordinances. This can put you in a precarious position, particularly if you're investing a lot of money in remodeling your home office.

Variances • •

Home Office Bill of Rights
www.businessmastery.us/
home-rights.php

If you're found in violation of a zoning ordinance, you're sent a notice ordering you to cease your business. You must file an appeal immediately or cease operations, because every day you continue to operate can be considered a separate violation. Remember that a decision from a zoning official isn't necessarily written in stone. You can often appeal that decision, get a conditional use permit or even obtain a zoning variance.

When meeting with any official, it's best to have garnered support from adjacent business owners, your neighbors (for home offices) and other members of the community. (This is an example of why it's important to be involved in your chamber of commerce, business networking organizations and local trade associations.)

If you need to alter the current zoning requirements to legally run your business, begin by meeting with city officials to ask for a zoning variance or "special exemption" permit. This requires the cooperation of neighbors or nearby businesses. Get letters or have them sign a petition that says they support your business use. If your business is already established, bring photographs that illustrate the scope of your business.

If this doesn't work, take your request to the zoning board. It is very helpful if you can get your neighbors or adjoining business owners to go with you and speak on your behalf. The next step would be appealing to the city council. If all else fails, you can take your case to court.

Wellness providers are often required to meet very stringent conditions founded upon antiquated regulations. I recommend that practitioners in each city get together and decide what requirements they feel are reasonable and submit them to the zoning board. Start a lobbying campaign now. Create a structure that you want—not one that's dictated by officials who may not understand your profession.

Office Design

The major elements involved in office design are ambiance, professionalism, visual stimuli, sensations (scent, touch and sound) and layout. Make this a space that is mutually healing to yourself and others. The basic tenet is: Appeal to the majority of your clients while being inoffensive to all. The main sources of offense are forcing your personal or professional beliefs on others and invading people's sense of smell, sight, sound and touch. Oftentimes people are affronted by things we don't even consider as potential problems.

For instance, you may hold strong spiritual or religious beliefs that are not shared by everyone. Most people would be fine with seeing one or two symbols in your office, but would probably feel ill at ease if they walked into a room filled with icons and artifacts. Your clients are much more comfortable if your office space is client-centered. In other words, create a space that's comfortable for them. This might not be your personal favorite decor; be sure to find some way to balance both your clients' needs and yours—after all, you're there day in and day out.

The first thing to do is review your client base and identify your major target markets. Next consider what would be an ideal space for them. You can also survey your clients and representatives of future target markets for direct feedback. After you've completed your research, the next stage is the actual creation of the session room. If you find the office atmosphere so abrades your natural tendencies, perhaps you should change your target market.

Your office design may need to be developed in stages. Begin by identifying the "must have" items and elements and include them as soon as possible. You don't have to own top-of-the-line equipment. Bigger, brighter, shinier isn't always better. Just make certain you have appropriate items in good condition for your specific target markets.

Consider hiring a feng shui consultant to enhance the energy flow and to create an overall sense of well-being throughout the office. Feng shui is the ancient Chinese art of creating harmonious environments. Although methods and schools of teaching vary, all are based on improving the flow of "chi" or life-force energy and aligning harmoniously with nature. Simply put, feng shui is all about a good flow of energy that supports well-being, vibrant health and prosperity.

When interviewing a potential feng shui consultant, ask to see an educational resume. Be careful of those who share only a biography of themselves. Pretty words can't compare to an in-depth education, no matter what feng shui method is practiced. Be aware that the current trendiness of feng shui has attracted some fly-by-night practitioners. Would you hire a doctor, lawyer or other professional who refused to answer your questions about their professional qualifications? Continue your search for the right consultant if your request for information is met with a less than an enthusiastic response or a lack of solid credentials.

Keep in mind that the foremost reason your clients come to you is for wellness services. Until you can establish your "ideal" office, make sure your space offers a warming energy with a tranquil ambiance—whatever shape that may take for you. Avoid letting clutter or other encumbrances creep into your space and detract from your desired image.

Sixty percent of healing is environment.

Feng Shui Your Life
by Jayme Barrett
and John Cooledge

Feng Shui and Health: Using Feng Shui to Disarm Illness, Accelerate Recovery, and Create Optimal Health
by Nancy SantoPietro

Interior Design with Feng Shui: New and Expanded
by Sarah Rossbach

10

Feng Shui Resources
www.fengshui-ii.org
www.fengshuidirectory.com

Ambiance ● ●

Ambiance is a rather amorphous concept. It is a special atmosphere created by your environment. It arises from all of the previously covered factors and impacts your image and the mood you set. Establishing the appropriate ambiance isn't always an easy feat; although an unlimited budget would certainly help.

You always create a mood—intentional or not. Consider the image you wish to portray and the characteristics associated with it. Do you want your office to project a clinical feeling (which would be appropriate if many of your clients are insurance referrals)? Do you want a calm, quiet, soothing atmosphere to appeal to those wanting stress reduction? Do you want a cheery room with toys and lots of color for infants? Do you want a high-tech look for executives?

Beware of "theme" rooms. They often have limited appeal and in time can become boring to both you and your clients.

Professionalism ● ●

A professional office establishes credibility and demonstrates concern for the client. You validate your credibility by conspicuously posting your business license, policies, educational certificates, awards, interview clippings, business cards, brochures and letters of appreciation and recommendation. These items represent the time you've invested in your career and the goodwill you've generated in your community.

You express concern for your clients by the ways in which you design your office to assist them in feeling comfortable, appreciated, and that they are the center of attention. Creating a sense of privacy is essential. You may need to be inventive to accomplish this. For instance, some massage therapists and estheticians work in beauty salons in which the walls don't even reach the ceiling or are paper thin. If remodeling isn't an option, it helps to pad the walls or enclose the room with a false ceiling or canopy.

Make your clients feel important by providing a special area for their belongings (e.g., a small closet, a shelf, a chair behind a screen, a hook with hangers); keeping supplies handy (e.g., linens, tissues, blankets, bolsters); and maintaining a comfortable temperature. If you don't have easy access to the temperature controls, place a portable heater and fan in the room. Keep notes about clients' preferences in their files, and refer to the file before the session so you can properly prepare the room.

Nothing detracts more from a pleasant atmosphere than a dirty office space, especially the bathroom. Keep your room clean and free of clutter. Make sure there are no product spills, trash cans overflowing with garbage, sinks filled with dirty dishes, soiled linens piled in a corner and dust-bunnies hiding under the furniture, on fan blades, in vents and around moldings.

Home Office Considerations ● ● ●

Home offices present a few additional challenges. The main things to consider in conveying professionalism are privacy, sounds, cleanliness and environment. First of all, make sure there's a separate workspace in your home. Ideally, this room would have a private entrance from the main house. The next best option would be to have a separate room. If you must meet with clients in the main living quarters, do your best to set up a private area. Room screens work well for this.

Sounds are a major concern. Make sure you can silence the telephone ringer. Pick a quiet area to answer phone calls from potential clients. I highly recommend a separate business telephone service, especially if you have children. You always want your phone to be answered in a professional manner.

Also, figure out a way to let others who may come to the door know that you cannot be interrupted. Be aware of ambient sounds, such as children playing. A major problem could arise when family members are in your home during a session. Set clear boundaries and rules with family members. Make sure they're quiet and never disturb you during a session. Pets are not always cooperative in honoring the silence rule. Extra steps may need to be taken to ensure quiet.

Cleanliness is imperative to your professional image. Pets can present a potential problem, because no matter how well you vacuum, dander is always present if they're allowed in the session area. Also take into consideration that many people are allergic to animals. Any area in your home that your clients may see needs to be kept clean and tidy.

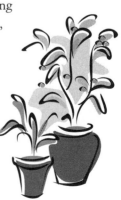

Consider adding a Permitted Incidental Occupancies endorsement to your homeowners policy that deletes liability exclusions for business activities conducted on the residence premises and modifies the business personal property limit.

Visual Stimuli ● ●

Designing the physical appearance of your treatment room can be fun. Most people are visually oriented and are affected by the colors, textures and artistry of your room.

Creativity specialists contend that the key to creativity is to get out of your normal frame of reference. One technique is to lie on your treatment table or sit on your chair and notice what you see. Include all positions: face up, face down and side to side. This is how your clients view your room. You might be surprised at what they can see at those angles. For example, if you have a bookshelf, note which shelves are at eye level and be sure to place appropriate books in that line of vision.

Simple changes to alter the visual impact of your ideal session room include painting the walls, texturizing the ceiling, suspending a mobile, hanging artwork and charts, furnishing the room stylishly, installing unique window coverings, and including potted plants or fresh cut flowers.

Make sure the floor covering is constructed of high-quality materials. Avoid light colors as they get dirty quickly. If the flooring is less than ideal, you can use throw rugs or an area carpet—just be certain they're skid-proof.

Lighting is another important element in the design of a session room. Ideally you would have a source of natural light from a window or a skylight. If not, place lamps in different areas of the room to give balanced, indirect illumination.

Sensations ● ●

We are all sensual beings. Incorporate as many of the senses as possible—particularly touch, smell and sound—into your design plans.

In terms of scent, a clean, crisp, barely discernible fragrance is usually preferred. If your office is in a salon, you must eliminate or conceal the harsh chemical odors from nail polish and hair treatment applications. Some solutions to odor problems are to insulate your room or mask the odors with air fresheners or essential oils. But be careful with fragrances, because your clients may suffer from allergies, or your next client may want the opposite results of the aromatherapy essence used by the current client.

Physical sensation plays an important role—especially in touch therapy practices. In addition to the actual hands-on treatment, are tactile sensations from your equipment and linens. A treatment table is one of the most important pieces of office equipment. Does it inspire feelings of safety and comfort? Can you make necessary adjustments? Is it wide enough? Is it well padded? Does it squeak? Do your clients need to pole vault to get onto it? Use a secure, well-padded table or futon, and make sure your sheets, towels and gowns are soft. You might also cover bolsters with a towel or sheet.

Most people like to touch things, so have items available for your clients to play with, such as a skeleton, a replica of the foot with reflexology points, a model of a muscle, samples of products you sell and books they can peruse.

Recorded sound, or the absence thereof, is the most commonly used means of creating a mood. Invest in a good system that's programmable. Purchase a wide variety of music and make sure you can easily adjust volume or change selection. Some settings might have piped-in music, but still you can often access the controls. I used to go to a dentist who played a style of music which I abhorred. I was always apprehensive about check-ups, not because I feared he might discover cavities, but because I dreaded listening to the music.

Regardless of the atmosphere you desire, it can be undermined if you don't block out external noise, so be sure you turn off the phone bell and soundproof thin walls. You can also create other auditory experiences with chimes, an aquarium, or even a specially designed indoor water fountain.

Layout ● ●

The most comfortable and inviting offices are organized, clean and free of clutter. Decorate the room with appropriate furniture and equipment. Don't put your favorite recliner in the corner if it takes up so much room that clients have to walk sideways to get to the table. Consider the ways in which you interact with your clients, and design your office accordingly. For instance, if you like to teach clients how to stretch, make sure there's adequate, obstruction-free floor space. Also, keep supplies such as tissues, blankets and water at hand.

My Ideal Session Room ● ●

My vision of the ideal session room is one in which I feel comfortable and pampered. The room is located in a small professional building that is nicely landscaped. I enter through the front door and find myself in the waiting room that's painted with pastel colors and the floors are tiled. There are several stuffed chairs, a couch, a magazine table, end tables with lamps on them, and vases of fresh flowers.

Directly to my left is a desk where the receptionist works. Next to the desk is a beautiful ficus tree. Against one wall is a bookshelf with brochures about the various practitioners and literature on well-being. Along an adjacent wall is a display case filled with unique health-related items such as books, essential oils, diffusers, hot and cold therapy packs, relaxation tools, ergonomic support devices and CDs. In the corner is a water dispenser and a stand with cups and a pot of herbal tea.

The actual session room inspires a sense of deep relaxation the moment I enter. The lighting is diffused, the temperature moderate, the walls are painted a soothing color, the ceilings are vaulted, and I can feel a soft breeze from an overhead fan. I experience a sense of total privacy—no outside noises whatsoever.

The practitioner guides me to a little alcove where I can get ready for my session. This dressing area has hangers for clothes, a shelf for belongings, a mirror and a chair. The natural sunlight gently streams through a skylight.

I proceed to get on the extremely comfortable table that is thickly padded and hydraulic with adjustable angles. I notice how good the soft linens feel, and appreciate that they're also fragrance-free. The table has a shelf that I can easily reach and on it I find tissues and a bottle of water. I look around the room and see certificates on one wall, artwork on another, and anatomical charts on the third wall. The window is covered with wooden shutters, and several large potted plants are positioned in the corners. The room is uncluttered, clean and exudes professionalism. Then I hear faint sounds emanating from the stereo, lulling me into a state of deep relaxation....

If people knew how hard I worked to get my mastery, it wouldn't seem so wonderful after all.
— Michelangelo

10

• Licenses and Permits •

State Guide for Licenses and Permits

www.smallbusiness.findlaw.com

www.sba.gov/hotlist/license.html

Business owners need to know the local, state and federal requirements that apply to starting or relocating a business. A useful online resource to simplify your research is the FindLaw for Small Business website, which provides extensive information about licenses and permits specific to each profession and the associated board regulations.

Your local City Hall, Secretary of State or the Consumer Affairs office can also provide you with information and resources. The following list provides an overview of the basic required licenses and permits, and who to contact for specific information and forms. This list doesn't cover every possible situation, as your business may have special site requirements or industry regulations.

Figure 10.7

Licenses & Permits — Quick Reference

Business License	Allows you the privilege of doing business. Contact your Business Licensing Bureau.
Occupational License	Allows you to work in a specific industry as long as you comply with that profession's regulations. Contact the State Agency of Consumer Affairs or the local Business Licensing Bureau.
Transaction Privilege Tax License	Allows you to collect (and remit) sales tax. Contact your State Department of Revenue.
Planning and Zoning Permits	These permits are issued after your location has been assessed and shows that the business operation conforms with area plans, has proper zoning and has adequate parking. Contact your City or County Hall Planning Department.
Building Safety Permit	This permit is issued after your location is inspected and has met the minimum safety requirements for you and your clients, and complies with fire and building codes. Contact the Fire Department.

• Insurance Coverage •

Determine which types of insurance are required by law and purchase those policies first.

Obtaining proper insurance coverage is imperative for any small business. Discuss your specific needs with an insurance agent (or three) to determine the types and amount of insurance appropriate for you and your business. You may need to have more than one insurance carrier, since very few companies offer all of the types of coverage. Check your office lease thoroughly. Your leaseholder may not be responsible for providing complete (if any) coverage. Also, if you work out of your home, be certain to review your homeowner's or apartment-dweller's policy. While the standard homeowner's policy protects you from personal liability, if a guest is injured at your home, it doesn't cover you if the visit is related to business.

Figure 10.8

Types of Insurance Coverage

Liability Insurance	Covers costs of injuries that occur to business-related visitors on your property. Don't assume that this is automatically covered in your office lease. Also, if you work out of your home, your homeowner's policy might not cover this either. Liability insurance doesn't cover you or employees.
General Liability Insurance	Covers negligence resulting in injury to clients, employees or the general public while you're on their premises. This is particularly important if you do office calls or teach classes.
Small Business Insurance	Offers umbrella coverage for business losses in terms of general liability, business interruption, errors and omissions, and product liability.
Malpractice Liability Insurance	Protects you from claims due to a loss incurred by your clients as a result of negligence or failure on your part to perform at a professional skill level.
Product Liability	Protects you from claims by clients who use products designed, manufactured or sold by you. Wellness providers rarely need this coverage.
Automobile Insurance	Very important, particularly if you use your car in your business. Be sure to carry full coverage including disability, business interruption and loss or damage to business-related items.
Fire and Theft Insurance	Covers business equipment, furniture, supplies and documents. If you work out of your home, you may need to purchase a rider to get adequate protection. You most likely need a separate policy for an outside office.
Business Interruption Insurance	Covers you if your business closes due to fire or other insurable causes. It pays you approximately what you would have earned.
Personal Disability Insurance	Safeguards you from loss of income if you cannot work due to illness or injury. You are paid a certain monthly amount if you're permanently disabled or a portion if you're partially disabled (can include long-term illness).
Medical Health Insurance	Helps cover medical bills, particularly for complicated illnesses, injuries and hospitalization.
Workers' Compensation Insurance	Required by law if you have employees. It covers all of the costs that you as an employer would be required to pay for any injury to an employee. It also provides the employee with disability and death benefits if injured or killed on the job. The employer is responsible for the cost of the insurance premium.
Partnership Insurance	Protects you against lawsuits arising from actions or omissions by any of your business partners.

10

• Setting Your Fees •

Fee structures vary greatly depending on the type of work you do and where you're located. Setting an appropriate fee structure and increase strategy is necessary in any business. No matter which method you choose for determining your rates, be certain your fee structure promotes credibility.

Figure 10.9

Four Major Fee-Setting Strategies

1. **High-end rate**   Set rate significantly higher than industry standard rate to target a small percentage of the population. This usually only works if your service is innovative, in demand and has no competition.

2. **Industry standard rate**   Determine the industry standard rate and align with it.

3. **Low-end rate**   Set rate significantly lower than the industry standard rate to attract a larger market share.

4. **Time-limited introductory rate**   Offer introductory rates for a limited time or package deals reflecting reduced rates. Beware of the tendency to overextend introductory rates.

Carefully consider all of the costs involved in running your business before you finalize your fee structure. This includes your fixed costs, such as rent, utilities, phone, equipment, loan payments, maintenance, insurance, licenses, promotion and staffing, as well as the amenities that vary depending on the number and type of clients (e.g., providing free samples and educational materials, taxes and supplies). Then there's your time: keeping client records, networking, planning, extended business hours, traveling, practice management, continuing your education and client follow-up.

Figure 10.10 illustrates how to determine your fees. It is based on a 40-hour workweek, which leaves a maximum of 25 billable hours per week. Since overhead varies greatly from one business to another, it isn't included in this breakdown.

Let's say that you want to earn $40,000 this year before taxes. If you plan on working 50 percent (billing 12.5 hours per week), then you need to charge $61.50 per hour. If you want to work 90 percent (bill 22.5 hours per week), then you only need to charge $34 per hour. But, you also must include the costs in running your business. Imagine that your fixed costs are $15,000 per year plus $6 per session. So, at a 50 percent workload, you need to cover $40,000 income, $15,000 fixed expenses, and $3,900 per session cost (650 sessions), which equals $58,900. Looking at the chart, you find that to bring in gross revenues of $60,000, you need to charge approximately $92 per hour. Yet, if you plan on billing 90 percent, then you need to cover $40,000 income, $15,000 fixed expenses, and $7,020 per session cost (1,170 sessions), which equals $62,020. In this instance, you only need to charge about $53 per hour. This chart can have an unsettling effect.

Figure 10.10

Time/Income Factor Analysis

One Year	=	365 days	–	104 days (weekends)
	=	261 days	–	8 days (holidays)
	=	253 days	–	10 days (health)
	=	243 days	–	10 days (vacation)
	=	233 days	x	8 hours per day
	=	1,864 hours per year		
	–	30% (promotion, operations, professional development)		
	=	approximately 1,300 hours		
	=	approximately 25 billable hours per week		

Annual Income*	50% 650 hrs (12.5 hrs/wk)	70% 910 hrs (17.5 hrs/wk)	90% 1170 hrs (22.5 hrs/wk)	100% 1300 hrs (25 hrs/wk)
$25,000	$38.50	$27.50	$21.50	$19.25
$30,000	$46.00	$33.00	$25.75	$23.00
$35,000	$54.00	$38.50	$30.00	$27.00
$40,000	$61.50	$44.00	$34.00	$31.00
$50,000	$77.00	$55.00	$42.75	$38.50
$60,000	$92.00	$66.00	$51.25	$46.00
$75,000	$115.50	$82.50	$64.00	$58.00
$100,000	$154.00	$110.00	$85.50	$77.00

* Does not include allowance for overhead and taxes

The difference between the top money winners on the PGA golf tour and the bottom money winners can be as little as one stroke a day.
— Steve Miller, former PGA tour player

You may be wondering how you can possibly earn the income you desire while charging a fair and equitable price. Several possibilities exist for increasing your income potential. First of all, you can increase the number of billable weekly hours by working more than 40 hours per week (which isn't uncommon with small business owners). Another alternative is to reduce your overhead costs—but be certain this doesn't cause clients to experience a decrease in benefits. You can also diversify your practice by selling products, subcontracting work (or hiring other practitioners to work for you) and leading seminars. Finally, one of the most viable options is to delegate some of your business activities, which frees you to increase the number of hours of direct client contact.

Determining your appropriate fee structure involves more than simply deciding what you want to charge per hour. You have to balance your desired income and requisite expenses with what's realistic. Set fees that you feel comfortable with and confident about that are also fair and instill trust. Even if you're considered to be the best practitioner in your field, it's futile to charge more than what the market will bear. Just because you desire a specific income level and feel you deserve to charge a certain rate doesn't necessarily mean people will pay it. Choose your market(s) carefully and strategize your fee structure.

10

Chapter 14, Page 298 for a Business Income and Expense Forecast.

When someone inquires about your fees, state them with confidence. If the client indicates in some way that he cannot manage that fee, you get to choose in that moment if you want to offer a lower fee to accommodate the client. You may want to offer a person-to-person sliding scale as you see fit and as your budget allows. Many practitioners know how many clients they need to see at full price and then how much room that leaves for other clients to pay less. I base my decision to lower a fee on necessity and desire to make positive change.

Money will not add to your self-esteem, it works the other way around.
— Phil Laut

Sliding Fee Scales •

A sliding fee scale allows people who cannot afford your full fee to pay a lower one. Sliding fee scales can be awkward and tough to set up in advance of the first session unless a client has said something to you while booking the appointment. I don't advocate advertising a sliding fee scale unless you know that your target market is going to need it (e.g., people on meager fixed incomes). Usually what works best is to give parameters. A frequently used model that seems least offensive and fair is determining fees based on income level. For example, your sliding scale statement might look like this:

> My standard rate is $55 per session. If this presents a hardship for you, then I accept a sliding scale fee based on your combined family annual income level. If the total annual income earned is less than $15,000 annually the fee per session is $25, $15,000-20,000 = $30, $20,000-25,000 = $40, $25,000+ = $55.

Chapter 17, Page 445

for additional ideas on client incentives.

Prepaid Package Plans •

Prepaid package plans encourage people to book sessions more frequently and infuse extra income into your bank account. Some ideas are: purchase three acupuncture treatments and get a $5 savings per treatment; seven counseling sessions qualify for a 20 percent discount; and purchase five massages and receive the sixth one free. Keep it simple—don't overwhelm yourself and your clients with too many options.

Raising Your Rates •

If you're a self-employed practitioner, you have ultimate control over when and how much to raise your fees. When you've determined a fee increase is required, be certain the amount is appropriate. You will probably lose credibility (and clients) if you raise your rates more than once per year. Do a one-year financial forecast. Ascertain the amount of money you need to charge per session should you experience no growth in your business. Raise your fees accordingly, with a caveat against an increase of greater than 15 percent.

Keep in mind that raising your rates isn't the only way to increase your income.

Inform your clients of your rate changes at least two weeks in advance via a personalized letter or pre-printed postcard. Springing a higher charge on them at the last moment, particularly right after a session, is disrespectful. If you offer series discounts, promote goodwill by allowing your clients the opportunity to sign up for a series at the "old" rates. Of course, they need to make this commitment before the new fee structure goes into effect.

Create a Dynamic Business Plan

• Overview •

If the thought of writing a business plan conjures up images of endless hours of drudgery, you aren't alone. Many business owners don't relish this time-consuming yet vital task. Several things can help ease the way. Keep in mind that building a business without a business plan is a lot like building a house without a blueprint. The house may get built, but the budget may go through the roof and the project may take a lot longer than expected. What's worse, "on the fly" construction doesn't lend itself to longevity. The house may look good for awhile but may not last as time and stress work their magic.

A business plan pinpoints what you aim to accomplish and how you intend to organize your resources to attain those goals. Creating a business plan makes good sense. Most importantly, it dramatically increases your chance of success. According to business expert David M. Anderson, "There is no single omission that bodes worse for a start-up's future than the lack of a comprehensive business plan."[1] In short, develop a business plan if you want to tilt the odds in favor of your success.

Although you may lack the financial resources to hire a highly paid business consultant to prepare a business plan—an ideal solution that many of us dream about—recognize that you don't have to approach this task alone. Those who have traveled the path before you have created numerous resources. You can find help through business organizations such as the Service Core of Retired Executives (SCORE), plan-writing software, local business school centers for entrepreneurs and some top-notch business books.

The first draft doesn't have to be perfect. Once you know the key ingredients of a business plan, you can start with a mission statement and let the rest flow from there. Think of your first few hours of work on a business plan as a brainstorming session. If you're having trouble getting started, plan an initial two-hour work session with a business advisor, colleague or business coach.

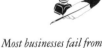

Most businesses fail from lack of imagination.
— Paul Hawken

Business Plan Fundamentals •

A business plan serves many functions. It is a powerful declaration of your goals and intentions, a written summary of what you aim to accomplish and an overview of how you intend to organize your resources to attain those goals. Developing an effective business plan generally requires a considerable amount of time. You have to do a lot of honest thinking in addition to some technical research. However, if you've completed the exercises throughout *Business Mastery*, you already have the groundwork for a business plan!

Efforts and courage are not enough without purpose and direction.
— John F. Kennedy

If you're opening a private practice or clinic, a business plan assists you to clarify your vision and values, evaluate the marketplace, identify your goals, calculate your costs, forecast your growth and identify your risks. For those of you who have been in business for a while, a new or updated plan can rejuvenate your practice.

A business plan addresses these issues: What are you offering? Who will your clients be? What needs do your services satisfy? How will your potential clients find you? How much money do you plan on making? What actions do you intend on taking to ensure success?

Although business plans vary in scope and content, the major components of a business plan are an owner's statement, executive summary, mission statement, business description, long-term and short-term goals, a financial forecast, operations overview, risk assessment, success strategies and a marketing plan.

As you navigate through your career, a business reminds you to celebrate important milestones.

Use your business plan to keep you inspired and on track. Many business owners get overwhelmed by the minutiae of running a business and miss valuable opportunities to plan strategies for future success. Clearly describing where you want to go and how you intend to get there encourages you to be more realistic. It also assists you to anticipate and avoid problems, or at least be prepared so that you can overcome them, thus minimizing your risks. Written goals give you solid criteria to evaluate progress. A financial forecast illustrates exactly what finances are required to launch and maintain a thriving business.

Schedule periodic "reality checks" with your business plan on a monthly, quarterly and annual basis to help you to adjust course when needed and identify new ways to grow your business. A business plan can help you discover vital steps to your success and happiness that you may have otherwise overlooked.

The rest of this chapter provides a business plan outline. Before you go to your journal or computer, scan through the chapter. It highlights the key components and scope of a business plan. Use this outline to refine what you've already written by completing the exercises from the other chapters, and to clarify the other details that are requisites for your success.

When your business plan is complete, print it and put it in a three-ring binder. This type of binder allows you to easily update your plan and add information (e.g., copies of reports and sample promotional materials) and keeps all major business documents in one place. If you're submitting the business plan for a loan, consider taking your documents to a print shop and having them copied and bound.

• Business Plan Outline •

The Basic Business Plan •

Cover Page • •

The cover page is simply the first page of the business plan. Include a title (e.g., "Business Plan for The Healthy Alternative"), and below it put your name, address, telephone numbers, fax number, website address and email address.

Table of Contents • •

The table of contents lists all of the business plan sections with corresponding page numbers. Title each document you include in the appendix.

Owner's Statement • •

This is a one-page description of the business and the owner. which includes: the business name, address, phone numbers, fax number, email address and website address; your name, home address, home phone number; a summary of your business experience and philosophy; and a brief business description (the year the business was established and current financial status).

Executive Summary • •

The executive summary consists of business plan highlights. This section critical if you apply for financial backing, as it must convince lenders and investors that your business will succeed. Although the summary appears at the beginning of the business plan, it's best to write it last (and keep it to three pages or less).

Mission Statement • •

A mission statement conveys the essence of your business—why your business exists and what values underpin everything you do. Values are beliefs that guide you and your organization. The best mission statements focus on the benefits your customers receive. For instance, an acupuncture clinic's mission may be: "We help clients achieve their wellness goals and enjoy vibrant health. We are committed as a team to values of integrity, compassion and excellent customer service." Approaches to writing mission statements vary. Some experts suggest keeping your mission statement short and memorable—a sentence or two at most. However, many owners and organizations like to say more, elaborating on who they are, why they do what they do, and what values and vision guide the company.

Business Plan Checklist
www.businessmastery.us/
biz-plan.php

Chapter 1, Pages 7-8
for more information
on values.

11

**How to Write a Mission
Statement**
www.successnet.org/articles/
mission130.htm

Purpose, Priorities and Goals ● ●

This section is a detailed description of your business activities and career plan in terms of short-term and long-term goals. State your overall career purpose and at least six priorities. List at least six long-term (three- to five-year time frame) priorities and at least two goals per priority. List at least six short-term (1-2 year time frame) priorities and at least three goals per priority. Many of these declarations assist you in being clear and motivated, and they can be quite personal. You may want to censor some of these statements if you're submitting this plan for a loan.

Business Description ● ●

Include photographs of your office in your business plan portfolio.

This section provides background about your practice. Begin by writing a brief history of your company and which business activities your company pursues to accomplish its mission. Describe the services you offer and products you sell; special products used; equipment; the physical location; and the unique features that distinguish your practice from others (e.g., experience, range of services, pricing, location, product sales, equipment, management abilities). If you sell products, include a product register with the suppliers' names and specify the types of clients who purchase products.

Marketing Plan ● ●

Marketing is the pivotal component of a business plan. Begin by depicting the image you wish to convey. Next describe your target markets and clarify your differential advantage. Follow with a competition analysis, including steps you'll take to meet any challenges. The major section is the strategic action plan. Outline your marketing goals for all four areas—promotion, advertising, publicity and community relations. Delineate a timeline, budget and rationale for each strategy. If you sell products, include a description and cost for the following: inside displays; additional sales staff (include training); equipment; and special promotions, discounts and sales. Set a marketing budget per year. Tabulate the cost to market your services and the cost to market your products. Determine the total marketing costs and calculate the actual cost per potential client. Close this section with a summary of how your marketing strategies will enable you to succeed.

Risk Assessment ● ●

Risk assessment is a demonstration of your ability to anticipate and manage risks. Detail the effects your competition has on all phases of your business. List possible external events that might occur to hamper your success, such as a recession, new competition, shifts in client demand, unfavorable industry trends, problems with suppliers and changes in legislation. Identify potential internal problems such as income projections not realized, long-term illness or serious injury. Then generate contingency plans to counteract the most significant risks.

Financial Analysis ● ●

This section consists of statements about your income potential, fees, current financial status and financial forecast. The financial analysis section differs if the plan is for a new or established business. For instance, financial data for a new business includes a projection of working capital for start-up expenses (e.g., equipment, office supplies, inventory), as well as an estimate of capital reserves required to keep the business afloat until it makes a profit.

For an established business, the financial analysis includes extensive historical data related to financial reports (e.g., balance sheets, profit and loss statements, cash flow projections, tax returns) and sales data.

The following guidelines focus on financial data for a new business. For more detail about a financial analysis for an established business, see the *Business Mastery* website for the extensive business plan checklist.

Genius begins great works, labor alone finsihes them.
— Joseph Joubert

Determining income potential for a new business can be tricky. Contact your professional society or several of the major teaching institutions (for your specific field) to get this information. You may have to do some informal research because this data has not been compiled for every profession. Describe the existing business conditions. Where do you stand in the current "state of the art"? Describe the projections and trends for your specific profession both nationally and locally. List the average income for practitioners in your specific field, both nationally and locally, for the first six months of practice, the first year, the second year and the third year. If possible, include the average number of clients for those same times.

List your service fees, including introductory offers, prepaid package discounts, professional courtesy discounts and sliding fee scales. Enumerate the amenities to be absorbed in pricing (e.g., credit offered, outcalls, parking, consultations, extended business hours, educational materials, samples and supplies). Describe your competition's effect on pricing.

Determine the equipment, supplies and inventory needed for next 12 months. Clarify your acquisition plan (buy, consign or lease), and prioritize the purchases. Calculate how much money is needed to open your business and the annual operations budget for each of the next three to five years. Generate this information from a computerized accounting program or the following forms found on www.businessmastery.us: Start-Up Costs Worksheet, Opening Balance Sheet, Business Income and Expense Forecast, Monthly Business Expense Worksheet, Monthly Personal Budget Worksheet, and Cash Flow Forecast. Put the actual worksheets in this section or in the business plan appendix.

List your potential funding sources, describe exactly how you anticipate spending the money received, and note how any loans are to be secured. Calculate a break-even analysis. Determine at what client (or sales) volume your business moves into the "black." This is the point at which total costs equal total income. You may need to update this every few months to accurately reflect your business growth.

11

Operations • •

This section is an overview of your business organization, procedures and policies. Identify the management qualifications needed to run the "business" part of your practice, and assess your strengths and challenges. Specify the legal form of ownership you've chosen and the reasons why. Cite the requisite licenses, permits and insurance coverage.

For businesses that have a staff, list the various functions and estimate the number of people needed for each function. Describe the training required, and state your compensation plan. If you have a group practice, describe the various functions and the person(s) responsible. Indicate the level of authority for each person (e.g., hiring, firing, scheduling and purchasing).

Write a brief overview of your company policies and procedures. Include details on safety precautions. Determine your security needs (consider client screening, location safety, ample lighting for the parking lot and night travel), and develop a plan to reduce these types of risks.

Close this section with an accounting and control summary. Clarify who does the bookkeeping (you or another). Set a production schedule (e.g., daily, weekly, monthly, quarterly, annually) for the following types of management reports: checking account balance; service reports such as the total number of return clients or the number of clients in relation to the time spent per client; product sales reports; balance sheets; profit and loss statements; condition of client accounts; expense reports; insurance reimbursement aging; forecasting; and inventory reports.

The Business Mastery Supplement by Sohnen-Moe Associates, Inc. This text-based CD for PC and MAC computers contains a 58-page sample massage therapy business plan in addition to the client correspondence and marketing letters.

Success Strategies • •

List your goals for developing your success strategies. Specify your methods for implementing your business plan and having a prosperous practice. Include activities, such as developing strategic plans, creating monthly flow charts, identifying decision points, reviewing and revising your plans, creating a business support system, networking and choosing appropriate advisors.

Appendix ● ●

The types of additional information or documents (if any at all) to be included in this section depend upon the nature of your business plan. If your business plan is mainly for your personal use, you may not need to add anything else. If you intend on using your business plan to obtain financial backing, consider including the following data. (Note: This list is only a guide. Check with the specific lending institutions or investors for their requirements.)

- Personal net worth statement.
- Copies of income statements and balance sheets from the last two years.
- List of client commitments.
- Copies of business legal agreements.
- Credit status reports.
- News articles about you or your business.
- Photographs of your location.
- Copies of promotional material.
- Letters of recommendation from your clients.
- Key employee resumés.
- Personal references.

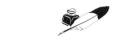

It's never too late, in fiction or in life, to revise.
— Nancy Thayer

Business Plan Supplement ●

If your business plan is for securing a loan, it's recommended to incorporate the following additional information into the previous sections of the business plan.

The Executive Summary ● ●

- State the type of business loan(s) you're seeking (e.g., line of credit or mortgage).
- Summarize the proposed use of the funds.
- Calculate the projected return on investment.
- Write a persuasive statement of why the venture is a good risk.

The Financial Analysis ● ●

- Describe the loan requirements: the amount, the terms, and the desired date.
- State the purpose of the loan, detailing the facets of the business to be financed.
- Provide a statement of the owner's equity.
- List any outstanding debts. Include the balance due, repayment terms, purpose of the loan and status.
- Document your current operating line of credit—the amount and security held.

References ● ●

- List all pertinent information regarding your current lending institution: branch, address, types of accounts and contact person(s).
- List the names, addresses and phone numbers of your attorney, accountant and business consultant.

11

❋ Getting Started ❋

Business Plans for Dummies
by Paul Tiffany
and Steven Peterson

Business Plan Resources

www.sba.gov/
smallbusinessplanner/
index.html

www.bplans.com

www.score.org/
business_toolbox.html

www.planware.org

Additional resources are available to assist you in writing a business plan. Browse an online or local bookstore and purchase a few books on business plan writing that catch your interest. Search the Internet for sample business plans and useful articles. Some tech-savvy business owners prefer to work with a business plan writing software that includes sample business plans, along with forecast and cash flow models.

Next consider contacting your local Chamber of Commerce or local chapter of SCORE. SCORE offers a reasonably priced online workshop "Develop Your Business Plan" and business plan templates. Advisors in local chapter offices meet with you to review your plan and can provide valuable feedback to fine-tune your rough draft. In addition, many local Chamber of Commerce organizations offer free consultations for new business owners as well as low-cost small business seminars.

Avoid getting stuck on attempting to create a perfect first draft of your business plan. Most business owners create a rough first draft and spend a good bit of time fine-tuning subsequent drafts. One of the toughest challenges in writing a business plan involves financial projections. Make informed estimates for sales, expenses and profits. Know that no one does it perfectly. Tend toward the conservative and include "wiggle room" for unexpected expenses.

Figure 11.1

Business Plan Tips & Insights

- Business plans for internal use average about 10 to 15 pages; business plans to raise funds typically span about 40 pages or more.
- Talk to other business owners about their business plans. Ask what they would do differently or what they found most valuable about the process.
- Consult with an accountant or CPA to look at your financials.
- Find an experienced business person and share your plan. Ask for feedback. Listen, but don't follow advice that doesn't ring true for you.
- Take your time and don't rush through the business plan process. The time you invest is well spent.
- Do your homework when it comes to competitive analysis and pricing. Gather as much supporting data as possible.
- Revisit your business plan quarterly to make sure you're on track.
- Celebrate when you've completed writing your business plan. It is the first key milestone of many to come.

Part V

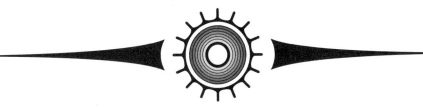

Business Operations

Part V of *Business Mastery* focuses on the nuts and bolts of business operations, and includes tips and information to help you run your business smoothly and efficiently. While much of the information in this part is geared toward practitioners who are self-employed, some of it is key to all practitioners.

Although not many people thrill at the thought of developing policies and procedures, Chapter 12 shows you they are like the frame of a house—a necessary part of building a house that lasts, and a business that thrives. You'll find tips on how to write policies and procedures, organize your office, make smart technology choices and comply with healthcare regulations. Also included are useful insights into contract basics, effective negotiation, conflict resolution, and insurance reimbursement.

Chapter 13 looks at those inevitable periods of change that every business encounters. Because even our best-laid plans can't protect us from the unexpected, this chapter first covers ideas on how to recession-proof your practice by diversifying into product sales and value-added services. But what if you want to change the direction your practice has taken? We help you recognize the signs that it's time to re-evaluate where you are and what options are open to you. For growing practices, you'll find insights into when and how to hire support or professional staff, as well as an overview of regulations regarding employees and independent contractors. For practitioners on the move, the chapter covers how to manage the relocation of your practice, near or far.

Chapter 14 presents the essentials of financial management. It provides concrete information to help you keep the books, prepare financial reports, and understand tax laws. You'll also learn how to use barter to exchange goods and services with others, and useful tips for efficient inventory control for wellness products. The chapter also looks at the variety of ways you can transfer or sell your practice and provides a step-by-step process for achieving the best outcome possible. Finally, the chapter covers the basics of retirement planning and offers a number of helpful resources to assist you in looking ahead.

Practice Management

❋ Policies and Procedures ❋

If you look behind the scenes of any smoothly running and successful business, you're likely to find clearly defined policies and procedures. A Policy and Procedure Manual provides a framework for your business by defining expectations, values and standard business practices. Policies direct your decisions and actions. They are built on the philosophy and values that guide your practice; procedures are specific steps that detail how you want to run your business day to day.

Formulate your policies and create a written manual, even if you're the only person in your business. By going through this process, you may discover conflicts or potentially risky situations, and thus address and resolve these issues before they actually arise. Also, if you decide to expand your practice and hire staff (or bring in an associate), the transition is easier if the operational guidelines are already established. If you work for someone else, discuss the current policies and procedures with your employer. You may find that you can add to or alter them.

We are what we repeatedly do, excellence then is not an act, but a habit.
— Aristotle

Policy Manual ❋

Policies are generally divided into two branches—internal company policies and client interaction policies. In designing a policy manual, begin with a statement of your company's purpose, priorities and goals. Next, clarify your employment policies.

Employment Policies ● ●

Employment policies cover the requirements and expectations of your staff.

Figure 12.1

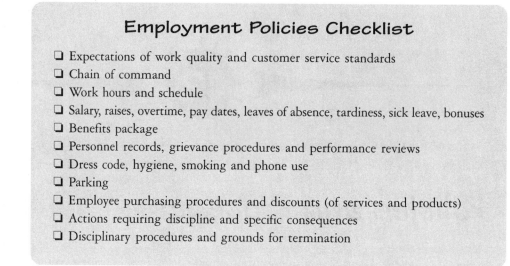

Employment Policies Checklist

❑ Expectations of work quality and customer service standards
❑ Chain of command
❑ Work hours and schedule
❑ Salary, raises, overtime, pay dates, leaves of absence, tardiness, sick leave, bonuses
❑ Benefits package
❑ Personnel records, grievance procedures and performance reviews
❑ Dress code, hygiene, smoking and phone use
❑ Parking
❑ Employee purchasing procedures and discounts (of services and products)
❑ Actions requiring discipline and specific consequences
❑ Disciplinary procedures and grounds for termination

Lots of folks confuse bad management with destiny.
— Kin Hubbard

www.businessmastery.us/
policy-checklist.php
for a detailed Policy and
Procedure Manual checklist.

Client Interaction Policies ● ●

Client policies are about setting boundaries that encourage trust, safety and comfort. Policies explicitly define the parameters of expectations for both clients and practitioners. They make running a business easier, circumvent potentially awkward situations, provide means for conflict resolution and demonstrate professionalism.

Figure 12.2

Client Policies Checklist

❑ Standard business hours
❑ Finances: fees, gift certificates, tips
❑ Product sales
❑ Guarantees
❑ Cancellation and lateness
❑ Mind-altering substances
❑ Inappropriate client behavior
❑ Hygiene requirements
❑ Ambiance: noise, children, food and beverages
❑ Communication
❑ Confidentiality
❑ Scope of practice
❑ HIPAA compliance
❑ Dual relationships

Client policy statements can take various forms, such as a letter, a page with bulleted items, or a combination of the two. The major areas to cover in your policies are finances, communication, scope of practice, etiquette and personal relationships.

Because change is a given, periodically review your policies to delete any outdated ones and clarify new requirements. It may be helpful to discuss potential changes with colleagues before updating the policy statement and sharing it with clients.

The main caveat with policies is: Don't create a policy you won't enforce. If you alter a policy for a client either on a one-time basis or if you change that specific policy permanently, make it clear to the client your intention is to address the specific situation and that you would appreciate her continued adherence to all other policies.

Written policy statements set a professional tone and help build positive relationships with clients, even if you don't have specific policies for every situation.

Finances • • •

When creating your financial policies, include the following: your fee structure; sliding scale schedules; package plans; credit terms; insurance reimbursement; product guarantees and returns; bounced checks; gift certificates; and barter.

Fee Structures vary greatly depending on the type of work you do and where you're located. Once you've determined your fees, it's important to communicate the following to your clients: your basic session rate and duration of the session; other alternatives such as longer sessions; options for other services (e.g., hydrotherapy, paraffin treatments, acupuncture, aromatherapy); and types of payments accepted (e.g., cash, check, credit cards).

Sliding Fee Scales can be awkward. It's tough to set one up in advance of the first session unless a client has said something to you while booking the appointment.

Package Plans encourage people to receive treatments more often and infuse extra income into your bank account.

Insurance Reimbursement is a time-consuming, detailed process. Many wellness providers prefer not to deal with it at all, some may help clients by filling out the forms (but require payment at time of service), while others will do direct billing. If you offer third-party billing, require the client to sign a statement saying that if a claim isn't paid within a specified time (e.g., 60 days), or if the claim is denied, the client is responsible for payment. Whichever method you choose, clearly state it in your policies.

Product Guarantees and Returns instill consumer confidence. Check with your suppliers to determine their return policies. Your customers may need to return defective or unwanted goods to the manufacturer. I recommend offering a money-back guarantee on all services and products. Of course, to take a stand such as this you need to carry quality products. You may want to include a time limit on returns, such as within 10 days of purchase.

Chapter 10, Page 214
for details on sliding fees
and package plans.

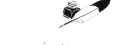

Common sense is not so common.
— Voltaire

12

Credit Terms are rare in service professions. The three most common reasons for extending credit are: the fees are billed to a third party, such as an insurance agency, attorney or a client's employer; a client forgets his checkbook; or a client has cash flow difficulties.

For those with a cash flow difficulty, create a formal IOU with a payment schedule. Let's say a regular client recently got laid off from work. She has another job lined up, but won't be starting for two months. She wants to continue receiving her biweekly treatments but is unable to afford them and doesn't have anything to barter. Ideally, she would pay a nominal fee with each session, but that might not be a viable option. For instance, a written payment agreement that both parties sign may state:

IOU

I, Darlene Dunning [client's name] agree to pay the sum of $70 per session for each acupuncture treatment I receive between May 1, 20__ [today's date] and July 11, 20__ [the week after her job resumes] in the following manner: Beginning July 14, 20__ I, Darlene Dunning, pay the sum of at least $30 every two weeks until the entire amount is repaid. This amount is in addition to any charges for treatments received after July 11, 20__ (which are payable in full at time of service).

In the event of nonpayment I, Darlene Dunning, agree to pay reasonable attorney's fees and costs for making such collection.

Bounced Checks happen to the best of us. Unfortunately, as the recipient, you must deal with the repercussions. In most states you can go to the bank where the check is drawn and obtain preferential status in getting the check cashed as soon as funds are deposited into the account. Many businesses charge a fee (ranging from $10 to triple the check's amount) for bounced checks to cover their bank's charges and time involved in settling the account. Note that this fee can be contested if it isn't stated in your policies.

Gift Certificates can be handled in various ways. Some people advocate assigning a three-month expiration date. Others recommend six months or a year, and some suggest no expiration date at all. All these options have pros and cons. Whichever you choose, make the conditions clear. Keep in mind that in many states you cannot put an expiration on a gift certificate that was purchased. I also suggest that the certificate be transferable. Clients often appreciate the added convenience and flexibility.

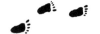

Chapter 16, Pages 397-400

for more on gift certificates and expiration dates.

Barter is one of the most commonly misused and abused areas of financial management. Although it isn't necessary to include barter in your written policy statement, it's important to set guidelines ahead of time for the types of bartering and the amount of bartering you allow. Keep accurate records, particularly if you aren't doing a direct trade.

Communication • • •

Policies relating to communication apply to the environment you intend to create, the language and terminology you use with clients, your attitudes toward clients, the types of questions you ask, the degree of honesty and self-disclosure you require of your clients, and your physical space boundaries.

Confidentiality • • •

Confidentiality must be maintained in a therapeutic relationship to promote an atmosphere of safety. Describe your procedures for maintaining confidentiality and the circumstances which require breaking confidentiality.

Business Hours and Availability • • •

Availability to your clients includes your business hours, location, and the time allotted before and after sessions to answer questions or offer support. Follow-up tends to be a weak area in most practices. While it's a good idea to place appointment reminder calls, it's also important to find out if your clients want you to call them, when they prefer to be contacted and where they want to receive the calls. Some practitioners call new clients within 48 hours of their first session just to check in with them. Others also like to call clients who've experienced a major shift during the session. Regardless of the type and frequency of follow-up, always discuss it first with your clients.

Scope of Practice • • •

These statements define the type of work you do and assist your clients in knowing what to expect. Consider prefacing your policies with a short paragraph describing your work, the types of clients you work with (or won't work with), your training and background, any conditions that are your specialty, and your procedures. Often these do not lend themselves to precise policies, yet are vital in setting the tone for a safe, enjoyable experience for both therapist and client. Some specific scope of practice policies cover draping, diagnosing and charting.

For detailed information on communication, policies, dual relationships, scope of practice, and confidentiality, refer to the book, *The Ethics of Touch* by Ben Benjamin, Ph.D., and Cherie Sohnen-Moe

Etiquette • • •

This topic concerns behaviors that generally fall under the heading of good manners. Policies need to address the following: late clients; clients who cancel appointments with less than 24 hours notice or don't show at all; hygiene (e.g., bathing and perfume); and personal habits, such as smoking on the premises, eating prior to a session or arriving in an altered state.

Personal Relationships • • •

Dual Relationships continue to be one of the most talked about subjects. As first mentioned in Chapter 5, the term dual relationships describes the overlapping of professional and social roles and interactions between two people. The classic depiction of a dual relationship is when two persons who interact professionally develop other roles of social interaction.

Some people claim that dual relationships should be avoided at all costs. But let's be real: they happen, especially in small towns or rural communities because of the limited numbers of people and choices for professional services. It's usually not a question of whether you'll have them, but how you'll handle them. And here is where policies come in.

Chapter 5, Page 85

for more information on Dual Relationships.

Think about who your first clients were—most likely friends and family. Many people find that at some point it becomes awkward juggling the roles of being a relative or friend as well as a wellness care provider. When I was in practice, one of my clients was my best friend. We had absolutely no problems for several years. Then the roles started blurring. We began chatting too much during sessions and discussing what occurred during a treatment when we were in a social setting. I created a simple ritual to transition our roles that proved to be extremely effective. Right before going into the treatment room, I would take a big step to the right and say, "Now I am your therapist and not your friend. And you are my client." After the session was over, I would take a big step to the left and say, "Now we are no longer therapist and client, but friends." That simple statement with the physical movement did the trick. Some people have very stringent policies about not working with friends or family members. There is no right or wrong here, although it's much easier if you don't have to accommodate dual relationships. You are the only one who can gauge your ability to keep clear boundaries. Even if you can work effectively in a dual relationship, you need to ask yourself if the other person can manage multiple roles.

Another aspect of working with family and friends is that they're more likely to test your policies and limits—although not always on purpose or consciously. Having clear policies makes enforcement less awkward.

Sexual Activity in a therapeutic context is never appropriate (unless you're a licensed sex therapist). Sexual inappropriateness on behalf of the client or practitioner isn't always easily defined. In addition to being clear with your own boundaries, it helps to set guidelines for your clients that include interactions and scope of practice.

Client Policies

- List your client interaction policies for finances, communication, scope of practice, etiquette and personal relationships.
- Specify what your clients can expect of you.
- Clarify how you will handle the "bending" of policies (e.g., a client forgets her checkbook or a client thought you were going to bill the insurance company).

Figure 12.3

Sample Client Interaction Policy Form

My requirements of clients:

1. Sessions begin and end at scheduled times. Sessions that begin late because the client arrived late end at the appointed time and are full price.
2. Be present (not under the influence of alcohol or drugs).
3. Clients provide a health history and update when necessary.
4. If cancellation is necessary, please give 24-hour notice or you are charged for the appointment unless it can be filled. Emergency cancellations are determined at the practitioner's discretion.
5. Payment is expected at the time service is rendered.
6. On outcall appointments if a client does not arrive within 15 minutes of the appointed time, he is charged for the appointment.
7. Sexual harassment is not tolerated. If the practitioner's safety feels compromised, the session is ended immediately.
8. This office is a nonsmoking environment.

For touch therapists, also include:

9. Be clean, having showered the same day as the treatment.
10. Do not eat a heavy meal less than two hours prior to the treatment.

What clients can expect from me:

1. I provide my clients with a competent and professional session each time they come for an appointment, addressing the client's specific needs for that session.
2. I am available to my clients between the hours of 8 a.m. and 6 p.m., and clients may reach me through my answering service on a 24-hour basis.
3. I return calls within 24 hours unless I am out of town.
4. Clients are treated with respect and dignity.
5. I charge a fair price for my services and offer a sliding fee scale when appropriate.
6. Payment is due at the time of service unless other arrangements have been made prior to treatment. I accept cash, checks and credit cards.
7. I do not provide direct billing for insurance. I will gladly assist clients in filling out the appropriate forms.
8. Appointments are confirmed the day before the session.
9. I perform services for which I am qualified (physically and emotionally) and able to do, and refer my clients to appropriate specialists when work is not within my scope of practice or not in the client's best interest.
10. I keep accurate records and review charts before each session.
11. I customize my treatment to meet the client's needs.
12. I stay current with information and techniques by reading, receiving regular sessions (of the same service I provide) and taking at least one workshop per year.
13. I respect all clients regardless of their age, gender, race, national origin, sexual orientation, religion, socioeconomic status, body type, political affiliation, state of health or personal habits.
14. Privacy and confidentiality are maintained at all times.
15. If I need to cancel an appointment, I do so within 24 hours whenever possible. If an emergency arises and I cannot keep an appointment, I provide a 50 percent discount on a client's next session. For nonemergency cancellations of less than 24 hours, the next session is at no charge.
16. My equipment and supplies are clean and safe.
17. Personal and professional boundaries are respected at all times.
18. If a client is dissatisfied with a treatment, and no other arrangement can be agreed upon, a 50 percent refund of the treatment is honored.
19. Clients may return for refund any unused products (in saleable condition) within 10 days of purchase.

For touch therapists, also include:

20. Clients are draped with a sheet or towel at all times during the session. Only the parts of the body being worked on are exposed at any time.

12

Procedure Manual •

A procedure manual defines operational best practices and methods to accomplish daily, weekly and monthly business tasks. Describe how you want to start each day (what needs to be done the moment the first person arrives to open the facility). Identify important daily activities. For instance, specify the following: phone etiquette; how to handle paperwork and client files; equipment operation and maintenance; how to write up sales; safety procedures and what to do in case of an emergency. Also define procedures for bookkeeping, routine business activities, client interactions (e.g., the way you want clients greeted, the forms they must fill out, financial arrangements, rescheduling, dispensing educational materials), and how to close the office at the end of the day.

Risk Management • •

Risk management activities minimize the risk a company may encounter for physical, emotional and mental liability involving its employees, clients, visitors and products. These activities also pertain to insurance liabilities for loss due to theft, fire, chemical hazards, neglect and misuse. Many large companies have Risk Management Departments, whose sole purpose is to analyze the physical layout of buildings, prepare ergonomically designed work space, assist employees in being comfortable (therefore more productive) in their working conditions, look for potential hazards, make sure comprehensive and liability insurance coverages are adequate, and assess and develop plans for any other problems that may put the company "at risk."

Within the realm of a small business, careful attention is required to manage and minimize risks. Implementing effective risk management practices and policies saves time and money, and may help to avoid costly lawsuits.

Figure 12.4

Risk Management Factors

- Condition of the building you're in
- Escape routes in case of fire
- How you position yourself as you work
- Ergonomic safeguards to avoid or minimize repetitive use syndrome
- Making sure you have adequate malpractice, liability and medical coverage
- Ample lighting (particularly if people work at night)
- Potential hazards for clients as they use your facilities
- Employee stress levels
- Proper use of equipment

After analyzing your working and client conditions at all levels, take care of any problems which can be eliminated, and make plans to minimize any that you cannot completely resolve. In a nutshell, manage your risks before they become crises.

www.businessmastery.us/
barrier-free.php
for information on a barrier-free practice.

For further information, contact the Occupational Safety and Health Administration (OSHA) which may be listed in the state government section of the phone book under the heading "Industrial Commission" or "State Compensation Fund, Legal Division"

Policy and Procedure Manual Draft

- Describe your philosophy toward your profession in general.
- Describe your philosophy and attitude toward your business in particular.
- Describe how you want to run your business.
- Sketch your procedure manual.
- Detail policies that apply to staff and clients.

• Make Smart Technology Choices •

Smart technology choices help simplify business logistics, reduce overhead and cost-effectively market your wellness services. From computers to copiers to cellular phones and answering systems, the tools you rely on each day to communicate with clients and operate your business can provide a competitive edge and boost productivity.

Especially for group practices, web-based capabilities such as online scheduling and marketing promotions are strong competitive differentiators. They can increase revenues and repeat business. In fact, studies show that customers who can serve themselves on a website are 30-40 percent more loyal.[1]

As with everything you purchase, check the warranties and keep all documentation.

Figure 12.5

Assessing Technology Needs

- Will it reduce my expenses?
- Will it increase my income?
- Will it save me time?
- How much does maintenance and supplies cost?
- How long will it take me, or how much will it cost to install?
- Am I willing to make the effort to learn how to properly use and maintain the equipment and software I need?

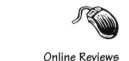

Online Reviews
www.consumersearch.com

12

Business Software *

Save time and energy in running the business side of your practice by using the right business software. Some programs are custom-designed for wellness practices, others are created for multipurpose business use. Listed below are some core business functions that you may want to automate using business software (Figure 12.6).

Figure 12.6

Software Capabilities

- Client scheduling
- Client database
- Client charting notes
- Accounting and taxes
- Human resources recordkeeping

- Insurance billing
- Project tracking
- Website setup and maintenance
- Automatic hard-drive backup
- Marketing materials design

First, decide what functions you want to computerize. Then expect to spend a few hours exploring options. One of the best ways to find user-friendly software is to ask other wellness practitioners what has worked well for them. Articles in trade magazines that focus on making smart technology choices are also a good source of practical tips and insights. You can also check out customer reviews on Internet sites such as amazon.com.

As you shop for software, make sure it's compatible with your computer's hardware, especially if you own an older model computer or handheld device. Check the minimum specifications of the software against the capabilities of your hardware.

Ideally, you would plan to attend hands-on training to learn new software. However, don't despair if this isn't possible or practical. Many software programs include online tutorials or help menus that you can use to master basic skills. Keep in mind that although your learning curve may seem steep in the beginning, hands-on practice—and a little coaching from tech-savvy friends or colleagues—is the key to mastery.

If you aren't computer savvy, consider hiring a technical expert to install the software on your computer and give you a basic tour of how it works. In most cases when you purchase software, install it and register it, updates are automatically downloaded to your computer.

Finally, explore options for automatic backup of your computer data to an external hard drive that doubles as a fully compatible replacement drive with a complete system image. In the event that your hard drive fails, this replacement drive can be installed in its place, avoiding many headaches and ensuring business continuity.

Before you purchase software or hardware, call the manufacturer's toll-free help line. How they handle your call (e.g., if you can't get through, are put on hold for what seems like an eternity or they don't promptly return messages) helps you determine whether you want to deal with them.

Business Software Capabilities ..

Accessing Information • • •

Utilize a database program to provide accurate analysis of any part of your business by setting up fields for the information, compiling them into reports and printing them out—all in a matter of minutes. For example, you can choose a single client or group of clients to contact with information (all based on certain criteria you select, such as locale or profession), analyze how often certain modalities are being requested, and evaluate marketing effectiveness (by setting fields to tell you which resources referred clients).

Recordkeeping and Financial Analysis • • •

Simplify your bookkeeping efforts and reduce the amount of time spent in recordkeeping. This type of software allows you to print checks from your computer and it automatically puts the information in all the appropriate places. You can examine expenses by category and do financial projections. Preparing taxes becomes a matter of a simple command stroke and voila, everything you or your accountant needs is in a printed report.

Personal Information Managers (PIMs) • • •

Computer calendars and address books help you manage your time and can automatically remind you about appointments, birthdays and follow-up calls.

Client Management • • •

These programs range in features from keeping client charts, preparing insurance billing forms, analyzing information, invoicing and sending follow-up correspondence.

Marketing Strategies • • •

Once you establish your marketing strategy, the computer can become your best ally in implementing your plan. With the ability to set criteria, select appropriate clients and handle functions such as mail merge and labeling, you can quickly get communications out to your target market(s).

Desktop Publishing • • •

Many programs can design business cards, brochures, fliers and newsletters. Some word processing software programs include basic desktop publishing, but most people purchase a separate program. The price (and commensurate features) range from less than $50 to nearly $1,000. Most of these programs come with templates, so all you need to do is type in the text. Several paper companies design products to work with these templates.

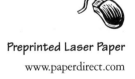

Preprinted Laser Paper
www.paperdirect.com

12

Online Scheduling • • •

Online scheduling is a great tool to enhance customer satisfaction and help you work smarter. It can minimize frustrating rounds of telephone tag, and save both you and your clients valuable time. Practitioners often find that online scheduling increases bookings from clients who appreciate the added convenience. It is an easy and affordable way to increase productivity and enhance customer service. Plus you can check and update your calendar from anywhere—home or office.

Using this software capability, clients can schedule appointments 24 hours a day at their convenience. Likewise, you can easily set single or standing appointments for customers when you see them in your office. If a customer needs to cancel or change an appointment, it's easy for them to do so online. In a spa or group practice environment, a receptionist can use the ease and flexibility of online scheduling to book and track appointments. You can also use online scheduling software to manage client contact information.

Another time-saving feature applies to tracking a client's package use. For instance, if your business sells packages, such as a package of 10 sessions, the software lets both staff and your clients know the number of remaining sessions. Usually the type of packages that can be set up are number of sessions, dollar amount or flat monthly fee.

Online Schedulers

www.bookingcalendar.com
www.appointment-plus.com
www.flashappointments.com
www.genbook.com

Setting up service is simple. You don't need to install any scheduling software on your computer to use the system. All you need is an Internet connection and some time to locate and evaluate service providers with a track record of success and outstanding customer service. Because your critical scheduling and operational data is stored on the company's remote server, it's important to evaluate what data security measures are in place to protect your data from harm—whether from natural disasters or data center events such as fire. Plus, the data needs to be secure to meet HIPAA regulations. Ask questions about these aspects of a service provider's operations before you sign on the dotted line.

Telephones •

What could possibly be said about a telephone besides the obvious: every business needs one. They've come a long way from the rotary dial, single line phone. Yesterday's optional phone services—such as caller ID, call waiting, call forwarding and voice messaging—are today's must haves. If you lean toward high-tech solutions, personal digital assistants (PDAs), such as BlackBerry, Treo and iPhone, offer mobile smart phones that combine access to phone, web browsing and email functionality.

Chapter 6, Pages 120-124

for ideas on telephone etiquette.

Headsets are handy when making lengthy calls or several calls in a row—either with a land line phone or a cell phone. This is far more comfortable than holding a phone to your ear. If you need to write while talking, a headset frees you from craning your neck to wedge a handset in place. It is also smart ergonomics, which means headsets may help to avoid muscle strain and headaches.

Not only are cell phones important for emergencies while traveling, they offer added convenience when scheduling, contacting clients and conducting business while in transit or in an area where a phone isn't available.

While cell phones offer convenience and safety, no one knows for sure what the long-term health effects on brain cells will be. The following are some simple safety precautions from George C. Carlo, Ph.D, researcher and cell phone safety advocate, from the Science and Public Policy Institute.

- Keep cell phone usage to a minimum, and turn off your phone when not in use.
- Use a nonmetal headset whenever possible to keep the phone out of direct contact with your body.
- Check to see if your phone has any type of noise-field technology, and if so, use it.

Your phone system is your primary link with clients, associates and vendors—in effect, all aspects of your business. Choosing the services and appropriate phone system is paramount. Research the different models and consult with a phone representative to assist you in making the best choices for your circumstances.

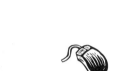

Caution!

Be careful if you drive and talk. It's a distraction and can cause an accident. It's also illegal in many places. Consider pulling over to make calls.

Cell Phone Safety

safewireless.org

Pagers

These relatively inexpensive gadgets have low monthly fees and provide you with 24-hour access nationwide. You can choose between numeric pagers and alphanumeric pagers that show you the phone number and a short message. There are two-way pagers that let you receive a message and respond directly from the unit. There are also voice pagers that serve as a portable answering machine and pager combination.

Message Systems

For those times in session or away from the office, there must be a system in place to receive your business calls. Some people use answering machines, others voice mail, and some use a combination of both. Many practitioners utilize answering services so their business contacts can speak with a person. Keep in mind that when people are trying to schedule a same-day appointment, they will often call different places until they get a live person to answer a phone. Ideally, have a live person who is knowledgeable and can schedule appointments.

Answering Machines

Answering machines vary in cost and capability. They provide a means to stay in communication with clients and business associates. Make sure you have a brief, warm, informational greeting (be aware of background noise) and that your machine works properly. There is nothing more annoying than a beep that is loud and shrill and goes on for what seems like forever. It is also handy to retrieve messages remotely by punching in an access code.

12

Answering Services ● ●

Answering services provides a human touch, which is often lacking in the business world, but they also leave things open to human error. Find a service that has a track record for accuracy, dependability and timeliness. Make sure to provide all pertinent information regarding your practice so questions can be answered correctly. Give your service up-to-date scheduling information and stay in communication with the service on a regular basis throughout your day.

Voice Mail Services ● ●

Voice mail is electronic messaging. Voice mail is usually more dependable and more easily accessible than an answering machine. One of the prime benefits is that many people can call at the same time and not receive a busy signal. Most services can receive at least 15 simultaneous calls. This type of service is available through your local or long distance carrier, and the monthly service fee is well worth the uninterrupted service and ease of retrieving messages. Be sure to create a welcoming greeting providing necessary information.

Fax Machines ●

Fax machines come in two major styles; a stand-alone model or a hardware/software combination you install on your computer. Even with the advent of the fax/modem, a stand-alone fax machine still comes in pretty handy. It is usually easier to put a document through the fax machine than to scan it into the computer, attach it to your fax and send it.

Photocopiers ●

Photocopiers range from very simple, relatively inexpensive desktop units to machines that do everything except go to the post office for you. You can spend a couple hundred dollars or many thousands depending on what you need. Having quick access to a copier can save time (not having to run out to make a few copies) and provide clients with important information without having them wait.

Choosing a copier can be an adventure since there are so many that do different tasks at varying speeds. Again, deciding on your needs will narrow the field. Copier companies are willing to bring machines to you for a trial period. Pick out several brands and see how they work. Compare features, cost per copy, maintenance agreement coverages and costs, trade-in allowances for the future, speed, and service availability. In many cases, having a full maintenance agreement covering all parts and labor is a good investment that saves you time and money.

You can get equipment that has copier, fax, scanning, and printing functions all in one!

Computers ●

Until the 1980s, most office documentation was done on a typewriter. Then word processing typewriters arrived on the scene, paving the way for the eventual emergence of personal computers (PCs) and Apple MacIntosh computers.

Despite advertising claims, computers aren't like toasters—they're more like automobiles. There is more to owning a computer than simply buying it and plugging it in the wall. You need to learn the special terminology (e.g., megabyte, RAM and hard disk), perform regular maintenance (e.g., file organization, cleaning and back-ups) and buy accessories. Fortunately, today's plug-and-play software makes it easier than ever for a computer novice to get up and running fairly easily.

While the Apple MacIntosh software and operating system still rules when it comes to graphics and is extremely user-friendly, it isn't as popular as the Microsoft Windows operating system for personal computers. Windows currently dominates the market, and the programs for PCs are generally less expensive than for MacIntosh. The system power and speed requirements depend on how you plan to use your computer.

First, determine what you want the computer to do. Decide which software you want. Software choices often determine computer choice due to many factors such as the amount of disk space the programs use and the speed you want. Some programs are only available for one platform.

Mail order is a source for saving on computer hardware and software costs. However, you need to be fairly computer literate to choose what you need, install additional hardware, load programs and learn how to use the software. If you aren't confident about your computer knowledge, establish a relationship with a local supplier who can furnish you with recommendations and continued support after purchases are made.

There are computer consultants available who design systems based on your needs, help you get the best prices, provide tutoring and troubleshoot problems. Of course, you're paying for their services in addition to the costs of hardware and software.

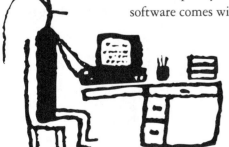

Once you know what you want, get supplier referrals from associates and friends. Call each one and explain your needs. Ask for price quotes, clarify what bundled software comes with the system (some include office software and games), determine warranty information and ascertain service time frames. Discuss purchasing and leasing options. Obtain pricing on each component of your system; ask for a package deal to include the entire system, training, maintenance agreement and support. Be sure to shop around to get the best price.

Once technology is out of the jar, you can't put it back in.
— Ervin L. Glaspy

12

Figure 12.7

Top 10 Reasons to Buy a Business Computer

1. Keep up with the Information Age.
2. Communicate with colleagues and the online public.
3. Access information and research.
4. Manage your business.
5. Maintain client files.
6. Bill insurance electronically.
7. Create documents with desktop publishing.
8. Archive data.
9. Educate yourself.
10. Market your practice.

Notebook Computers ● ●

Today's notebooks offer many of the same features as a desktop computer with added mobility. Most people adjust easily to the smaller keyboard of a notebook computer and don't mind using a touch pad instead of a mouse. If you travel outside of your office often, a notebook may be a good choice. Owning both a desktop and notebook computer is ideal, if you can afford it.

Features to Consider ● ● ●

Additional Batteries: You need an additional battery if you plan to use your portable on a plane or in an area with no electrical outlet. The following are battery types in order of longevity: lithium ion, nickel-metal hydride and nickel-cadmium.

Battery Life: Your battery will usually last two to four hours with constant access to the hard drive. However, most portables come with software that helps manage power use to maximize battery usage, generally doubling the minimum time.

Pointing Device: Your choices include trackballs, trackpads or keyboard buttons called trackpoints. The trackpad is the most popular (utilizing your finger as the means to get around the screen). Next are trackpoints and then the trackball. The standard mouse is awkward on the lap.

Power Supply: While most portables come with external AC adapters, some have built-in power supplies, which means all you need is a power cord and an AC outlet.

Weight: You are looking at carrying around about six pounds plus the weight of an adapter, a cord, batteries, carrying case, disks and whatever else fits in your case. There are "sub-notebooks" available weighing about four pounds plus paraphernalia.

Personal Digital Assistants (PDAs) *

For many business people, notebook computers are unwieldy. PDAs are compact (handheld) and travel easily. These units provide limited computing and electronic communication. You can connect them to your computer or electronic notebook and transfer information. These lightweight assistants can help you schedule meetings while on the run, take notes during meetings, track expenses, write letters, make airline reservations, check your email and do market research on the Internet. The most popular PDAs are the Palm Pilot, Apple Newton, BlackBerry and the PocketPC. Newer models also have both color screens and audio capabilities, enabling them to be used as mobile phones (smartphones), web browsers, or portable media players.

Printers *

The two most widely used printers are laser and inkjet printers. Inkjet printers spray tiny droplets of ink into patterns on a page. Inkjet printers are primarily used for color and can be purchased for under $100. If you mainly use your printer for black-and-white printing (e.g., correspondence and basic marketing materials), consider the laser printer. Laser printers use a laser to electrostatically imprint information on a page (this eliminates the smudging problems often encountered with inkjet printers). They are faster, quieter and provide the clearest print. Color laser printers are becoming more popular, although the cost is usually prohibitive for most businesses—with the exception of the graphics industry.

The Internet *

The Internet offers a wealth of resources for your business. First, you need to set up an Internet Digital Subscriber Line (DSL) or cable account with a local cable or telephone company. Monthly service fees and access vary, so it's a good idea to shop around. Once you get your high-speed DSL or cable connection in place, you can connect to the Internet via browser software such as Apple® Safari, Opera Software® Opera, Mozilla® Firefox or Microsoft Internet Explorer®.

Through email software—either installed on your computer or through an Internet service provider such as Yahoo or Google—you can easily and quickly communicate with clients and co-workers. Whether your email contact is in your hometown or halfway around the world in India on vacation, you can seamlessly coordinate business logistics or share insights into challenging case studies. You can also use the Internet to order supplies, manage online banking and bill paying tasks, access trade journal articles, locate the latest research, register for continuing education seminars, and post job openings.

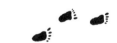

Chapter 16, Page 401-409
for online marketing tips.

12

• Office Organization •

While it might take some time to organize your office for maximum productivity, once you get the systems in place, you're free to concentrate on working with clients. The major areas involve planning, managing paper and operations. Two keys to avoiding clutter are: designate a proper place for keeping your records; and establish a routine for when and how you attend to specific tasks.

The Paperless Office •

The paperless office is still a dream for most of us. Even with the advent of PCs, scanners and email, a lot of paper passes through our hands on a daily basis. Many practitioners rely on paper for their client records and financial management. Use a laptop or desktop computer as much as possible. Time is the most important commodity practitioners possess. The increased productivity, time savings and enhanced service that technology provides more than compensate for your learning-curve efforts and expenditures.

First review your files and purge outdated or irrelevant materials. Discard instruction manuals on equipment you no longer use. A common contributor to clutter is keeping numerous copies of the same item. Usually one copy is enough, although you might keep a duplicate if the item has an artistic value (e.g., a beautifully designed, multicolored brochure). Use a paper shredder if the information to be disposed of is related to clients or finances. Put inactive files and past records in storage boxes. Label the boxes and put them in a secure place. Archived files should be kept in a separate filing cabinet or storage box. Store your critical financial records in a fireproof case, or take them to a place that specializes in archiving documents (this also holds true for computer files).

Get Organized Now! •

The first step to getting organized is to establish a space that's dedicated exclusively to your business. This area would include: a writing surface (preferably a desk), an ergonomic chair, a desk lamp, a filing drawer or cabinet, and a collection of office supplies.

Having difficulty finding needed information is the most common form of office inefficiency. This applies to paper systems as well as computers. Consider the various business activities you engage in and design a structure to deal with them.

Minimize handling of paper. Begin by dividing all paperwork into four initial categories: take action; file; get rid of it; read or review later. The primary purpose of a filing system is easy retrieval, not storage. Ideally you would have at least three separate filing drawers: client records; current projects, upcoming events and financial management; and resources.

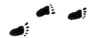

Chapter 14, Page 287

for a list of how long records should be kept.

Mail ● ●

We spend an incredible amount of time dealing with mail. Set a specific time of day to open mail. Avoid going through your mail if you do not have the time to appropriately process it. The goal is to handle mail once. First, choose a place for opening mail that's next to a filing center, trash can and paper-recycling bin. Use a letter opener—it saves time, keeps things neat, and, most importantly, alleviates paper cuts. Whenever possible, take immediate action such as write a return letter, file the information in resources, or trash it.

Phone Calls and Messages ● ●

The key to managing the telephone is to be prepared logistically and mentally. You don't want to keep callers waiting while you search for supplies or information. Store needed provisions (e.g., paper, pen, appointment book, and new client checklist) within reach. Keep a message pad next to the phone and return calls within 24 hours.

Contacts ● ●

Keep track of contacts and potential business resources. Use your computer contact manager or place sheets (purchase predesigned forms or make your own) in a binder with alphabetical dividers. Give each contact a separate sheet. Some of the information to include is the person's name, company, title, work address and phone number, home address and phone number, email address, who referred you, where you met, any personal or professional information that you want, and action to be taken. Transfer the items from the action to be taken section to your tickler file or appointment book. You might also want to list the dates and times of any actions directly onto the contact form. This is particularly helpful as a document to record business interactions. For example, you get a bid for supplies over the phone and you place an order. Then you get your bill, and it's for a different price. You are more likely to resolve the difference in your favor if you can say, "I talked with Ann Alleby on Tuesday, August 17th, at 3:20 p.m. and was told...."

Storing business cards can be frustrating. They can be filed by name, company, or type of business. Choose a method and stick to it. Otherwise, you'll spend a lot of time attempting to remember which way you filed that specific card. If you have extra cards, then you can file by each category (the downside to this option is that your business card holder gets filled extremely quickly). Options for storing business cards include using a Rolodex® type of system, inserting cards in binder sleeves or stapling the cards to contact sheets.

Client Files ● ●

Keep client files in alphabetical order. Determine what client information and forms you want included in each client folder. Design a one-page checklist and staple it to the left side of the folder. On the top of the form put the client contact information. Then include other details that you deem important, such as who referred the client; insurance data; and physician contact information.

Contact/Referral Record
www.businessmastery.us/
forms.php#busman

Chapter 16, Pages 357-360
for Networking Tips.

Review your contacts at least every two months.

Designate a section that lists filled-out forms to be put in the folder (e.g., client intake, insurance verification, treatment plan and HIPAA forms). Be sure to leave space next to each item to put the date when the form was placed in the file. If you do not have a computerized tickler file, consider putting a follow-up section on the bottom of the page so you can easily see when you last made contact.

Review all client files at least twice a year. See if you can re-establish connections and if not, consider these inactive files and archive them. There is no federal guideline for how long client records must be kept, although some states do have specific laws. In general, keep all records at least 10 years (indefinitely is ideal).

If you do a lot of work on the road, purchase a portable file carrier. Stock it with your promotional materials, client materials, a receipt envelope, and supplies (e.g., a calculator, receipts, pens, and paper clips). Each morning, go to your master filing system, pull the client files on the specific clients you'll be seeing that day, and add those files to the portable carrier.

Projects • •

Create a separate file for every project you work on. Whenever you come across information pertaining to a particular project, immediately put it in the proper folder. Once the project is complete, sort through the file and put into your resource folders any information that could be useful in the future. Then archive or throw away (if possible, recycle) the rest of the file's contents.

Upcoming Events • •

Develop a tickler file for upcoming events. A tickler file reminds you of your commitments and assists in follow-through. Essentially, it contains 12 separate sections (one for each month) and a set of dividers numbered 1-31, for each day of the month. You can put these in a three-ring binder, an accordion file or hanging files. Place the 31 dividers in the "Current Month" section. Then, if someone asks you to contact them in two weeks, you go to your tickler file, turn to the corresponding date, and make a note to call that person. Check your tickler file daily. Look at the current day and possibly the next two days. If you own a computer, you can purchase planning software programs that include tickler systems.

The true beauty of a tickler file is for keeping track of future events. For example, a client is going out of town for the summer and asks you to call back on September 12th. You put a note in the September section of your file. When it's the end of August and you transfer your 31 dividers to September, you would put the note under 12. Using this system helps ensure that you won't forget your commitments. Various computer programs do this automatically. Even if you use a computerized tickler system, a physical tickler folder is handy for keeping paperwork associated with the activities on the various dates.

Financial Management ● ●

The rule of thumb for financial recordkeeping is: Keep all receipts. A corollary is: Jot down expenses when receipts are unavailable. Keep all receipts in one place, and post them on either a weekly or monthly basis to ease the paperwork burden at income tax time.

The two major ways for keeping financial receipts are: by the category (place receipts in separate folders according to type, such as "Marketing Expenses"or "Supplies"); or by the date (one file folder for each month of the year). Keep in mind that even though you do your bookkeeping on a computer, you still need to keep receipts.

Resources ● ●

This group of files can easily get unwieldy. What may work well is to store magazines and journals on a shelf, and put newsletters into a binder. Sort loose papers by subject. Oftentimes an article or piece of information could go in several places. A solution is to make copies and put them in the various places. A paper-conserving idea is to put the information in one folder, and then make a note on the inside of the other folders referencing the folder where the information is stored. Significantly reduce the amount of paper you accumulate (such as magazine articles), by scanning them into your computer using a good cross-indexing program. If you need materials from your master files to go into a project folder, either make a copy or note in the master folder as to where the resource material has been moved.

Figure 12.8

Filing Tips

Managing Paper:
- File materials immediately with the most current materials in the front.
- Files should be in use or put away.
- Label and color code file folders.
- Separate active files from archive files.
- Don't overstuff folders—create subfiles.
- Ease filing by reducing oversized documents to letter size.
- When a project is finished or a client is inactive, remove extraneous material from the file and archive the rest.

Organizing Computer Information:
- Use the same names for computer directories, folders and files that you label your paper documentation storage.
- Back up your files regularly and store them in a fireproof box or off premises.
- Eliminate inactive files on a monthly basis.

Protecting Your Records ✳

Any number of mishaps and catastrophes can occur in a place of business. One of the most common is damaged or lost computer data due to viruses, hard drive failures, spilling liquids or food onto the computer, or energy spikes. Other culprits are theft or property damage due to vandalism, critter infestation, broken water pipes, fire, smoke and acts of nature. The good news is that you can take proactive measures to limit damages caused by an unforeseen catastrophe and speed recovery.

Figure 12.9

How to Protect Your Records

Emergency Contact List	Keep a list of who should be notified in the event of a disaster: insurance agent; lawyer; clients; colleagues; suppliers; employees; property manager or owner.
Key Documents	Maintain a copy of key documents (e.g., bank account, loan papers, client files, tax records, accounts receivables, back-up files) off-site.
Computer Back-Up	Regularly back up your computer information onto a CD or back-up tape and archive off-site or in a fire-proof box (a bank safety deposit box is good for this).
Insurance Recordkeeping	Store insurance related information such as photographs, major receipts, and identifying information of your insured assets (e.g., model numbers and year purchased) in a fire-proof box or off-site.

✳ Health Insurance Portability and Accountability Act ✳

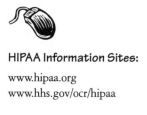

HIPAA Information Sites:

www.hipaa.org
www.hhs.gov/ocr/hipaa

In 1996, the Health Insurance Portability and Accountability Act (HIPAA), was passed, and healthcare providers (and other agents) were mandated to comply with its requirements as of April 2003. HIPAA has three major purposes: (1) to protect and enhance the rights of consumers by providing them access to their health information and controlling the inappropriate use of that information; (2) to improve the quality of healthcare in the United States by restoring trust in the healthcare system among consumers, healthcare professionals, and the multitude of organizations and individuals committed to the delivery of care; and (3) to improve the efficiency and effectiveness of heathcare delivery by creating a national framework for health privacy protection that builds on efforts by states, health systems, individual organizations and individuals.

The Four Facets of HIPAA

1. **Electronic Health Transactions Standards:** When billing insurance, practitioners are required to use the Standard Code Sets of the International Classification of Disease (ICD-10) codes and the Current Procedural Terminology (CPT) codes.
2. **Unique Identifiers for Providers, Employers, Health Plans and Clients:** Each practitioner who transmits information electronically is assigned a National Provider Identifier (NPI).
3. **Security of Health Information and Electronic Signature Standards:** All practitioners must provide uniform levels of protection of all health information that is stored or transmitted electronically. This includes your computer, along with any faxes and email messages sent. An electronic signature is required for all HIPAA transactions.
4. **Privacy and Confidentiality:** Limits the nonconsensual use and release of private health information; gives clients new rights to access their medical records and to know who else has accessed them; restricts most disclosure of health information to the minimum needed for the intended purpose; institutes criminal and civil sanctions for improper use or disclosure; and establishes new requirements for access to records by researchers and others.

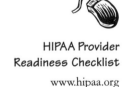

Get your Assigned National Provider Identifier

www.cms.hhs.gov/ NProvidentStand

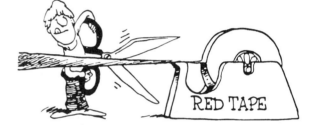

Who Must Comply with HIPAA Regulations? •

Unfortunately, the answer is not straightforward. In the December 2, 2002 issue of the *Atlanta Business Chronicle*, journalist Julie Bryant stated, "What was to be a simple federal rule, designed to lift the healthcare industry out of antiquated paper-based systems and into the bright, organized world of high-speed technology, has instead spawned hysteria, predatory opportunists and outright befuddlement."

Many companies are charging thousands of dollars to provide businesses with training, guidelines and forms to ensure HIPAA compliance. Caution is advised before investing in these programs, particularly since it's still not clear exactly what is required of all wellness practitioners.

HIPAA Provider Readiness Checklist

www.hipaa.org

The current emphasis of HIPAA compliance centers on electronic transmission of a client's Protected Health Information (PHI). When you go to the HIPAA site, review the readiness checklist to determine if you're a Covered Entity. Many wellness practitioners (unless they bill insurance) will find that indeed they are not required to be HIPAA compliant. Unfortunately, this is misleading, because there are still the privacy considerations that apply to many wellness practitioners.

12

Following the HIPAA guidelines actually makes good business sense, and the requirements are fairly easy to implement. Consumers are used to receiving privacy policy statements from other healthcare providers as well as from a myriad of other business such as insurance carriers and credit card companies. Your clients might find it disconcerting if you don't follow suit.

Note that even if you do not need to be HIPAA compliant for your own practice, you still need to be compliant if you work with other covered entities. The term for this is a "chain of trust." If you're a Business Associate, you must meet the same requirements for privacy and security as if you were a covered entity.

Chapter 6, Pages 110-112 for information on charting.

According to the HIPAA regulations, a Business Associate is defined as: persons, companies or entities hired by the practitioner to perform duties, requiring access, the use of, or disclosure of a client's PHI. Thus, if a primary care provider refers a client to you or you send a client's progress report to her doctor, then you're considered a Business Associate. There is a form that Business Associates must sign. If you currently work with other providers and haven't received one of these forms, you will soon! Also, be aware that your state regulations might be more stringent than the federal requirements.

Myths

www.businessmastery.us/ forms.php#hipaa_form for sample HIPAA forms.

Some of the confusion about client privacy has led to unnecessary changes. Myths abound regarding using a client's name and client paperwork such as sign-in sheets and files. It is fine to greet your client by name even if others are in the waiting room. You can still have client sign-in sheets as long as they don't disclose any PHI. You can put clients' charts on the treatment room doors as long as the clients' names don't show and unauthorized people can't have access to the charts. For instance, if people have to walk past a treatment room to get to the bathroom, then it might not be wise to put a chart on that treatment room door.

Penalties for Noncompliance

Failure to heed the HIPAA regulations can result in civil and criminal penalties, starting at $100 per person per violation and not exceeding $25,000 per year per person. The penalties get worse for knowingly violating HIPAA, especially if the offense is "under false pretenses" in which case there's a potential fine of up to $100,000 and/or imprisonment up to five years. If the offense is with intent to sell a client's information, the penalty is up to $250,000 and 10 years' imprisonment.

Steps to Implement Now

If you work with insurance reimbursement, it's wise to immediately follow the HIPAA compliancy guidelines. If you're a covered entity, compliance is mandatory. Regardless of insurance issues, it's vital that you take appropriate measures to ensure the privacy, confidentiality and security of clients' personal health information and records. More clarity will emerge as the remaining HIPAA guidelines go into effect over the next few years. (See Figure 12.10.)

Figure 12.10

HIPAA Tips

- Designate someone in your office (or hire an outside party) as a Privacy Officer. This person is responsible for creating a process to handle PHI. If you work alone, you are the privacy officer.
- Train office staff on how to handle PHI, including what circumstances PHI may be disclosed.
- Use consent or authorization documents that clients sign.
- Do not discuss any medical information with any third parties unless written consent or authorization has been obtained.
- Be careful when discussing a client's PHI with office staff. Be aware of who may overhear conversations.
- Assign User IDs and passwords to anyone with access to electronic information.
- Verify that your software is HIPAA compliant.
- Use passwords and security programs to protect and maintain computer and PDA files.
- For email, obtain written consent from the client and use secure transfer methods (encryption). Use electronic signatures to authenticate who sent the email.
- Use auditing software to monitor who sent what and when.
- Develop a policy and procedure manual that delineates how you handle all aspects of HIPAA compliance. Also designate your policy for the destruction or retention of client records that include email communications.
- Design a client information sheet that explains the following: how you use clients' information; the storage method for client files; the circumstances under which you may disclose client information; and the procedure for clients to see or obtain copies of their files.
- Store all client files in a locked room or in a locked cabinet. Only allow authorized employees access to these files.
- Do not leave files in an area that is accessible by clients or unauthorized staff.
- Keep appointment books from view of anyone except those directly dealing with client care.
- Get authorization from clients about marketing (including greeting cards, fliers and newsletters).
- Present each client with a "Notice of Privacy Policies" form.
- New clients must sign a separate form indicating that they've received the Notice of Privacy Policies.
- Each client must sign a form giving consent for treatment, payment and healthcare operations.
- When applicable, have clients sign an authorization for any and all releases of PHI.
- Put confidentiality notices on all faxes and emails.

• The Anatomy of a Contract •

Legal forms and agreements are an integral part of any business relationship, yet all too often people avoid written contracts. Whether you're interested in a one-time only interaction or a long-term affiliation, it's wise to delineate in writing your roles and expectations. Clear written agreements serve several purposes: they keep you focused on your goals, help avoid problems, and provide a predetermined method for resolving conflicts.

A verbal contract isn't worth the paper it's written on.
— Samuel Goldwyn

Figure 12.11 is a contract checklist to help you make informed choices and protect yourself legally. It defines the major elements of any contract. Sometimes this information may appear in separate documents, although it's best to combine it in one contract signed by all parties. Too many horror stories abound about people terminating business relationships and filing lawsuits due to misunderstandings that could have been averted with a solid contract. Your contracts should reflect the specific nature of your business and clearly define the expectations of all parties involved. Keep in mind that contracts are negotiable.

Ideally, you would come to the negotiating process with a sample of your own contract and the checklist, review the other party's contract, and create a contract mutually agreeable to both of you. If the other party insists on only using their contract, make sure you have responses (preferably in writing) to all the items in the checklist.

Although the contract checklist is quite substantial, most issues can be addressed in a one or two-page contract document. Sometimes an informal letter of agreement serves the same purpose, sans legalese. You may be tempted not to use a contract for presumably simple transactions, particularly if it's just a "one-time" deal. Yet it's usually those seemingly negligible events that you live to regret! Invest the time in clarifying what is truly important to you in a business relationship. Even if you're currently involved in a business relationship and don't have a contract, you can always design one now. Each situation is unique, and one contract doesn't suit all situations. Once you've crafted a basic contract, you will find it much simpler to alter any subsequent contract.

Figure 12.11

Contract Checklist

- ❏ Names and addresses of all parties involved.
- ❏ A short description and mission statement of the companies involved.
- ❏ A statement summarizing the desired role of the contracted party.
- ❏ A classification of the business relationship.
- ❏ A detailed description of what each party agrees to provide.
- ❏ A timetable for the work to be performed.
- ❏ Location of where work is to be performed.
- ❏ The duration of the contract.

  Contracts may be for a single specific event, a series of events (e.g., providing wellness care at all the bike races for a particular team for the next six months), or ongoing until either party decides to terminate the contract.

- ❏ Payment method and schedule.
- ❏ Additional benefits. (This is mainly for an employment contract. Items to consider are health insurance coverage, facilities privileges, sick time, paid vacation and discounts on products and services.)
- ❏ Opportunities for increases in financial remuneration.
- ❏ Insurance coverage provided.

  If the contract is for providing wellness services, find out if the hiring company provides workers' compensation, premise liability insurance, fire and theft insurance and medical health insurance. If you provide services as an independent contractor, it's wise to also obtain general liability insurance. It covers negligence toward clients, employees and the general public while you're on their premises. General liability insurance is good to have anyway—particularly if you do any on-site work or even public demonstrations. Unfortunately, none of these policies cover you personally, so be sure your medical health and personal disability insurance provides adequate protection.

- ❏ Insurance coverage required.

  If this contract is for wellness services, most companies require practitioners to provide their own malpractice/professional liability insurance. Malpractice insurance is usually limited to protecting you against claims due to loss incurred by your clients as a result of negligence or failure on your part to perform at a professional skill level.

- ❏ Guarantees.
- ❏ Financial obligations of the contracted party.

  This is usually included when the contract involves subcontracting and is mainly to protect the hiring party in case you do not perform your services adequately. For example, let's say a convention coordinator contracts a local company to provide 10 massage therapists for their convention. The local company hires you as a subcontractor, but for some reason you don't show up. The convention coordinator could require compensation from the local hiring party, and then the local hiring party would pass that charge onto you.

12

❑ Conditions for termination of the agreement.

Some conditions to consider are violation of the hiring company's policies and procedures, poor or nonwork performance, mismanagement of funds and untimely payment of fees due.

❑ Guidelines for transfer of the contract.

The ability to transfer your contract to another person or company is always desirable, although it won't work in all cases. Since wellness is such personal work, the hiring party may be reluctant to have a different practitioner provide the service. You can most likely include a transfer clause if you are truly an independent contractor. For example, let's say you were hired by a company to provide their staff with on-site yoga classes for eight hours per week. After a while you decide that it isn't in your best interest to do this anymore (perhaps you've moved or the other aspects of your practice are requiring all of your time). Since you were the one responsible for getting the contract (marketing, negotiating the original contract and providing the services for a time), you could easily charge a fee to another practitioner for the privilege of taking over the contract.

❑ Arbitration. This clause usually states that if an irreconcilable problem arises, the parties will take the matter before a mutually agreed upon mediator.

❑ Designate who is responsible for legal fees if a breach of contract occurs. Most often contracts state that the party who breaches the contract is responsible for the other party's legal costs.

❑ The location and contact to send communications regarding the contract.

❑ Signature lines and date the contract is signed.

• Negotiations •

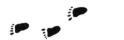

Chapter 6, Pages 107-109
for information on
active listening.

Throughout your career as a wellness practitioner, you will experience situations in which negotiation skills serve you well—such as negotiating an employment contract, vendor agreement or working arrangements with team members. On the client side, you may encounter problematic situations such as repeated cancellations, bounced checks or an unhappy customer for whom you must set boundaries and negotiate a solution agreeable to all parties.

When it comes to unhappy clients, do your best to appreciate their feedback—even it lacks tact or diplomacy. Many times you garner a kernel of useful information that may help you retain that client, or perhaps another in a similar situation. At other times, clients may be unreasonable or inconsolable due to causes beyond your control, and you must set clear and firm boundaries for what you will or will not do in response to their discontent. In all cases, be sure to thank clients for their feedback, listen carefully, and explore solutions that may work best.

The goal of all negotiations is to find a rewarding and mutually satisfying outcome for all parties. For this to occur, each person must feel truly heard and valued as an individual. Sooner or later you may run into thorny situations and unpleasant characters—such as the bully, screamer or a less than honest person—that require special skills. Fine-tune your skills by reading books about the art of negotiation. You may also find trade magazine articles that offer useful and practical insights. Like any skill, the more you practice, the more your expertise grows. Following are some tips to keep in mind when you're negotiating.

Fearless Negotiating
by Michael C. Donaldson

Beyond Reason: Using Emotions as You Negotiate
by Roger Fisher
and Daniel Shapiro

Figure 12.12

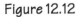

Negotiating Tips

Logistics Count
- Give careful thought to choosing the right time and the right place.

Prepare
- Get crystal clear on what you want.
- Practice stating your key points concisely.
- Get a sense of what the other party wants and how he or she will push for results.
- Determine where you will draw the line you will not cross.
- Know when to talk; know when to listen.

Negotiating Styles and Personality Dynamics
- Spend some time learning about personality types so you can adjust your communication style and better understand the person you're negotiating with.
- Seek to develop an appreciation for the healthy differences we all have.

Use Active Listening Skills
- Listen carefully to the other person and restate what he or she has said, using your own words. This helps the other party to feel heard and prevents misunderstandings.

Walk Away for Awhile
- If you come to an impasse, don't hesitate to take a break. You can say something like, "It looks like we're both bogged down here, so let's take a break to do more homework and talk again in a day or two."
- Avoid appearing overeager to come to an agreement.

Set Time Limits for Complex Negotiations
- Hearing each other's view (20 minutes).
- Brainstorming solutions (20 minutes).
- Finalizing a solution (20 minutes).

Pause and Reflect
- Before you sign on the dotted line, take a couple of hours or a few days to think things over, especially when signing contracts or agreements that involve large dollar amounts or time commitments.

12

• Conflict Management •

Honest disagreement is often a good sign of progress.
— Mahatma Ghandi

Most people hate conflict, some seem to thrive on it. Conflict can be a good thing. It can bring sensitive and controversial issues—and subtle counterproductive behaviors—to the surface so they can be resolved. The ability to skillfully navigate frustrating situations and people offers many benefits—such as more self-confidence, less anger and greater enjoyment of life. Learning conflict resolution skills is like turning on the light in a dark room. You can see your way more clearly and get to where you're going much faster.

Conflict occurs when individuals or groups aren't getting what they need or want. Sometimes an individual isn't aware of an unmet need and unconsciously starts to act out by exhibiting annoying or counterproductive behaviors. The highly effective individual is aware of what she wants and then acts to achieve a goal—using clear communication and mutual give-and-take to find a solution that satisfies all parties.

Figure 12.13

Common Sources of Conflict

- Poor communication
- Not involving people in decision-making that directly affects them
- Clashes in chemistry—rooted in either conflicting values or personality styles
- Inconsistent leadership
- Broken promises
- Lack of fairness (e.g., favoritism toward certain employees or family members)
- Lack of openness
- Violated expectations
- Poor behavior (e.g., boundary violations, not honoring commitments, disrespect)

Although uncomfortable at times, confrontation is necessary to hold people accountable for actions or inactions. Whether it's a difficult employee or co-worker, or a family member slacking off on chores, learning how to generate a positive outcome from confrontation helps strengthen relationships while solving problems. The following are tips and techniques from well-known conflict resolution experts to help build your knowledge, skills and confidence.

Figure 12.14

Dealing With Upset People

- Carefully listen to the person's concern. Also listen for the emotion behind the words.
- Refrain from venting at the person with anger or frustration. Stay centered.
- Acknowledge and reflect back the person's concern and feelings. For example, "It sounds like you're really frustrated right now. If I understand correctly...."
- Don't pacify or over-apologize. Upset people respond much better to a genuine apology that comes from strength not weakness.
- Focus on the core issues and solutions. Don't get sidetracked by unimportant details.

Figure 12.15

Effective Ways to Manage Conflict

- Agree to a mutual give-and-take in which both parties create a mind-set focused on finding a solution that meets the needs of both parties.
- Take time to gain some perspective on the conflict before entering into a conversation about the conflict.
- Identify the issue, including what you want that you aren't getting.
- Explore the conflict by talking to a friend or putting your thoughts in writing. Does the issue bother you because you're tired or angry about something else? What's your role in the conflict?
- Identify one thing you can do about the conflict.
- After you take a good look at the conflict and potential solutions, wait at least a day before you do something to address the conflict.
- Use "I statements." Avoid the use of "you statements" that place blame.
- Give your full attention to the other person when they're speaking. Do not interrupt or judge what is said.
- Practice "active listening." Ask the other person to rephrase what they heard you say. Rephrase what you hear the other person say.
- Talk in terms of the present as much as possible.
- Identify the things on which you agree and disagree.
- Focus on the issue, not the person.
- Ask: "What can we do to fix the problem?"
- If possible, identify at least one action that each of you can take to move closer to a solution
- Ask for a "cooling off period" if you come to an impasse.
- In business situations, consider seeking a third party to mediate if you have difficulty resolving a conflict.

Coward's Guide to Conflict: Empowering Solutions for Those Who Would Rather Run Than Fight
by Tim Ursiny

Crucial Conversations: Tools for Talking When Stakes are High
by K. Patterson, J. Grenny, R. McMillan, A. Switzler

Mediation and Arbitration ●

Mediation is a popular method small businesses choose to resolve business disputes. It is cheaper and faster than litigation, and oftentimes leads to a settlement that all parties find agreeable. Although some disputes wind up in arbitration, mediation is popular among those who prefer to find quick and cost-effective solutions to their problems. By relying on expert mediators trained to negotiate many types of disputes, business owners can avoid costly, time-consuming lawsuits and achieve more win-win results. Due to the growing popularity of mediation, you can easily find local, national and online resources.

Arbitration usually takes place when a business dispute or contract negotiation comes to an impasse or when mediation fails. Typically, each side takes a turn to present their case to an arbitrator, who makes a final decision. There are two kinds of arbitration—binding and nonbinding. In binding arbitration, both parties agree to accept the arbitrators final judgment. In nonbinding arbitration, both parties are free to go to court if one or other disagrees with the result. Typically, an arbitrator is a neutral third party.

Mediation Resources
www.mediate.com
www.nolopress.com

Arbitration Resources
www. adr.org
www.arb-forum.com

12

• Insurance Reimbursement •

Accepting insurance can be an incredible boon to your business. However, if not properly managed, it can bring extra stress and negatively impact your profitability. For this reason, many practitioners who accept insurance hire outside help to handle this part of the business. That way they can stay focused on clients doing what they love to do, and they don't get bogged down by the mounds of paperwork that inevitably accompany insurance processing.

Oftentimes your policy on accepting insurance can be the determining factor in whether a potential client chooses you as her wellness provider. In addition, during economic downturns, clients with insurance can help keep your income stream steady. Carefully consider these points when you evaluate whether to accept insurance.

Words have the power to both destroy and heal. When words are both true and kind, they can change our world.
— Buddha

Many practitioners are pinning a lot of hopes on the insurance industry. Look what it has done to enhance the medical profession in terms of recognition and financial compensation. The most recent example of this benefit is evidenced in the chiropractic field. We've all heard people say how much other wellness providers' credibility increases as more and more insurance companies cover their services. Perhaps so, but at what cost?

If these services become acceptable billable modalities under all third-party insurance coverage, then it makes this field a much more viable career path, because more money will be available to cover these services. And truthfully, we know that many people only utilize wellness services that are covered by insurance.

Keep in mind that the "cost of doing business" for a non-insurance case is less than that for a medically related case. A medical case involves far more time spent on documentation, processing paperwork, coordinating payment conditions, tracking payment and appealing rejected claims. When determining fees for medically related sessions, it's best to consult a business advisor or reference manual.

When it comes to determining best treatment options for clients, you will find that insurance companies are increasingly dictating to the healthcare community the types of treatments they can perform. Since the insurance companies are paying for these procedures, they're imposing stricter guidelines about what they consider acceptable care and under what conditions.

As we progress in this arena, we must strive to keep the integrity and diversity of our work intact. I think it's possible to have the whole spectrum of allied wellness covered by insurance and to provide varied techniques. To accomplish this, we must make a concerted effort to educate the primary care providers and the members of the insurance industry as well as employer groups about the different therapies, techniques and their specific benefits.

This section provides an overview of insurance processing, insights into the pros and cons of accepting insurance as payment, descriptions of the types of insurance, key definitions, and the basic steps for submitting a claim. Because this vast topic could span thousands of pages, if you decide to accept insurance, it's best to seek specialized training—either by attending a course, working with a consultant or studying a reference manual.

Insurance Claim Processing Overview ●

Let's look at the insurance industry itself. From a consumer's point of view, most of us think about health insurance as a way to ensure that our healthcare costs are covered in case of a serious illness or accident and as a means to assist in the payment for our well-being to prevent major illness. What we tend to forget is that insurance companies are just that—companies. And as such, one of their major priorities is to make a profit. Very few insurance companies hold altruistic beliefs as their main purpose for being in business; we must always remember that motivation when contemplating the role of the insurance industry.

The three main types of insurance claims are: third party (general medical health), Workers' Compensation and personal injury. Unfortunately, because insurance companies do not recognize most wellness practitioners who aren't physicians or physical therapists as "primary" healthcare providers, the insurance billing process can sometimes be cumbersome. Workers' Compensation and personal injury claims also have unique aspects that are important to understand before jumping into claim processing. The classic advice "look before you leap" certainly applies to all types of insurance reimbursement.

Third-Party Insurance Claims ● ●

Currently, insurance reimbursement is a bit erratic, particularly with third-party claims. A lot seems to depend upon the unique perspective of the claims adjustor as well as the policies of the specific insurance company. A company might honor a claim one time and refuse payment on the next. Each company has different general rules that apply to coverage and payment. Each insurance company offers a variety of insurance coverage policies, and each of those policies has its own rules and benefits. As a result, you may have conflicting experiences from the same carrier due to a difference in the terms of the policies.

In short, you can't always predict if an insurance company will authorize payments, the total amount it will cover or the number of sessions it will allow. Worse, verifying the coverage of a specific policy doesn't always guarantee payment. I know of several instances in which a massage therapist obtained verbal pre-approval for massage treatment complete with an approval code number, only to have the claim later rejected.

In view of the uncertainties surrounding insurance reimbursement, it's wise to create a statement of financial responsibility for all new clients. This clearly communicates that even with insurance, a client is ultimately responsible for any unpaid balance for sessions. This approach may not apply in certain cases, such as Workers' Compensation.

Determine how much credit you're willing to extend to a client, and over what period of time, before requiring the client to provide payment for a specified amount of the outstanding balance. Some practitioners require the client to pay up front and provide the appropriate documentation for the client to submit to his insurance company.

12

Workers' Compensation and Personal Injury Claims ••

Workers' Compensation claims account for a significant amount of money that goes toward healthcare. If you decide to accept clients with Workers' Compensation insurance, the easiest way to find the agency for your state is to look under the state government section in the phone book for a category titled either "State Compensation Fund," "Industrial Workers' Insurance" or "Workers' Compensation Board or Division." If you still are unable to locate the appropriate agency, call the general information number. The state agency can provide information about required procedures for filling out paperwork.

Personal injury claims are handled differently than most other types of insurance cases. Typically, you submit the bill directly to the claims adjustor or the attorney. In most instances, they cover everything unless the injured party's insurance requires a co-pay or deductible. Again, if you are not the primary care provider, you need a prescription from one.

To Bill or Not to Bill •

Choosing whether to accept insurance reimbursement clients (or even developing associations with primary care providers to gain referrals) is a major decision. Sometimes it becomes a spontaneous decision if a potential client comes to you with a prescription in hand; you must decide right then if you will help this client and possibly earn extra income from this source, or to refuse to work with the client's insurance.

The potential advantages are higher fees and an increased number of client sessions. The disadvantages include masses of paperwork, possible regimentation, the potential of not receiving compensation for your work and the time lag between provided service and remittance (payment). This can pretty much be alleviated by knowing what you're doing and by having proper training in working with insurance.

Keep in mind that you or your staff could spend a lot of time in verifying policies and filling out paperwork. That is why many practitioners don't accept insurance claims. They require the client to pay them directly for the services, and then the client must submit a voucher to his own insurance company (or attorney) for reimbursement. This can pose a problem in those cases in which you would in fact be reimbursed but the client may be unable to pay for the two to three treatment sessions a week that the referring physician prescribed.

In the best of all possible worlds, all wellness practitioners would be fairly and promptly reimbursed for delivering a competent service of proven effectiveness. Until (and even after) we reach that stage, you must weigh the tradeoffs inherent with the insurance bureaucracy, realizing that as your business grows, you may change your mind.

Points for Profit
by Honora Wolfe,
Eric Strand, Marilyn Allen

The Comprehensive Guide to Insurance Billing
by Vivian Madison-Mahoney

Hands Heal
by Diana L. Thompson

The following insights into insurance reimbursement are based on information provided by Vivian Madison-Mahoney, author of the *Manipulate Your Future* manual and home study course. Her expertise stems from 18 years experience operating a medically oriented massage therapy practice. Contact her at: www.massageinsurancebilling.com or by 865-436-3573.

Figure 12.16

Types of Insurance

Fee for Service: General health insurance coverage offered by an employer or other entity to an individual or a group. With this type of coverage, an insurance provider reimburses directly to the healthcare provider as long as they accept an assignment of benefits to the provider (you) from the insured person. The amount of reimbursement to a healthcare provider is based on what is termed "usual, customary and reasonable" charges.

Workers' Compensation: This insurance coverage is required in almost every state. Most employers must carry this coverage to protect employees in case of injuries on the job.

Personal Injury: Covers a multitude of situations. For the most part it means that someone was injured in an automobile accident or during a slip-and-fall accident.

No-Fault: This is referred to as personal injury protection. What this means is that in No-Fault states, if one is injured, the injured party can obtain medical treatment and have the bills submitted to her own insurance company for bills for remittance regardless of who is at fault.

Med-Pay: Refers to medical payment. This is additional coverage a person can purchase when first purchasing or renewing an auto insurance policy. This is coverage above and beyond the usual $10,000 coverage that is on a no-fault policy.

Uninsured Motorist (UM): If an uninsured driver injured the party, the injured party must have previously purchased "uninsured motorist protection" (UM) on her policy to be covered for the injury the uninsured person caused.

Medicare: A federal program that provides health benefits for those 65 years of age or over, and for those under 65 who are permanently disabled prior to age 65.

Medicaid: Medical coverage for those unable to pay for medical services due to financial hardships. Medicaid is run by both the state and federal government, with the federal government covering 55 percent and the state paying the remainder. Some states such as Tennessee do not utilize the Medicaid System. These states offer other methods of providing medical coverage.

Types of Insurance Providers ✱

To help you get acquainted with some common terminology, listed below are descriptions of the major types of insurance providers. Arrangements made between insurance companies and employers must comply with state regulations. In addition, some states now require individuals with Workers' Compensation claims to be processed through Managed Care Organizations.

Managed Care Organizations (MCOs) ✱ ✱

These entities manage costs by contracting with providers who agree to charge predetermined fees. They are administered by a *gatekeeper*, a physician who oversees the services supplied by the organization. All providers must be contracted by the MCO and approved by the gatekeeper prior to providing services to the patients. Some MCOs include complementary wellness providers.

12

Health Maintenance Organizations (HMOs) ••

A type of MCO, HMOs provide healthcare services for a fixed fee to subscribers in a specific geographic location. Plans usually cover preventive services with little or no out of pocket expenses. In most cases members must use the physicians and facilities authorized by the HMO. They typically don't reimburse complementary wellness providers unless it's written in the state law.

Preferred Provider Organizations (PPOs) ••

A type of MCO. A PPO contracts with a group of preferred providers to deliver healthcare to members. Unlike HMO members, PPO members are free to choose any physician or hospital for services, but they receive more benefits (or pay less of the cost themselves) if they choose a preferred provider. A PPO plan usually requires filing claims and paying deductibles and co-payments.

Licensing Regulations •

An **occupational license** is a license required by a city or county to sell a product or perform a service for money at a certain location. A **licensed provider** of healthcare services is a professional who obtains a state license by passing a state examination and has received a license to operate by his state professional board. Most wellness providers are allowed to see a client without a physician referral or prescription. However, for the service to be reimbursed by an insurance company, it must be considered medically necessary. Additionally, you must have a physician's diagnosis written on the prescription as well as the frequency and duration of treatment.

Unlicensed states often have restrictions and requirements to operate within their cities or counties. It is strictly up to the person providing treatment for compensation to know the specific state licensing laws, rules and regulations. In these unlicensed states, practitioners can sometimes provide services if they hold a certification in their profession. When it comes to licensing requirements, it's best to ask the insurance company what its requirements are, and to check the state statutes for both automobile and Workers' Compensation cases.

Procedure and Modality Codes •

Procedure and modality codes are critical pieces of the insurance puzzle. All insurance carriers require these codes to process insurance claims. Procedure codes are also known as Current Procedural Terminology (CPT) Codes. They indicate the type of services performed during the session to improve function. These codes are defined and maintained by the American Medical Association.

A *procedure* is the main service you provide, such as massage therapy. A *modality* is an adjunct to that procedure, such as a hot or cold pack. For example, CPT Code 97124 refers to massage therapy, each 15 minutes; CPT Code 97140 is for manual therapy techniques, each 15 minutes. CPT Code 97010 (hot and cold packs) is a modality code and can only be used one time per session. In an acupuncture scenario, CPT Code 97810 is for a basic acupuncture treatment of 15-minutes duration. Thus, if your session is 60 minutes and you included a hot pack, then you list the main procedure code three times and the modality code once (e.g., 97810, 97810, 97810, 97010)

Diagnostic Codes • •

The diagnostic codes for licensed healthcare providers are listed in an ICD-10-CM (*International Classification of Diseases-Tenth Revision-Clinical Modification*) Code Book. The diagnostic codes are used by physicians to indicate a medical condition for diagnosing and prescribing treatment and therapies for their patients. A nonphysician provider cannot diagnose a medical condition. Be sure to check with your state professional board for detailed requirements for your profession.

The Physicians' Current Procedural Terminology (CPT)™ Code Book by The American Medical Association

Basic Steps for Submitting Claims •

1. **If you aren't considered a primary care provider, you must have a written prescription from a referring physician.** The prescription must indicate the following: the procedures or modalities to be performed; the number of visits per prescription, (e.g., how many times per week for how many weeks, or the total number of visits allowed); the diagnosis, (e.g., 847.2: lumbar strain and sprain).
2. **Verify coverage.** During the call to the adjuster, confirm the following: the client does indeed have insurance; what, if any, are the deductibles; has the deductible been met, and if not, when is it due; does the patient have co-payments that need to be collected, and if so, how much.
3. **Prepare the claim form.** A new claim form now referred to as a "1500 Insurance Claim Form" has been developed. This form replaces the CMS1500 or HCFA1500 Claim forms.
4. **Submit the completed claim form.**
5. **Record the treatment session, amount billed and total amount due.**
6. **Copy all checks when received, record payment and balances due.** In instances of a personal injury case, bill the client for any amounts due if you haven't agreed to send balances to the attorney for payment at time of settlement.

Coding Resources
www.cdc.gov/nchs/about/
otheract/icd9/abticd10.htm

www.ama-assn.org/ama/pub/
category/3113.html

Ensure Efficient Claim Processing • •

When processing an insurance claim, it's advisable to check with the insurance carrier or adjuster for each client. When a client arrives to complete his initial evaluation and intake form, he should provide this contact information for you. If not, it can be obtained from the treating physician.

Obtaining verification for services can be very helpful in receiving payment. Always note the name of the insurance company representative you talk with and (if possible) get a code for verified service. Obtaining written insurance verification provides you with the most protection. When it comes to Workers' Compensation claims, you must obtain authorization from the insurance adjuster to treat the client.

Medical Forms Processing

http://officeally.com

Figure 12.17

Reasons for Denials, Delays or Reductions

1. Prescription is outdated or not included in the claim
2. Documentation not accurately or timely performed
3. Claim not submitted in a timely manner
4. CPT Codes not in scope of practice
5. Fees are more than usual, reasonable and customary
6. Accepting a type of case that would not be covered by the policy
7. Pertinent information not included on the claim form

If you aren't HIPAA compliant, don't submit claims electronically.

Pages 246-249

for details on HIPAA.

Electronic Billing

The best reason to utilize electronic billing is that this type of insurance claim gets processed and paid much more quickly. It can simplify recordkeeping and decrease the time spent processing claims. Those who submit electronic claims have fewer denials, reductions and disputes. In short, electronic billing can save you time, money and enhance your cash flow.

To date, nearly 90 percent of all insurance companies have implemented electronic claims submission to streamline operations and lower costs. Some commercial carriers don't yet accept electronic billing, even though they do accept electronic claims reports for notice of injuries. In most cases, electronic billing involves submitting a claim to an insurance provider through a clearinghouse. Many practitioners find this speeds up claim processing and minimizes errors. An electronic claim is typically submitted to the insurance provider in a digital format via a tape or diskette, or as a digital fax.

Figure 12.18

Top 10 Billing Tips

1. Submit your claims "personal & confidential" to the adjuster in charge.
2. Check your prescriptions often to make sure they haven't expired.
3. Be sure the client has provided a completed history form with all required contacts.
4. The best time to contact insurance companies for verification or authorization is during the middle of the week and not around lunch or closing time.
5. Have a pre-printed prescription so the physician knows which services you provide.
6. Ask the client to advise you whenever a new physician or attorney is involved in his case.
7. Use black or blue ink for all documentation or claim forms if not typed.
8. Know that medical cases are legal cases, so document them accordingly.
9. "If it isn't documented, it wasn't done."
10. Document and submit claims for only that which is written on the prescription.

Take Your Practice to the Next Level

• Recession-Proof Your Practice •

A substantial number of talented and dedicated wellness practitioners find it difficult to earn enough money to adequately support their families. One of the biggest drawbacks is the finite number of hours you can work directly with clients. Depending on the type of work you do, you may only have the physical and emotional stamina to work directly with clients for 25-30 hours per week. Imagine that you see 25 clients per week, 50 weeks per year. At $50 per session, that's $62,500 per year. Not bad, except that figure is before expenses. Depending on your setup, you may clear less than $25,000 per year after deducting business expenses.

It is hazardous (physically, emotionally and financially) to rely on your hands-on work as the sole source of your livelihood—particularly if your work requires intensity. You can increase your income potential in several ways: reduce your overhead, increase your number of billable hours, hire support staff to free up your time, raise your rates or diversify your practice.

Diversification is the key to long-term financial success. The most common methods of diversification are to vary the scope of your practice by incorporating additional billable modalities, hiring other practitioners, teaching and selling products.

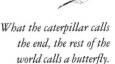

What the caterpillar calls the end, the rest of the world calls a butterfly.
— Lao Tzu

Product Sales •

Of all the above diversification techniques, selling products has the potential for being the most lucrative. Some disciplines discourage (or even prohibit) their members from selling products. I can understand their concern: as a wellness provider, a power differential exists between you and your clients. Clients assume that you are the authority, and they may feel influenced to purchase products out of a need to please you or because they think you know best. Even if you take great care not to exploit this power differential, it still exists. You must not manipulate or coerce your clients.

Ethical sales are based upon educating your clients on the benefits of certain products and then allowing them the opportunity to purchase them from you. Only sell products that you know are reliable, are suitable for use by your clients and are a natural extension of your business. For instance, if local statutes permit, it's totally appropriate for a massage therapist to sell healthcare products that are designed to assist in the relief of pain and promote well-being. Examples of these items are hot and cold packs, ice pillows, relaxation tools, support pillows and similar ergonomic devices, herbs, supplements, remedies, essential oils, sports creams, self-health books and videos. A counselor might sell books, hypnosis tapes and batakas. A reflexologist might carry pain erasure balls, wallet-sized reflexology cards, specialty lotions, tea tree oil, aromatherapy oils, foot sprays, pumice stones, loofah pads, foot bath equipment or products, and arch supports.

Selling products is not about hype or "hard-sell" tactics. The income you receive from the items your clients purchase is not going to make you rich, but it can be a decent source of supplemental (passive) income. The point is providing your clients with easy access to high-quality products that help enrich their well-being.

Focus on products that fit into the type of work you do. The following examples demonstrate how to incorporate different products into your practice:

- Display your products and promotional literature in the waiting area. If you carry self-health videos, play them before and after sessions.
- Utilize products during the treatment: play a CD (just be sure that it doesn't zone you out); apply a hot or cold pack (be aware of contraindications—and while you're at it, tell your client about what they may be); give your client an appropriate formula such as Bach Flower Remedies; or include aromatherapy applications.
- Print fliers that describe all the products you carry. Give these to your clients and mail them for special promotions.
- Offer specials on products and promote them in your newsletters and on your website.
- In the post-interview, recommend any reference materials, relaxation tools, support devices, books and other items that are appropriate to the client's goals. Be certain to demonstrate any products and explain all procedures.

As a wellness provider, your clients depend on you to give them accurate information. You must know every one of your products well and can convey that information to your clients. Let's say your client really enjoyed the cervical hot pack you used during the session and wants to purchase one. You need to educate the client about how to use the pack and when not to use it. Your clients will lose faith in you (and then no longer be your clients, not to mention the loss of goodwill) if you fail to adequately inform them about the appropriate use, benefits, limitations and possible side effects or contraindications of products sold.

Just carrying a product isn't going to sell it. Because people are more inclined to buy something they've experienced, remember to incorporate your products into your practice and take the time to educate your clients. Always keep in mind that the major focus of product sales is to enhance your clients' health and well-being.

Ultimately, selling products is like "selling" your services—simply share your enthusiasm about them. If you make your products visible, accessible, attractive and affordable, your clients will buy them when it's appropriate.

Nutritional Supplements • •

In the quest to diversify their practices, many practitioners are selling nutritional supplements. The major concern is that practitioners may be working beyond their scope of practice, unless they are a nutritionist or herbologist (or extremely well versed in this subject).

The use of herbs and vitamins has expanded so much that an industry term of "nutriceuticals" has been coined. And given that it sounds like medical-ese, you can be sure that the government has its eye on regulating it. The Food and Drug Administration (FDA) has attempted to reclassify certain herbs as narcotics, and, on more than one occasion, has said that certain supplements are not safe.

Rumors cycle through about pending legislation to require these types of nutritional supplements to be prescribed by a physician. These bills haven't come to fruition, but the idea is frightening. Most consumers don't want anyone to take away their freedom to choose and purchase supplements from wherever or whomever they desire. Unfortunately, the more that people haphazardly sell products without proper education, the more likely the government will intercede.

Chapter 5, Page 84
for information of the
Power Differential.

I have been in some wellness practitioners' offices where the waiting room looks like a small health food store. I'm willing to wager that those practitioners know little about all the various products they carry. You might be thinking that store clerks don't know that information either, so what's the problem? Essentially, the problem is that you have a client/therapist relationship, which differs from a consumer/retailer relationship.

But what happens when you've taken a product that changes your life or someone you know has experienced profound change? How can you not sell it? After all, your role is to support your clients in their overall wellness. If there's a product that you really believe in and want to make available to your clients, educate yourself on the product: the contents, suggested applications, possible adverse reactions and contraindications. Keep in mind that just because something works for you doesn't mean it's beneficial to the next person. Also, "works" is a tricky word. Results aren't always proven or reliable. The possibility exists that the product could even be harmful to someone else. When discussing nutritional supplements with clients, you need to discuss the potential side effects (such as a healing crisis) in addition to explaining the benefits.

The more informed you are about the products you carry, the less risk there is for you and your clients. If you are interested in herbs and vitamins, consider taking courses on the subject—or even pursue a degree in nutrition or herbology. Another option to help ensure that you are providing your clients with information and products that are in their best interest is to team up with a nutritionist or herbologist.

The U.S. market is flooded with nutritional supplements, and the general public is looking for direction. As wellness providers, your clients naturally rely upon you to provide them with information, products and services to enhance their well-being. Proceed cautiously when it comes to incorporating nutritional supplements into your practice.

13

Value-Added Service

Most wellness providers have a rather extensive repertoire of techniques and services they use on a regular basis. Even though these modalities may usually be incorporated into treatments without additional charge to clients, you may want to consider expanding some of those services and charging a fee. For instance, instead of doing a three-minute energy balancing technique at the end of a treatment, you could do a full 20-minute energy balancing session.

Using massage therapy as an example, other techniques that can be full sessions in and of themselves are: modalities such as reflexology, acupuncture and craniosacral therapy; crystal or stone therapy; sound treatments; chakra clearing and balancing; breathwork; stretching and exercise; biofeedback; and vibrational treatments. Many complementary services such as facials, pedicures, hypnotherapy and ear-coning can be performed after the massage or even at the same time by another practitioner.

It is common sense to take a method and try it. If it fails, admit it frankly and try another. But above all, try something.
— Franklin D. Roosevelt

Another arena to consider is the use of products or equipment that take very little of your time yet are of immense benefit to your clients. This includes hydrocollator packs, hot pads, ice packs, ginger fomentations, herbal compresses, paraffin treatments, aromatherapy, heated gloves and booties, as well as special equipment such as steam units, passive movement tables, anti-gravity machines, flotation tanks and "brain-gym" equipment. Again, some of these treatments can be part of your primary treatment or done before or after the session.

A terrific advantage to utilizing these products and equipment is your ability to be doing other things such as paperwork, phone calls or exercising while your client is receiving the treatment. They provide you with an innovative means to serve your clients' well-being and earn money without much of your hands-on time. Also, most of these items are a pure profit-generator after the original cost of the equipment. For instance, you can purchase a paraffin unit for $150. It would only take between 15-20 sessions to recoup your initial outlay for the cost of the unit plus the extra wax. A great side benefit is that you can utilize the equipment to take care of your own hands and feet. A steam canopy is another example of a tool which provides a profitable adjunct service to your practice. For less than $1,000, you can own a piece of equipment that virtually costs nothing to use and takes very little of your time. This is my idea of working smarter—not harder.

You have to gauge what is a billable modality and what isn't. For instance, some massage therapists charge extra for using aromatherapy oils or hot packs while others don't—they consider it a way of differentiating themselves from other therapists. The questions to ask yourself to determine whether to charge an additional fee for a service are: Does this cost me much in time or money? Are others charging for this service? Will my clients easily perceive the benefits? Does this make my job easier (e.g., a hot pack loosens muscles so I don't have to put in as much effort or pressure to achieve the same results)? Will offering this service at no extra charge increase the number of referrals and enhance client retention? Is incorporating this service the most effective use of my time?

Figure 13.1

Package Example

Francine Feelgoode is a massage therapist who is trained in several energy balancing techniques and aromatherapy. In addition to her massage equipment, Francine has a steam canopy, a paraffin unit and a set of heated gloves and booties. She offers several different packages to her clients:

- 1-hour Massage $60
- 90-minute Massage $80
- 20-minute Steam Treatment $15
- 20-minute Aromatherapy Steam Treatment $20
- 30-minute Energy Balancing Treatment $30
- Hand and Foot Paraffin Treatment $20
- Deluxe Session (1-hour Massage and Aroma-Steam) $70
- Mini-Spa Session (90-minute Massage, Aroma-Steam and Paraffin) $95
- Total Health Session (90-minute Massage, Aroma-Steam, Energy Balancing and Paraffin) $125

As you can see, the discounts increase with the number of services included in the package. The beauty of this customer service-based marketing approach is that the client receives a wide variety of services without costing the therapist much in time or product (the steam treatment is done without the therapist needing to be present, and the paraffin treatment can be done during the massage). Using the Total Health Session as an example, the time required for Francine to be directly working with a client is approximately two hours. She is earning more than her standard hourly massage rate, and the client receives an incredible treatment. This is what win-win is all about.

Offering adjunct services and treatments to your primary service is beneficial to both you and your clients. It increases your clients' awareness of the scope of available modalities and gives them the power to take more responsibility for their wellness by designing their ideal treatment sessions. Keep in mind that most people appreciate options as long as the list of choices isn't too overwhelming. It also helps you avoid burnout from doing one session after another, gives you a competitive edge and increases your income potential.

• Choose Your Direction •

Businesses take on a life of their own. Throughout the life of your business, you may encounter pivotal moments when it's necessary to reassess your direction. For instance, one day you may look around and ask yourself, *"Just how did I get here? This wasn't exactly what I had in mind."* Even though you may have an elaborate business plan with specific goals, sometimes things snowball. Consider the following scenario.

> Robin Smith is a massage therapist who has been in practice for 18 months. The majority of her work is deep-tissue and sports massage. She decides to get training in chair massage so she can diversify her practice and because she sees it as a way to increase her visibility in the community and thus enlarge her clientele base. After a while, she secures a corporate account to provide chair massage once a week for ACME, Inc. employees.
>
> All is going well, and after several months, the company's director asks her to come in two days each week. Smith is ecstatic! She enjoys the change of pace of working part time at the company and is relieved to have a steady income source.
>
> Soon Acme, Inc. expands exponentially. Smith finds herself working more and more there and less and less at her own practice. A year passes, and she is in the position of needing to hire additional therapists to fulfill the massage needs at Acme, Inc. The prospect is exciting to her, yet she is also experiencing a vague sense of uneasiness. At first, she dismisses her discomfort as fear. Upon further reflection, she discovers that the uneasiness stems from the fact that although she is very "successful" with her corporate massage, she isn't really doing much of the type of work she truly enjoys.

Often, changes are so subtle that you don't even notice them until something forces you to evaluate your situation and life. In this scenario, Smith easily adapted her practice to include the corporate work when it was part time. Not until she was required to make a major shift did she even question the direction her career was taking. At this point Smith has many options. Her choice need not be an all-or-nothing proposition. The following ideas cover the major ones. Many sublevels of activities can be developed within these four career positions.

Chapter 3, Page 34
for Success Markers.

- Devote herself completely to managing the corporate account. This includes hiring and managing staff, directly working with clients, marketing the service within the corporation and overseeing all aspects of the operation.
- Do most of the steps above and hire enough staff so she can still work on private clients one or two days per week.
- Manage the account, not do any chair massages, and work on private clients two to four days per week.
- Sell her corporate contract to another therapist, invest the money, and go back to working with private clients. She might include a clause in the sales agreement that she be retained as a consultant.

Decision-Making Pinnacles ✸

It can be difficult to change career direction when you are experiencing the outward manifestations of success. Some common indicators that point to the need to re-evaluate your practice's growth may include:

- Working too many hours, yet not having enough billable hours.
- Developing the practice to where there's too much work to do by yourself.
- Outgrowing the physical space.
- Needing to better serve your clientele.
- Attempting to appeal to too many target markets.
- Offering too wide a range of services.
- Restlessness or vague dissatisfaction.

Exploration and Evaluation ✸

The first step in determining your best course is a thorough evaluation of your wants, needs and values. Start this exploration process by putting aside your career. Focus on the bigger picture of your life. Are you satisfied in most areas? Are you living the life you choose, or have you acquiesced to what has come your way?

After you've identified the elements of life that are truly important to you now, examine how your career fits into that picture. How does your business support your life vision, and how does it detract from it? Once this groundwork is established, you can more easily be objective in your business direction decision-making process.

Business Evaluation

Write a business description that includes the following:

- Brief history of your practice with opening date, major achievements and mission statement.
- Facilities description.
- Summary of services, products sold and fees collected.
- Client overview, including their profiles and their total number.
- Financial statement, including the average number of sessions per week, gross income and net profit.
- Staff and associate job descriptions.
- Activity synopsis of a typical week.

13

After you've composed your business description, compare it to your original business vision. If you don't have a written business plan, take a few moments to remember why you chose this career and recall your aspirations. Then compare your original vision to your current status. Notice your feelings and thoughts during this process.

Options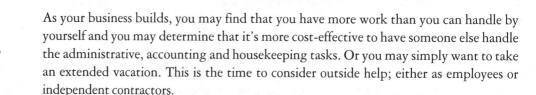

Ultimately, there are no right or wrong answers when it comes to making a choice to either stay on a path or change. The only true factor is what is the best decision for you in terms of your overall needs, wants and goals. Keep in mind that bigger is not always better. Also, you don't have to pursue each of your talents or abilities. Note that it isn't always easy to see all your options by yourself, as in not seeing the forest for the trees. You might consider working on this process with a colleague, counselor or coach.

• Hiring Help •

This information can also help if you desire to work for someone else.

As your business builds, you may find that you have more work than you can handle by yourself and you may determine that it's more cost-effective to have someone else handle the administrative, accounting and housekeeping tasks. Or you may simply want to take an extended vacation. This is the time to consider outside help; either as employees or independent contractors.

Expanding your practice by bringing in other practitioners or support staff can free you to focus on what you do best. This relates to honoring yourself and valuing your time; often we do everything ourselves instead of delegating tasks. Usually this isn't the wisest use of our time. For example, let's say you charge $60 an hour for your services and it takes you three hours per week to clean your office. Most cleaning services charge about $20 per hour. If you were to hire a service rather than do the cleaning yourself, you could spend those three hours working with clients. It would cost you approximately one hour's worth of service ($60). This leaves you with two extra hours in which to make a profit of $120.

I realize this isn't as simple as it sounds. Often it means taking a risk, because you might not get those extra appointments. Consider, though, that the more you focus on income-producing activities, the more profitable your practice becomes.

Hiring office support staff can free you up to spend more time with clients or focus on marketing tasks to help grow your business. Administrative tasks, such as scheduling and confirming appointments, organizing client records, and purchasing supplies, can usually be handled efficiently and cost-effectively by someone other than yourself.

Financial matters, such as bookkeeping, tax preparation, payroll and filing insurance claims, can easily be assigned to another person or firm. Many of the operational duties in your practice can be handled by janitorial and laundry services.

Some wellness providers hire a marketing consultant to coordinate their promotions and advertising, organize special events, oversee the graphic design and printing of promotional materials, and schedule speaking engagements.

The most common manner in which practitioners enlist additional help is by including other wellness providers in their business. This usually occurs when a practice has grown to the point at which there is a client overflow or the owner wants to expand the scope of modalities and services offered to current clients.

IRS publication 15, (Circular E) Employer's Tax Guide
www.irs.gov/pub/irs-pdf/ p15.pdf

Administrative Support Staff

Administrative support staff are key team members in any small business. They are often the first point of contact that a potential client has with your business. In those first few minutes (as well as in the continuing relationship with established clients), your support staff establishes the persona of your business, its image and philosophy. Therefore, hiring the right type of person with the proper skills for your particular job requirements and client service is critical.

The first step is to identify what type of support you need. What are the job duties? Are you looking for a receptionist, secretary, bookkeeper, administrative assistant or operations manager? Each type of position has differing job duties and responsibilities. Some common office tasks are typing, filing, answering the phones, taking messages, producing monthly reports, filing insurance claims, analyzing data, marketing, maintaining databases, managing inventory and proofreading. Determine whether the position is part or full time, the hours you require, and the wage rate according to the demands of the position and the skill level required.

U.S. state and federal law requires all employers to report each new hired employee to the State Directory of New Hires.

Schedule ample time to screen candidates, interview effectively and hire intelligently. The better you can clearly and concisely communicate job requirements to an applicant, the better prepared the applicant will be to realistically assess if the job is a right fit.

Once you have established the position's duties, responsibilities and the personality you need to project the persona of your business, design your interview questions to elicit the most information about your candidates and whether they fit into the mold you have established for the job. Consider the following (true) story:

Employee Interview Questions
www.businessmastery.us/ interview-questions.php

> A manager had gone through five secretaries in one year. She finally admitted that obviously something was amiss, otherwise, why would five different secretaries quit within a one-year period? The manager established that she needed to know what would make an individual person quit. Hence, in the interview, one of the questions she asked was simply, "What would make you quit a job?" She also got feedback from her previous employees and established a certain "personality" that she knew was needed to work together effectively and harmoniously.

Therefore, by identifying your position well and designing your interview effectively, you enable yourself to choose the best possible support staff—not just for yourself and your business persona, but for those you serve.

Sources for Finding Help ●

There are many options to explore when looking for quality people to assist you with your business. You can hire independent contractors, consultants or employees. You may even find someone to work as an intern or apprentice. You can contract with a company that provides specific business services (e.g., secretarial, answering service, laundry, bookkeeping, janitorial). Or you may hire a "temporary employee" through an employment agency or even an employee leasing company—then you won't have to worry about all the paperwork, because those agencies are responsible for withholding taxes, paying appropriate fees such as workers' compensation and filing all the governmental forms. Another option is to form associations with other business owners to share tasks and expenses.

As for where to find good people, many cities have an online employment resource such as Craig's List, an Internet website and virtual online village with a wide variety of community resources. You may also want to check your local Chamber of Commerce for resource listings and tap into local business networking groups. Often, local or regional industry trade association websites or trade publications include job listings, particularly useful if you are looking for a wellness practitioner or independent contractor. Many times, community newspapers are a good source for finding cleaning and laundry services. If you're looking for part-time help, check with career centers or job boards at local colleges and universities. Lastly, you may want to search the Internet using key words, as each city offers different types of resources.

Employment Regulations ●

Deciding whether to hire an employee or subcontract for the services you need can be a difficult decision. You may want to incorporate a variety of people and service providers in your business support team. Most small businesses prefer to hire independent contractors, consultants or service firms rather than employees.

The IRS guidelines for determining employment status are fairly clear when it comes to administrative staff: in most instances, an office support person is an employee. A gray area exists in hiring other wellness providers.

When you hire an employee, your status changes from simply being a practitioner to also being a manager. It takes considerable time and excellent communication skills to be a good boss. You have to train your staff so they understand the type of work you do so they can explain it to potential clients. You need to organize your business to make certain there's enough work to be done, hold staff meetings, give employees regular feedback and be willing to delegate.

Generally, it's much easier and less risky to terminate a contract than to fire an employee. Also, your liability is reduced in terms of malpractice if you hire independent contractors, because you can require they carry their own insurance. The potential pitfalls of working with non-employees include paying a higher price for their services and not having control over their work in terms of timeliness and quality.

I may seem to be making a strong case for not hiring employees. *Au contraire!* Many practitioners and clinic owners claim they could not be where they are without employees. It can be extremely helpful and comforting to know that someone is going to be at your office every day taking care of business. A strong bond tends to develop between employees and the business owner, particularly in a small business. The peace of mind and sense of stability this creates is invaluable. You also receive the other benefits as previously mentioned when you can focus on your high priority activities.

I've interviewed and consulted with many business owners, and the majority prefer to have practitioners work as employees rather than independent contractors. The benefits far outweigh the drawbacks. Practitioners who are employees tend to be more committed, and there's a heightened sense of camaraderie. Employees are there to help build your business, while independent contractors are attempting to build their own businesses. If you decide to hire an employee but are concerned about the regulations and paperwork, you can pay an accountant or payroll service to do it for you.

Give me a stock clerk with a goal and I'll give you a man who will make history. Give me a man with no goals and I'll give you a stock clerk.
— J.C. Penney

In addition to the responsibility of having enough money for employee paychecks, you need to comply with various payroll requirements. You must match their FICA (Social Security and Medicare) deductions; pay FUTA (Federal Unemployment Tax Act), pay state unemployment taxes; provide workers' compensation; withhold state and federal taxes; deposit withheld taxes; file regular returns; and send W-2 forms to employees annually. In most instances, to stay competitive with other employers, you need to offer benefits such as health insurance, paid time off, sick leave and retirement plans.

Two of the employment forms you need are SS-4, Application for Employer Identification Number, and Form W-4, Employee's Withholding Allowance Certificate. Check with your state employment department for requirements, fees and forms. In addition to a Federal Employer's Identification Number (EIN), you need a state EIN. All employees must also fill out Form I-9, Employment Eligibility Verification (from the U.S. Department of Justice, Immigration and Naturalization Service).

You don't have to withhold income tax or Social Security tax from independent contractors. But if you pay an independent contractor $600 or more during the year in the course of your trade or business, you must file a form 1099-MISC at the end of the year. That form is optional if you've contracted with a service company.

Independent Contractor Status •

As an employer, you take a considerable risk by deeming a worker an independent contractor. If the IRS determines that your independent contractors are (or were) indeed employees, you may be required to pay fines of up to 100 percent of the tax, in addition to the back income taxes and Social Security taxes. This easily adds up to a sizable amount. In the eyes of the IRS, it makes no difference if you signed an agreement that states you are contracting with an independent contractor—although a written agreement is advisable. Many spas, clinics and group practices walk a very thin legal line. A significant number of the so-called independent contractors they have working for them would most likely be classified as employees under the IRS guidelines. Just calling someone an independent contractor doesn't make it so.

13

You can minimize the risks of your independent contractors being reclassified as employees by taking the following steps: make certain independent contractors have multiple sources of income; sign "independent contractor" contracts which clearly state the requirements of all parties while making it clear the contractors are free to pursue other clients; require contractors to provide their own tables, linens, products, music and other supplies; allow contractors to set their own schedules (ideally, no more than 10 hours per week or on an as-needed basis for special events); have clients pay contractors directly; request copies of the contractors' tax returns; and require contractors to provide their own insurance and workers' compensation coverage.

Complying to these suggestions still doesn't guarantee independent contractor status. If in doubt, you can have the IRS determine whether a worker is an employee by filing Form SS-8. Get legal counsel to develop an independent contractor agreement. Include a work description for each subcontracting assignment along with a policy and procedure statement.

IRS Publication 937— Business Reporting ••

Under common-law rules, anyone who performs services subject to the will and control of an employer, as to both what must be done and how it must be done, is an employee. It doesn't matter that the employer allows the employee discretion and freedom of action, so long as the employer has the legal right to control both the method and result of the services.

In general, it's wise to consider an individual as an employee until you can prove otherwise.

Two primary characteristics of an employer-employee relationship are:

1. An employer has the right to discharge an employee.
2. An employer supplies the employee with tools and a place to work.

Be careful not to assume that this can be skirted by the practitioner providing his own specific supplies. "Tools" is a broad term that can include the equipment required in running a practice, such as telephones and copiers.

From an IRS viewpoint, if there is an employer-employee relationship, it's irrelevant how it's described. It doesn't matter if the employee is called an employee, associate, partner or independent contractor. It also doesn't matter how the payments are measured, made or what they are called. Nor does it matter whether the individual is employed full time or part time.

The Internal Revenue Service Guidelines ••

To assist business owners in complying with IRS regulations, the IRS has developed a list of 20 factors that determine whether the status of employee or independent contractor applies. See Figure 13.2. The degree of importance of each factor varies according to the profession and the conditions in which the services are performed. The most important factor is control. If the business owner has the right to control how and when a person works, then that person is most likely an employee.

You can still qualify as an independent contractor even if some of these factors are present in your working relationship. The key elements that differentiate between employee status and independent contractor status in the wellness industry are listed in Figure 13.3.

Other Government Agency Guidelines ● ●

State workers' compensation, unemployment compensation and tax agencies use various tests to determine worker status. Many use the common-law right of control test, but emphasize different factors than the IRS. Each agency is concerned with worker classification for different reasons, and has different biases and practices. Thus, it's possible for one agency to view an individual as an employee, while another agency may view the same individual as an independent contractor.

Figure 13.2

IRS 20-Point Checklist for Determining Employee Status

An individual is likely to be considered an employee if he or she:

1. Is required to comply with company instructions about when, where and how to work.
2. Has been trained by the company to perform services in a particular manner.
3. Has her services integrated into the company's operations because the services are critical to the success of the business.
4. Must render services personally.
5. Utilizes assistants provided by the company.
6. Has an ongoing, continuing relationship with the company.
7. Has set work hours established by the employer.
8. Is required to work the equivalent of full time.
9. Works on the company's designated premises.
10. Must perform services in the order or sequence determined by the employer.
11. Must submit regular progress reports.
12. Is paid in regular intervals, such as by the hour, week or month.
13. Is reimbursed for all business and travel expenses.
14. Uses tools and materials furnished by the employer.
15. Has no significant investment in the facilities that are used.
16. Has no risk of loss.
17. Works for only one person or company.
18. Does not offer services to the general public.
19. Can be discharged by the company.
20. Can terminate the relationship without incurring liability.

Figure 13.3

Wellness Industry Key Independent Contractor Elements

- Who regulates the type of work done and how it's performed
- Where and when the sessions occur
- Who determines the fee structure
- Who receives the money from the clients
- Who provides the equipment and supplies
- Who pays for client-related expenses
- Who generates the clientele

13

This sample agreement is for illustrative purposes only and not intended for use as legal document. Please confer with an attorney before finalizing any legal agreements to specify financial arrangements and to ensure the document meets IRS guidelines.

Figure 13.4

Massage Therapy Independent Contractor Agreement

This agreement, dated July 4, 2020, is by and between Mobile Holistic Health Services ("Company"), with principal office located at 1776 Independence Way, Washington, D.C., and Frank Benjamin ("Contractor"), with principal office located at 1912 Thomas Jefferson Blvd., Washington, D.C.

Status as Independent Contractor

Contractor is an independent contractor and not an employee of the Company. As an independent contractor, Company and Contractor agree to the following:

a. Contractor has control of the means, manner and method by which services are provided.
b. Contractor furnishes all necessary supplies and materials used in the performance of services (e.g., oils, lotions, linens and music).
c. Contractor has the right to perform services for others during the term of this Agreement. Contractor shall not solicit services to Company's clients for private practice during the term of this Agreement or for one year after termination. Upon termination of Agreement, Contractor and Company shall discuss which clients, under what conditions and with what compensation Contractor may maintain continuity of service. All client records shall remain the property of the Company unless otherwise agreed.
d. Contractor shall indemnify and hold Company harmless from any loss or liability arising from services provided under this agreement.
e. Contractor is responsible for maintaining appropriate certification and licensure, including all costs thereof.

Services to Be Provided by Contractor

Contractor agrees to provide massage therapy services within the scope of Contractor's licensure. Contractor agrees to dress in a style consistent with the Company's image. Contractor shall maintain client records in a mutually agreed manner.

Services to Be Provided by Company

Company shall provide the following: a safe, clean environment; appointment scheduling according to Contractor's stipulated hours; and marketing.

Other Provisions

All Contractor's marketing materials which include any information about Company must be approved in advance.

Fees and Terms of Payment

Company shall pay the Contractor $35 per massage.
Contractor acknowledges that Contractor is not eligible to receive any employee benefits.

Local, State and Federal Taxes

Contractor is responsible for paying and filing all applicable local, state and federal withholding, Social Security and Medicare taxes.

Workers' Compensation and Unemployment Insurance

Company is not responsible for payment of Workers' Compensation and Unemployment Insurance. If Company is a corporation, Contractor must provide Company with a certificate of Workers' Compensation Insurance prior to performing services.

Unemployment Compensation

Company shall make no state or federal unemployment compensation payments on behalf of Contractor. Contractor isn't entitled to these benefits in connection with work performed under this Agreement.

Insurance

During the term of this agreement, Contractor shall maintain a malpractice insurance policy of at least $2,000,000 aggregate annual and $1,000,000 per incident.

Term of Agreement

Either party may terminate this agreement, given reasonable cause, as provided below, or by giving 30 days written notice to the other party of the intention to terminate this Agreement:

a. Material violation of the provisions of this Agreement.
b. Action by either party exposing the other to liability for property damage or personal injury.
c. Violation of ethical standards as defined by local, state and/or national associations and governing bodies.
d. Loss of licensure for services provided.
e. Contractor engages in any pattern or course of conduct on a continuing basis which adversely affects Contractor's ability to perform services.
f. Contractor engages in any pattern or course of conduct on a continuing basis which adversely affects Company's or Company's associates' ability to perform services.
g. It is agreed that any unresolved disputes are to be settled by mediation. Any costs and fees other than attorney fees associated with the mediation shall be shared equally by the parties. If the dispute is not resolved within 30 days after it is referred to the mediator, any party may pursue further action.

This constitutes the entire agreement between Contractor and Company and supersedes any and all prior written or verbal agreements. Should any part of this agreement be deemed unenforceable, the remainder of the agreement continues in effect. This agreement is governed by the laws of the District of Columbia.

Signatures

Employee: _Frank Benjamin_ Date: _July 4, 2020_

Employer: _Marshall Taylor_ Date: _July 4, 2020_

Witness: _Joy Cronkite_ Date: _July 4, 2020_

13

Managing Your Staff •

As a manager or owner, you're responsible for "supporting" all the members of your team, including your support staff. Simply establishing positions and hiring the appropriate people isn't the end, it's the beginning of a working relationship. One of the most important concepts to grasp is that you're working "with" your staff, not managing your staff from an ivory tower. This establishes a sense of teamwork and camaraderie. Quality intercommunication is essential, since you work with your staff many hours during the work week. If issues arise regarding job performance, they need to be handled diplomatically and quickly.

Be certain to carefully listen to all team members' input, as they're the ones who deal with daily tasks and generally have some very creative, imaginative and efficient methods of conducting their work. Never underestimate your staff. They are one of the greatest assets to your business. While they may not all have college degrees or be versed in the intricacies of your profession, they may provide valuable insights and practical solutions to everyday problems.

When managing your business, allow plenty of individual autonomy; avoid micro-management (i.e., an overcontrolling approach to things). Don't hesitate to give your staff the authority to make decisions. Make certain your team understands company policies and procedures, and knows when to take initiative and when to confer with you before taking action. It is important to oversee your staff and review their actions, yet refrain from monitoring their every move. Identify and eliminate barriers to effective teamwork.

Motivate employees, train them, care about them, and make winners of them. At Marriott we know that if we treat our employees correctly, they'll treat the customers right. And if the customers are treated right, they'll come back.
— Bill Marriott Jr.

Performance Reviews • •

Institute annual performance reviews which not only evaluate job performance, but also establish goals and objectives for the coming year. Review the position duties and responsibilities and make adjustments according to the changing needs of your office operations. Make this performance review a two-way communication. Ask your staff members to clarify:

1. What are their perceptions of their duties and responsibilities?
2. What are the contributions they've made to the position other than the mechanics of the job?
3. What are their goals and objectives for the coming year?
4. What additional seminars, lectures or outside activities would they like to participate in?

Answer these questions from your own perspective and then sit down together to review them. This allows each of you to jointly assess the previous year, while lessening the opportunity for misunderstanding and poor communication about each of your expectations and needs. Included in this performance evaluation should be an objective review of performance (e.g., quality of work, quantity of work, communication, timeliness).

A well-designed performance evaluation is an excellent management tool that promotes effective, clear communication and establishes a sense of teamwork. This helps form a satisfying working relationship.

Don't wait until the end of the coming year to informally discuss progress and concerns. Conduct informal reviews quarterly, if not monthly. This provides an occasion for you to affirm exceptional performance, correct minor difficulties before they become major problems and initiate changes in operational needs in a timely manner. It also allows your staff the opportunity to discuss those matters of concern they may have in their working relationship with you or your clients.

Cultivate Camaraderie • •

In addition to reviews, hold regular staff meetings. These should be at least once per month and preferably once per week. These meetings serve to build camaraderie as well as provide a forum to discuss problems, learn new skills, brainstorm ideas and set goals. It also keeps everyone informed and fosters better understanding and teamwork when people are aware of each other's projects and deadlines.

Every business has the "Jobs That Nobody Wants To Do." These tasks are either boring, unpleasant or difficult to accomplish. It isn't uncommon for resentments to arise around these noxious tasks. As a manager, you need to find a way to balance these duties among your staff. This can be difficult when you only have one employee or if you're the only person in your business. If you're lucky, you will find someone who loves to do those tasks that everyone else hates. Alas, such people are rare. So, the next best option is to hold a staff meeting and brainstorm ideas for dealing with these tasks. Conducting brainstorming sessions and including your staff in some of the decision-making processes enhances teamwork. When people feel that they're working as a team, they're less apt to feel resentful over having to do those "awful" assignments.

One of the outcomes of a brainstorming session might be a change in the company's operations and procedures. Sometimes a slight alteration in the execution of a task can alleviate the dread associated with it. Frequently, tasks can be simplified or even eliminated. Changes don't occur very often because people rarely take the time to evaluate policies, procedures and goals. Another outcome of the brainstorming session may be that the staff decides to rotate these unpleasant tasks. Whatever the results of this session are, it's imperative that you follow through by monitoring progress.

People are motivated most by recognition, appreciation and participation. Each person on your team requires a different type of encouragement. Get input from your staff and develop incentive programs.

By skillfully managing your staff, you create a happy and harmonious team, an efficient workplace and an environment that fosters good relationships with both employees and clients—all of which adds up to a healthy bottom line.

One of the reasons people stop learning is that they become less and less willing to risk failure.
— John W. Gardner

13

• Relocating Your Practice •

At some point over the course of your business you will most likely need to relocate. Regardless of whether it's down the street, to the other side of town or across the country, moving can be a stressful event. Before you actually relocate, set a foundation for success and ease your stress level by establishing a network of professional resources in the new community, thoroughly researching regulations and becoming well informed about any unique aspects of the new locale. Any move provides you with an opportunity to re-evaluate your life and business, implement changes, meet new people and revitalize your practice.

Moving Within the Same City •

One of the most important factors to consider in choosing a new location is the potential impact on your clients. Whenever you move more than several blocks from your current location, you risk losing clients. This chance is heightened if a large portion of your clientele is based on geography. Let's say your office is in a downtown skyscraper and the majority of your clients are attorneys who work in that building. Attorneys tend to keep chaotic schedules, and, most likely, one of the reasons they utilize your services is that you're convenient. If they can't simply take the elevator to your office (or at the most, walk across the street), they may not see you as frequently—if at all.

Regardless of how good a practitioner you are, many people won't travel far to see you, especially on a regular basis. Who wants to drive 45 minutes through traffic after getting relaxed? Other people may only have a limited amount of time they can take from work and thus need to schedule after hours or find another practitioner.

Figure 13.5

Moving Checklist

❏ Send moving notification (three weeks prior to moving date).
❏ Review files.
❏ Organize paperwork into active and archival boxes.
❏ Make an inventory list.
❏ Clean and organize the new office before moving.
❏ Hire movers.
❏ Schedule an open house.
❏ Send a second announcement (one week prior to move).
❏ Call current clients.
❏ Introduce yourself to your new neighbors.
❏ Forge alliances with businesses.
❏ Gain visibility in the local community.
❏ Post new address at previous location.

Retain Clients by Communicating Benefits • •

Help retain clients and foster goodwill by taking the time to communicate the benefits of your office relocation to your clients. Do this by sending a promotional mailing or welcome letter offering special pricing.

An office move may result in the following: more space; improved ambiance; a location adjacent to other wellness providers; proximity to public transportation; an office away from the hustle and bustle of the city or closer to the center of town. In some cases a move may provide: a more intimate, relaxed, private space (good way to describe downsizing); a safer location; a greater variety of practitioners in the same office; space for classes; more convenient parking; lower overhead to keep prices down. Whatever the case may be, when clients feel valued and the location is convenient, a move to a better locale is usually welcomed by clients.

Revitalize Your Practice • •

Moving provides you with an excellent opportunity to reconnect with your clients, particularly those you haven't seen lately. Many wellness practitioners avoid contacting inactive clients due to the time involved in reviewing their files and writing individualized letters. A form letter without something specific to each client is usually ineffective in generating interest. But moving announcements don't require personalization! You can even offer an incentive for them to come back.

After you have relocated, go through your client files and send out one letter or postcard each day.

Take the time to go through your files as you box them. Note who hasn't been in for a while and send them a special letter (if they don't attend your open house). Think about what you could do to provide further service to each client. For instance, a client has been diagnosed with fibromyalgia. You haven't worked with her in more than a year. Several months ago you read an excellent book on the subject and could share some information with her. Place a reminder in your tickler file to send her a note about the book and invite her to your new facilities.

Notification • •

Notify all of your clients, colleagues and associates as soon as possible. Send out announcements or fliers at least three weeks before the move. Include the date of the move, your new address and phone numbers, any changes in hours and a map detailing directions to your new facilities. Consider sending your active contacts another notice closer to the moving date. If your office accepts last-minute appointments or walk-in clients, call your current client list one week before the actual move to inform them of your new address.

Once you relocate, post a note on the door of your previous office with the address, phone number and directions to your new location. If that option isn't available, perhaps you can leave a stack of fliers with the new tenants. Be sure to confirm all appointments and remind clients of the address change. To keep track of who has been reminded about the new location, code your clients' files with colored dots (or if you're computerized, create a special field).

Most phone companies wait three to twelve months before reassigning business numbers. Right before that time comes, call your old number and tell the new holder your phone number and address. Send a thank-you card and a gift (flowers, plant or gift certificate) to thank them in advance for forwarding your calls. Deliver additional thank-you notes as long as they continue to forward your information.

Figure 13.6 We're Moving Flier

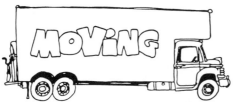

STRESSBusters

We're moving!

StressBusters is moving to larger facilities on November 1st.
Our new location will be at:

**123 Breeze Court
Sea City, NJ 07094
908-555-5555
www.stressbusters.com**

Come celebrate with us at our grand opening on Saturday, November 1st from 10 a.m. to 2 p.m. We will be serving refreshments, providing mini-workshops on stress reduction techniques and offering complimentary auricular acupuncture treatments. Please join in the fun. Bring a friend.

Redeem this invitation for $10 off your next session!

Sally Smith

Generating New Clientele • •

Relocation furnishes you with a splendid opportunity to generate new clientele. Survey the surrounding area for other businesses that could be a source of referrals (mutual referrals are even better). Get to know your neighbors. Hand-deliver fliers or brochures to adjacent businesses, hold a special open house just for the people nearby, and make yourself visible in the community. Get involved in local business association meetings (e.g., the Downtown Business Owners Alliance). If there's a local publication, advertise in it or offer to write a health column.

Most large buildings have a newsstand or coffee booth in the lobby. Ask to place your cards and flyers near the counter. Perhaps you can leave a container in which tenants place their business cards to win a free session. In addition to generating visibility, this provides a means to obtaining the tenants' names for future marketing ventures. If you're a somatic practitioner, you can offer the stand owner a free weekly 15-minute session (preferably right in the stand area) in exchange for displaying your materials.

Forge alliances with other business owners for the purpose of cooperative marketing. Let's go back to the attorney example. You are a massage therapist who wants to increase the number of attorneys in your client pool. To heighten your differential advantage, you decide to relocate to a building that is populated mainly with attorneys. A restaurant down the block offers free delivery service to tenants in your building. Together, you could plan several marketing activities that would increase the range of people you reach and reduce the cost of reaching them:

1. Share the cost of hiring someone to hand-deliver your brochures and the restaurant's menus to each office.
2. Offer a joint special, such as "Receive a certificate for a free 15-minute chair massage with your 10th delivery" and "Receive a 10 percent food purchase discount coupon with every massage."
3. Keep a stack of menus by your office door. At the restaurant, place your cards and brochures (in a plastic holder) near the cash register.
4. Get the restaurant to cater your open houses (at cost or for free). Offer free massages for special events hosted by the restaurant.
5. Have monthly drawings at the restaurant for a free massage and at your office for a free dinner for two.

Moving to a New City

For most people, moving to a new city means starting a business from scratch. You can create a smoother transition and actually develop a strong referral base and network by doing legwork before the actual move.

Research • •

Research your new location to determine what it has to offer economically, socially, politically, culturally and climatically. Start by asking the Chamber of Commerce to send you a relocation packet with information on the city, population, demographics and major industries. Request that they send you the following: the Yellow Pages on your specific service, health services, stress reduction and holistic wellness providers; listings of business and professional associations; and anything else that piques your interest. Not all chambers are so accommodating—you may need to order a phone book from the telephone company. You can also do some of this research at the library and over the Internet.

Another method for gathering information about the community and your specific profession is talking with people in that city. If you're a member of any professional association, contact members in the area. If you aren't a member or if no other members live there, contact the officers or directors of allied professional associations. Send letters or call several people in your same profession. Request information from any local allied wellness schools.

Some questions to ask are: What position does your type of service hold in this community? What are the attitudes toward the profession and the practitioners? How much publicity does this profession garner? What is the range of fees charged and what is the scope of practice? What is the average annual yearly income for a practitioner in your specific profession?

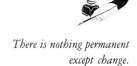

There is nothing permanent except change.
— Heraclitus

Librarians excell at searching for information and it's usually a favorite aspect of their job.

13

Call the relevant business, zoning and health licensing agencies to ascertain their requirements and obtain the number of licensed or registered wellness practitioners in the area. You may need to contact state agencies to learn the specific regulations for wellness providers. Get in touch with a commercial real estate agent to obtain information on the types of available office space and the going rates. Order copies of the local newspapers(s), holistic magazines and special interest publications—all of which provide valuable information about your new city.

Network ● ●

Begin to network even before you move. Ask your friends, relatives and colleagues if they know anyone in that city. Send a letter of introduction to allied professionals such as physicians, counselors, chiropractors, massage therapists and other healthcare providers. Let them know who you are and what you do, including your abilities and qualifications. Address the potential mutual benefits of your association. Close the letter by telling them how to contact you and inform them that you will be calling them within the next few weeks. When you do, ask for any advice, suggestions or contacts they might recommend. Be sure to thank them for their time and consideration with a follow-up note.

Scouting Expedition ● ●

If you're considering a place for relocation and it isn't definite that you will actually move there, visit the city during the worst (hottest, coldest, wettest, driest, most crowded) part of the year to see whether you can tolerate it. This is also a good time to meet with colleagues and explore potential associations.

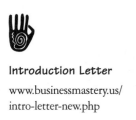

Introduction Letter

www.businessmastery.us/
intro-letter-new.php

Financial Management

• Money, Money, Money •

Some people naturally handle money well while others find it difficult to balance their checkbooks. For many of us, money matters get tangled in a web of emotions because we don't know how to relate to money in a healthy way, or because we didn't have the opportunity to learn money smarts when we were growing up.

In fact, many passionate and talented wellness practitioners struggle financially. Whether they own their own business or work as an employee, they find it a challenge to get ahead. According to many money management experts, the first step to enhancing your financial prosperity is to transform your attitude toward money. As Suze Orman, author of *The 9 Steps to Financial Freedom*, so aptly states: "Before we can get control of our finances, we must get control of our attitudes about money, feelings that were shaped by our earliest experiences with it. Opening ourselves to abundance—not only of the pocketbook but also of the heart—is what's necessary for true balance and freedom."[1]

An odd phenomenon sometimes happens in the helping professions. This takes the shape of practitioners who proudly wear the "poor but pure" badge because they're uncomfortable with money or fear that financial prosperity will somehow corrupt them. Besides contributing to financial insecurity, this attitude can lead to questionable business practices. These same practitioners can experience difficulty in charging appropriate fees for their services and many are uncomfortable charging anything at all.

On the flip side, employees can become resentful over the disparity in their wages versus the charged fee. This misconception can occur because they haven't factored in the true costs the business owner incurs in setting up and running the business. They only look at the $100 the company charges per session and the $35 they receive. They forget about the thousands or even millions of dollars the facility cost.

The universe operates through dynamic exchange...giving and receiving are different aspects of the flow of energy in the universe. In our willingness to give that which we seek, we keep the abundance of the universe circulating in our lives.
— Deepak Chopra

Chapter 10, Pages 212-214 for information on setting your fees.

www.businessmastery.us/
forms.php#finman
for sample financial
worksheets.

Rich Dad, Poor Dad, by
Robert Kiyosaki

*The 9 Steps to Financial
Freedom*, by Suze Orman

Disclaimer!

This is not an accounting
book. The material in
this chapter is provided
to assist you in
developing your
bookkeeping system and
inform you about basic
Internal Revenue Service
(IRS) tax regulations. It
has been streamlined to
highlight key points. For
more detailed
information please visit
the IRS website or read
accounting books.

The next step to financial freedom is to know where you stand. With the fast pace of life and the many demands on our time, it's easy to be in denial about finances. A simple and time-tested antidote to this common experience is to develop and work with a budget. A personal monthly budget can prevent a lot of financial stress and build a solid financial future. A budget gives you a realistic picture of what you need to earn to cover your expenses. Use your budget as a tool to forecast your daily, monthly and annual expenses and plan accordingly. If you intend to be self-employed, you need to do similar estimating and forecasting for your business.

Forecasting is a great tool to help keep expenses on track. Be aware of a tendency to let "extra cash" slip away. For instance, it's natural for many people to spend "extra cash" when they experience an unexpected windfall such as having a higher than usual number of clients for the week. Avoid this pitfall by checking your cash flow forecast before spending that extra income, as you might have a large one-time expense coming up soon. Another useful strategy is to put at least half of the extra money into a savings account.

Although we may wish money didn't play such a central role in our lives, money skills are crucial to creating personal and professional success. By working with this book you can easily master the basics of money management—and pave the way to your future success.

• Financial Recordkeeping •

Financial recordkeeping, particularly bookkeeping, is often viewed as an evil chore or an arcane art designed to deaden the psyche. Since most people will do almost anything to avoid chores, many practitioners keep minimal records if they keep any records at all. Thus they miss numerous legitimate tax deductions. Keeping records is a habit that must be developed. It is highly recommended that prior to setting up your books you consult with a bookkeeper or an accountant, and most definitely confer with an advisor when it's time to file tax returns. The manner in which you keep your records can be simple and straightforward despite complex tax laws that seem to change every other week.

Maintaining accurate records is vital for any small business. Bookkeeping entails more than keeping a ledger for tax purposes. The information you glean from your records assists in running your business smoothly and achieving optimal profits. It is difficult to make prudent decisions without all of the facts. The checkbook alone doesn't always give an accurate account of the business' financial standing. Many business owners make the mistake of believing they're generating a profit because they have plenty of funds in their checking account, while unpaid bills accumulate and upcoming expenses are forgotten.

In addition, many people find themselves in a precarious financial position come tax time because they haven't set aside money for taxes. I advocate opening an interest-bearing business savings or money market account and regularly depositing money into that account. Accountant Robert Decker, says, "The two most common mistakes that people make are doing their own taxes, and not setting aside money to pay for taxes." He suggests putting away 20 to 30 percent of the amount you pay yourself. For instance, every time you write yourself a check for $1,000, immediately write another check for at least $200, and deposit it into a savings account that you designate specifically for paying taxes.

What Types of Records Should I Keep? •

Your bookkeeping can be quite simple if you operate a small sole proprietorship with no employees. All you really need is a bank account, a ledger system with income and expenditure sheets, and a file to store receipts. It isn't necessary to spend a fortune on a bookkeeping system. Sometimes simple columnar sheets from an office supply store suffice (or use sample ledger sheets we provide). The records required and the complexity involved escalate with added business dimensions such as employees, product sales, partnerships and corporations.

Some people use hand-posted ledgers for all their bookkeeping activities. I highly recommend using a computer as much as possible. Several inexpensive, user-friendly accounting programs are available for personal computers. These software programs can print your checks and post the information in the appropriate places. The software usually includes a tutorial that walks you through setting up your accounts—it poses questions, and your responses enable the computer to determine how to organize your files.

It is so much easier to know where you stand and to plan the future because the information is right there. You simply go to the "Reports" icon where it lists all the major standard reports. All you do is highlight the dates (e.g., "Last Month" or "Current Fiscal Year to Date"), and, in a matter of seconds, a report is prepared—one that could easily take hours by hand. You can also examine expenses by category, such as creating a report of all your automobile expenses for the year. The reports can combine information from all of your accounts (e.g., checking, credit cards and petty cash). Let's say that XYZ Supplies sends you a notice for an outstanding invoice. You're fairly sure you paid for it, but you don't remember the payment method. If you only kept manual files, it could take you 20 minutes (or more) to sort through all the various ledger sheets and receipts. It takes moments with a computerized accounting package.

IRS Guidlines

www.irs.gov/businesses/
small/index.html

www.irs.gov/publications/
p583/index.html

Small-Time Operator
by Bernard Kamoroff, CPA

Minding Her Own Business
by Jan Zobel, EA

Figure 14.1

How Long Do I Need to Keep My Records?

Document	Retention
General correspondence	5 years
Bank statements	7 years
Receipts	7 years
Canceled checks	7 years for most
Ledger sheets	7 years
Year-end financial statements	Indefinitely
Contracts	Indefinitely
Licenses and permits	Indefinitely
Insurance claims	Indefinitely
Tax returns	Indefinitely

Record Retention Schedule

www.businessmastery.us/
records.php

IRS regulations require taxpayers to keep records and receipts for as long as they may be applicable to the enforcement of tax law. For income and expenses this is usually the later of three years from the date the return was filed or two years after the tax was paid.

Bank statements and other documents, such as inventory records, canceled checks, expense records, and payroll records, should be kept at least seven years. Tax returns and records related to the basis (cost) of property should be kept indefinitely (e.g., papers related to the purchase of real estate and equipment).

Creating a Separate Identity

A separate business identity is important for personal and financial reasons. Corporations have regulations that require financial divisions between the business and the business owners, many sole proprietors are lax about setting business boundaries. One of the best ways to set boundaries is to keep business and personal finances separate. Open a business bank account. This can be a "personal" account with your name (e.g., Mary Jones, D.C.), although it's best to establish yourself with a "business" account. Deposit all income (checks and cash) into the business checking account. If you accept credit cards, the monies collected should be directly transferred to the business checking account.

Pay your business bills by check or credit card. This provides better documentation than cash. If you use credit cards for purchases, note the charges on a ledger sheet and pay the monthly statement with a business check. Avoid paying for business expenses with cash or personal checks. If you find yourself in a store with only a personal check, don't worry. Just make sure that when you return to the office, you post the expense under Petty Cash and note which checking account was used and the check number. Then write a check to "petty cash" for the same amount to cash.

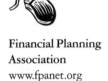

Financial Planning Association
www.fpanet.org

Figure 14.2

Recordkeeping Tips

- Keep all business-related receipts.
- Pay bills when they're due—unless you receive a discount for early payment.
- Have a separate business checking account.
- Keep financial records according to the above guidelines.
- Keep lists of inventory, equipment and furniture.
- Maintain thorough and professional client files.
- Make cash flow projections.
- Keep automobile mileage logs.
- Maintain daily records: appointment book, cash expenses, activity tracking sheets.
- Prepare monthly bank reconciliations.

Figure 14.3

Accounting Definitions

Assets   The total resources (current, fixed or other) of the sole practitioner or business—tangible and intangible. Assets may include cash in the bank, inventory, equipment, goodwill, accounts receivable and equipment.

Liabilities   Current and long-term debts of the practitioner or business. Liabilities may include accounts payable, long-term debts, (e.g., a car loan), payroll taxes and credit card balances.

Capital   Essentially it's the net worth of a business—the difference between the assets and the liabilities.

Accounts Receivable   The amounts owed to you by another person or business.

Accounts Payable   The amounts you owe another person or business.

Capital Account   The total money invested by the owner.

Shareholders' Equity   The amount owners invested in the company's stock plus or minus the company's earnings or losses since inception.

Journal   A book for recording complete information on all transactions as they incurred (e.g., Monthly Expense Disbursements Journal).

Ledger   Summary sheets—final entry.

Debits   Entries conventionally made on the "left side" of an account. Debits increase Asset and Expense Accounts, and reduce Liability, Capital and Income Accounts.

Credits   Entries conventionally made on the "right side" of an account. Credits reduce Asset and Expense Accounts, and increase Liability, Capital and Income Accounts.

Drawing Account   Sole proprietors may withdraw cash for personal use. It is similar to a salary except you don't take out withholding taxes (instead you pay self-employment taxes). Withdrawals can reduce the owner's equity.

Petty Cash Fund   Cash on hand to pay for incidental expenses. Put a voucher in the petty cash drawer and record each transaction. Do not put cash received from a client into the petty cash fund. When the fund is low, write a check (and cash it) to bring the fund back to the desired level (most likely between $20 and $100). Be sure to transfer the transactions to your Petty Cash or Disbursements Journals.

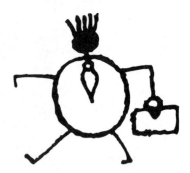

Business Income

Business income includes all monies received: cash, checks, credit cards and barter. Record income at least twice a week; daily is preferred.

Credit Cards

We live in a society that relies heavily on credit, and many clients appreciate the convenience of this payment option. From a business standpoint, the advantages of accepting payment cards usually outweigh the disadvantages. In fact, marketing research shows that people are often are willing to spend more if they can pay with a credit card—plus there's the impulse buy factor. Advantages that come with accepting this form of payment are added convenience for your regular clients, increased appeal for your gift certificate program, more high dollar product purchases and an increased likelihood of clients purchasing a package deal for a series of sessions. In many instances, you don't even need special equipment—you can call in the transaction or process it over the Internet.

Set-up fees can range from $25 to $250, the charges range from 1.79 percent to seven percent of the gross sales (plus with some systems, you pay 15 to 70 cents each time you process a charge), there is usually a delay (up to seven days) in getting access to the money, and the client has up to six months to refute a charge.

Managing Gift Certificate Finances

I recommend that you put at least half of all gift certificate revenue into a savings account and transfer the funds into your checking account when the certificate is redeemed. Otherwise, if you sell a lot of gift certificates, you could find yourself in the position of working for an extended period of time without receiving "new" income.

Keeping track of gift certificates is easy when you design a system and stick with it. This can be done on a computer in a spreadsheet program, accounting software or client management software. You can also use a manual register system (see Figure 14.4).

Make sure your bank and credit card processor properly code your business. For instance, massage therapists should use the SIC/MCC code 8099 (Health and Allied Services, Not Elsewhere Classified). The NAICS code for massage is 621399 (Offices of All Other Miscellaneous Health Practitioners).

Merchant Credit Card Services

www.PayPal.com
www.cardservice.com
www.chargeamerica.com
www.cellcharge.com
www.merchantseek.com

Chapter 16, Pages 399-400

for tips on marketing gift certificates.

Figure 14.4

Sample Gift Certificate Register									
Date Sold	Amount Paid	Purchased by	Phone Number	Issued to	Phone Number	Services	Products	Dollar Amount	Date Redeemed
10/12	$45	S. Smith	555-1111	P. Jones	555-2222	5 yoga classes			
10/14	$60	T. Silver	555-1234	???		1-hr massage			
10/15	$75	L. Gold	555-5555	J. Dowd	555-3333			$75	

Gratuities • •

The topic of accepting tips is complex. Some professions would never consider it because of the problems inherent with transference: since there is no guarantee that a client is feeling equal in power in the relationship, it's unwise and often unethical to take extra money. This includes extravagant gifts such as the use of a vacation home. The gray area concerns gifts that are more symbolic, such as garden produce or homemade cookies. Graciousness is a delightful skill. It recognizes and affirms positive intentions. The acceptance of a flower can be a healing moment. However, if a client were to always bring something extra for you or offer you an expensive gift, it would be prudent to state that you're well compensated for your time and nothing else is needed.

Most people feel awkward about tipping. They aren't certain when it's appropriate or how much to give. Are you supposed to tip mail carriers, hair stylists, pet groomers, auto mechanics, estheticians, gardeners and physicians? Do you tip them if they work for someone else, but not if they're the owners of the business?

Remember that tips and most gifts are considered taxable income.

Unfortunately, practitioners who work in settings such as spas usually receive minimal remuneration and rely on tips. To complicate matters, many spas are expanding their services and employ a wide variety of practitioners including acupuncturists, nutritionists, massage therapists, movement specialists and physical therapists. This puts clients in a quandary about tipping protocol. Of course, if the practitioners were receiving appropriate fees for their work in these settings, tips wouldn't be an issue. Clients, however, are usually unaware of the arrangements between the spa and the practitioner.

Many spas provide envelopes printed with the word "gratuity" for clients to leave tips for the practitioners. The manner in which this is handled makes all the difference. It is one thing to tastefully display the envelopes at the front counter; it's another to post a sign by the envelopes that says, "I've helped make your day, now help make mine (hint, hint)."

Another downside to accepting tips is that it creates expectations: you don't want clients worrying about whether to give you a tip. Even worse is the anxiety clients might experience if they give you a tip one time and not the next. Will you think they didn't like the session as much? Will they receive the same level of service next time? This tension defeats the therapeutic value of the work.

If you decide that in your setting a professional doesn't accept tips, you can make a clear choice. If someone asks you about tipping, you can say something like, "I appreciate the acknowledgment, but a tip isn't expected in a therapeutic relationship." You can also give the client options such as donating the tip to your favorite charity or starting a scholarship fund for people who normally could not afford your services. Another idea is to thank the client and ask her instead to tell her friends about your services. Remind the client that gift certificates are a wonderful way to introduce individuals to your services.

Gratuities can make you feel appreciated, yet money is not the only way to express appreciation. Given that many people have money issues, it is not necessarily the best form of gratitude. Encourage people to simply say, "Thank you!" and have that mean something.

Business Deductions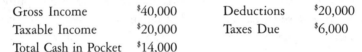

Business deductions reduce your net profit which in turn reduces your tax liability. Business owners are entitled to numerous deductions. Most of these expenses (except for those such as draw) are recognized as full deductions on Schedule C—although some of these allowances have strict guidelines and ceilings.

Business 2000 Magazine reported a CPA study showing that in 1999, America's small businesses overpaid their income taxes by over $2 billion. According to Bernard Kamaroff, author of *Small Time Operator* and *422 Tax Deductions For Businesses & Self-Employed Individuals*, "The overpayments were made because the businesses failed to take tax deductions they were legally entitled to take. Many of these businesses are still unaware of their errors. They overpaid their taxes and don't even know it."[1]

According to the IRS, a legitimate expense must meet the following guidelines: it must be incurred in connection with your business; be ordinary (similar expense to others in your profession); and be necessary.

Consider the following example for a sole practitioner's business that generates $40,000 in income from client sessions and product sales and has $20,000 in expenses from items such as rent, supplies, marketing and inventory.

422 Tax Deductions For Businesses & Self-Employed Individuals
by Bernard Kamaroff

Gross Income	$40,000	Deductions	$20,000
Taxable Income	$20,000	Taxes Due	$6,000
Total Cash in Pocket	$14,000		

Depending on your tax bracket, the combined tax rate of your Federal, State and Self-Employment Tax rates can vary from 20 percent to well over 50 percent. Thus, in this example, the taxes due would be between $4,000 and $10,000! Now you can see why every penny counts. Even just an additional $1,000 in expenses saves you between $200-$500 in taxes. However, to reap these benefits you must develop a system to accurately track your expenses.

As of 2007, office furniture, computers or other equipment may be written off up to a maximum of $112,000 per year (keep in mind that this may decrease in future years), or else they need to be depreciated.

Page 306
for Education Tax Credits.

Educational expenses can only be deducted if they relate to improving your current line of work. In general, you cannot deduct education expenses for starting a new career. For instance, if you're a physical therapist or a chiropractor and you want to expand your practice by offering massage, it would most likely be deductible. But if you're an artist and want to sculpt muscles instead of clay—it would not be deductible.

Expenses most often questioned during an audit are claimed expenses that are not usually associated with your profession, as well as extravagant travel, entertainment and transportation expenses. The latter are also areas that rarely receive full expense deductions.

Figure 14.5

Common Fully Deductible Business Expenses

- Bank Service Charges
- Business Books and Trade Publications
- Business Insurance
- Credit Card Fees
- Dues
- Education
- Furnishings, Decorations & Equipment
- Interest on Business Debt
- Insurance
- Inventory Cost of Goods
- Linen Service

- Maintenance and Repairs
- Marketing
- Office Supplies
- Online Fees
- Postage
- Printing and Copying
- Professional Fees
- Rent
- Sales and Excise Tax
- Samples
- Telephone & Utilities

Business Use of Home • •

You can deduct expenses related to using a part of your home regularly and exclusively as either a principal place of business or as a place to meet clients. The percentage of business use of a home is determined by dividing the square feet of the business space by the total square feet of the home. If the space was used for less than a full year, you must prorate expenses for the number of months used for the business.

One hundred percent of the cost of decorating, furnishing, repairs and maintenance of the business-use space is deductible or depreciable. The business percentage of permanent improvements that benefit the entire home (e.g., new roof or temperature control unit) are depreciable. Deductions for the business use of a home may not be used to create a business loss or increase a net loss from a business. Deductions in excess of that limit may be carried forward to later years (subject to the income limits in those years). Also, if you deduct office space in your home, you may be subject to a capital gains tax upon the sale of your house.

To claim a home office expense, you must file Form 8829 (Expenses for Business Use of Your Home) with your Schedule C.

Travel, Entertainment and Gifts • •

Keep accurate records to substantiate travel and entertainment expenses. In addition to receipts, keep a journal that denotes the following for each expense: a description of the expense; the amount spent; date, time and place; business purpose; names and business relationship of person(s) entertained or gifted; and any other pertinent information. In regard to gifts for clients, you're allowed to declare $25 per client per year. The deduction for business-related meals and entertainment is limited to a maximum of 50 percent (the IRS frowns upon lavish meals that include magnums of Dom Pérignon). If you must travel any distance for business, the transportation and lodging costs are usually wholly deductible (although an unusual number of trips to exotic locales might spark an audit).

Transportation ● ●

The customary and necessary expenses incurred on operating and maintaining a vehicle for business purposes are deductible according to the actual percentage of business use. The two methods for computing allowable expenses are the actual expenses (at the business-use percentage) or the total business mileage (using the IRS determined allowance). You must use actual costs if you use more than one vehicle in your business. The best evidence to support a transportation deduction is a logbook or journal that shows the date, business purpose, destination and mileage of all business travel.

Business Mileage Sheet
www.businessmastery.us/
forms.php#busman

Assets Owned Prior to Business Establishment ● ●

A common question asked by new business owners is, "Can I deduct the expenses of the equipment and books I bought while I was a student?" If you're a sole proprietor, anything that was your personal property and is now being used solely for your business can be declared as owner's equity (e.g., inventory, merchandise, supplies) or as a fixed asset (e.g., massage table, office furniture, stereo equipment), which then gets depreciated as of the date you place it in service in your business. The basis used for depreciation is the lower of the actual cost or the fair market value of the item when placed into service, not the original cost.

Pro Bono Work ● ●

Many people wonder if they can legally take a deduction for their pro bono work. Alas, no. Such work doesn't "cost" you money. What it does cost is your time. Even though we know time is money, the IRS doesn't view it in those terms. So choose wisely to whom you give your pro bono work, be it for an individual, organization or event. Most people do pro bono work to help a needy individual, support a specific cause or group, or to further establish themselves in the community. The services you give to charity should be considered an act of goodwill, motivated by compassion.

Depreciation ● ●

Depreciation is a tax term that describes the loss in value of an asset over time. An asset is a tangible commodity that will last for more than one year (e.g., a computer or a building). When you purchase more than a certain dollar amount of assets in any given year, the IRS requires the cost to be deducted over years (since the asset's life is greater than one year). The amount of depreciation allowed depends on the category of the asset and its value. Depreciation rules change almost every year and can be quite complicated to calculate. This is a prime example of why you need an accountant.

Figure 14.6

Common Estimated Business Expenses

Initial Expenses:	Estimated Cost:
Opening Business Checking Account	$100
Telephone Installation/Activation	$200
Equipment	$1,500
First & Last Month's Rent & Security Deposit	$1,000
Business Cards	$100
Stationery & Envelopes	$200
Brochure	$250
Logo	$250
Opening Promotion Package	$1,000
Fliers, Announcements, Ads in local papers, magazines, radio	
Decorations	$250
Office Supplies	$500
Furniture, Music System, CDs, Clothes	$1,000

Annual Expenses:

Property Insurance	$175
Business License	$100
Liability Insurance	$250
Professional Society Membership	$300
Legal & Accounting Fees	$400

Average Monthly Expenses:

Rent	$400
Utilities	$50
Telephone	$75
Bank fees	$10
Supplies	$75
Networking Club Dues	$40
Education (seminars, books, journals)	$50
Promotion	$100
Postage	$25
Entertainment	$50
Repair & Maintenance (also cleaning service)	$70
Travel Expenses	$30
Yellow Pages	$30
Inventory	$150
Business Loan Payments	$?
Staff Salaries	$?
Personal Draw/Salary	$?

Financial Statements

Financial statements are formal records of the financial activities of a business. They provide an overview of a practice's profitability. They show where a company's money came from, where it went and where it is now (e.g., assets and profits).

Income and Disbursement Ledger Sheets: They provide detailed, categorized information on income and expenses. These ledger sheets can be recorded manually or by using accounting software. It is ideal to update them daily. (See Figures 14.7 and 14.8.)

Business Income and Expense Forecasts: These forecasts project the income derived from an estimated number of clients you expect to utilize your services, how often they will schedule appointments, as well as how many will also purchase products and the amount of product they will purchase. (See Figure 14.9.)

Profit and Loss Statements: Also called Income Statements, they tell you how much a company earned or lost over a specific period of time (usually for a quarter or a year). They show how much money a company generated over a specific time period, as well as the costs and expenses associated with earning that money. (See Figure 14.10.)

Balance Sheets: Provide summary information about a company's assets, liabilities and net equity as of a given point in time. A company's assets must equal, or "balance," the sum of its liabilities and shareholders' equity. (See Figure 14.11.) The following formula summarizes what a balance sheet shows: Assets = Liabilities + Equity

Cash Flow Statements: Cash flow statements document the timing of how income and expenses occur throughout a year. They are best used as a forecasting tool so you can gauge how to manage your finances. For instance, if you discover every April your income decreases by 30 percent, then you can either save money to cover your expenses for that month or increase your marketing efforts in February and March to boost April's revenues. Using another example, let's say you've completed your forecasting for the next year and discover a one-time $2,000 expense in June. You then go back to the forecast and add another category titled "Savings for June Expense" and split up the $2,000 over the previous five months (and, of course, actually put that money into a savings account). (See Figure 14.12.)

www.businessmastery.us/
forms.php#finman
for blank financial forms.

The reaction of weak management to weak operations is often weak accounting.
— Warren Buffett

Figure 14.7

	Sample Weekly Income Ledger Sheet								

Month __April__ Week __1__ Year __2020__ Page __1__

Date	Client Name	Amt Paid	Ck #	Services	Products	Type	Location	Company	Notes
4/2	Perry Winkle	20	911	20	0	O	Outcall Office	ABC Corp	
4/2	Astria Ames	20	123	20	0	O	Outcall Office	ABC Corp	
4/2	Sandy Lott	35	709	25	10	O	Outcall Office	ABC Corp	
4/2	Maureen Dock	25	312	25	0	O	Outcall Office	ABC Corp	
4/2	Brad Jones	35	1947	25	10	O	Outcall Office	ABC Corp	
4/2	Amy Allen	50	417	50	0	N	Office	Humane Society	
4/2	Bill Peters	0	Prepay	0	0	O	Outcall Home	Attorney	Prepaid Services
4/3	Warren Piece	55	Cash	55	0	N	Office	Evans & Assoc	
4/3	Shirley Ujest	0	Prepay	0	0	N	Office	T&J Accounting	Gift Certificate
4/3	Weldon Rod	75	Cash	40	35	O	Office	Artist	
4/3	Les Moore	0	Promo	0	0	N	Office	Stars R Us	Knows many people
4/3	Helena Montana	55	653	55	0	N	Office	Thornton Co.	
4/4	Gail Windser	47	712	7	40	O	Outcall Home	Mattson Corp.	Prepaid Services
4/4	Hope Esperanza	0	Prepay	0	0	O	Outcall Home	N/A	
4/4	Holly Fields	100	211	60	40	N	Office	N/A	
4/5	Morris Katz	55	506	55	0	O	Office	School District	
4/5	Grover Funk	45	614	35	10	O	Office	TMJ Corp.	
4/5	Butch Smalls	55	430	55	0	O	Office	Allied Assoc.	
4/5	Truly Scrumptious	60	Cash	40	20	O	Office	Carpenter	
4/5	Harry Beardsley	55	Barter	55	0	N	Office	N/A	Barter for bookcase
4/6	Sam Iyams	0	Prepay	0	0	O	Outcall Home		Prepaid Services
4/6	Somer Days	90	347	35	55	N	Office	Model	Referred by Moore
4/6	Clyde Dales	220	940	220	0	O	Office	Burns & Assoc	Series of 5
4/6	Penny Cash	55	Cash	55	0	O	Office		
4/6	Sylvia Goldsmith	65	810	45	20	N	Office	Data Tech	
4/6	May Springman	55	Cash	55	0	O	Office	M&M Inc.	

Total Income: $1,272   Service Income: $1,032   Product Income: $240   # Sessions: 26   New Clients: 9   Ongoing: 17

Figure 14.8

	Sample Monthly Disbursement Ledger Sheet													

Month __April__ Year __2020__ Page __1__

Date	Description	Amt Pd	Ck #	Rent Util	Maint Phone	Suppl Postage	Promo Fees	Travel Auto	Furn Equip	License Dues	Educ Ins	Books Inv	Bank Fees Ent.	Misc. Draw
4/2	ABA	250	140							D 250				
4/2	Jones Cleaning	27	141		M 27									
4/2	Paul 'd Auto	17.30	142					A 17.30						
4/2	Sunset Bld	350	143	R 350										
4/3	Gas To Go	9	Cash					A 9						
4/4	RJ Office	6.21	144			S 6.21								
4/4	Pace Printer	29.50	145				P 29.50							
4/4	Last Cafe	12.70	Cash										E 12.70	
4/10	The Garden	18.40	146										E 18.40	
4/12	Phone Co.	65.90	147		T 65.90									
4/12	Success 1st	20	148							D 20				
4/17	Career Sem	50	149								E 50			
4/17	Draw	800	150											D 800
4/18	Discount Sup	8.14	Cash			S 8.14								
4/19	Western Bank	8.20											B 8.20	
4/20	Ace Ins.	200	151								I 200			
4/21	USPS	25	152			P 25								
4/25	Earth Time	60	153				P 60							
4/25	AAA Util	50	154	U 50										
4/26	Discount Sup	20	155			S 20								
	Total	2027.35		400.00	92.90	59.35	89.50	26.30	0.00	270.00	250.00		39.30	800.00

Please note that not all expenses are 100% deductible. Please consult current tax laws.

Figure 14.9

Sample Business Income and Expense Forecast

One Year Estimate Ending <u>12</u> / <u>31</u> / <u>2020</u>
month day year

— PROJECTED NUMBER OF CLIENTS —

For Your Services Only	30
For Your Products Only	15
For Your Services and Products	55
Total Number of Clients	**100**

— SESSION FREQUENCY —

Weekly	5	X	52	=	Yearly total =	260
Twice per Month	20	X	24	=	Yearly total =	480
Monthly	30	X	12	=	Yearly total =	360
Quarterly	30	X	4	=	Yearly total =	120
Other						15
Total Number of Sessions						**1235**

— PROJECTED INCOME —

Sessions (at $55 per session)		$	67,925
Product Sales		$	4,000
Other (workshops)		$	1,000
Total Income	(A)	$	**72,925**

— PROJECTED EXPENSES —

Start-up Costs		$	10,000
Monthly Expenses (x 12)		$	18,000
Annual Expenses		$	3,000
Total Expenses	(B)	$	**31,000**
Total Operating Profit (Or Loss)	(A – B)	$	**41,925**
Capital Required for the next 12 Months		$	*

Depends on how much money you need for your personal expenses.

Figure 14.10

Sample Abbreviated Profit and Loss Statement	

This Report Covers June 1, 2020 to June 30, 2020

Income

Sessions	$4,000
Product Sales	300
Workshops	400
Room Rental to Associate	300
Total Income	**$5,000**

Expenses

Rent	$ 800
Inventory	200
Utilities	50
Supplies	120
Phone	80
Marketing	200
Misc (see Figure 14.6)	350
Total Expenses	**$1,800**
Net Profit	$3,200 *

*Note: this does not include income tax and self-employment tax.

Figure 14.11

Sample Abbreviated Balance Sheet	

Balance Sheet as of December 31, 2020

Assets

Current Assets	
Cash/Bank Balance	$5,000
Accounts Receivable	500
Inventory	1,000
Supplies	1,000
Fixed Assets	
Property	-0-
Equipment	3,500
Total Assets $11,000	

Liabilities

Current Liabilities	
Accounts Payable	500
Credit Card Charges	500
Long-Term Liabilities	
Bank Loans	$3.000
Total Liabilities	**$4,000**

Ner Worth (Owner's Equity)	**$7,000**

Figure 14.12

Sample Cash Flow Projections Sheet

	May	June	July	Totals
Beginning Cash	1,000	2,690	1,890	1,000
Plus Monthly Income From:				
Fees	3,000	2,400	3,200	8,600
Sales	300	200	300	800
Loans	0	0	0	0
Other	0	0	0	0
Total Cash and Income	4,300	5,290	5,390	10,400
Expenses:				
Rent	400	400	400	1,200
Utilities	50	55	50	155
Telephone	75	75	75	225
Bank Fees	10	10	10	30
Supplies	75	10	65	150
Stationery & Business Cards	0	150	0	150
Insurance	0	650	0	650
Dues	75	0	325	400
Education	25	200	0	225
Advertising & Promotion	100	150	250	500
Postage	25	0	40	65
Entertainment	40	30	60	130
Repair & Maintenance	80	50	80	210
Travel	0	70	0	70
Business Loan Payments	0	0	0	0
Licenses & Permits	0	0	75	75
Salary/Draw	500	1,000	500	2,000
Staff Salaries	0	0	0	0
Taxes	0	0	600	600
Professional Fees	35	50	25	110
Decorations	20	0	0	20
Furniture & Fixtures	50	0	0	50
Equipment	0	0	425	425
Inventory	50	500	0	550
Other Expenses	0	0	0	0
Total Expenses	1,610	3,400	2,980	7,990
Ending Cash (+ or -)	2,690	1,890	2,410	2,410

• Taxes •

The information provided here is a general overview. Tax laws change regularly, so keep apprised of current regulations. IRS Publication 334 (Tax Guide for Small Business) is published annually and contains comprehensive tax information for sole proprietors, partnerships and corporations.

I highly recommend you consult with an accountant regarding tax matters. Unless your financial affairs are extremely simple, chances are that you will overlook deductions and credits to which you're entitled. A professional tax preparer knows what to look for and what's available to reduce your tax bill. While it's important for you to be familiar with the general workings of tax planning and the tax law—leave the technical details to your accountant.

Think of this in terms of your own practice. The general public might adequately handle their well-being on their own, but they come to you because you offer a higher degree of knowledge, experience, objectivity and techniques than they possess. Similarly, it makes sense to rely upon the expertise of a tax professional and other business experts.

Common Tax-Cutting Strategies •

The topic of taxation has become enshrouded in an aura of mystique. For instance, some people believe that cutting taxes means hiring high-priced experts to find "loopholes" in the law (an option only for rich people). In fact, the law is the same for everyone, and tax-cutting strategies are available to all.

No one is required to pay more tax than the law demands. Some of the more common tax-cutting strategies are:

- Splitting income among several family members (age 14 and older) or between legal entities to get more of the income taxed at lower brackets.
- Shifting income from one year to another so that it falls where it is taxed at lower rates.
- Shifting deductions from one year to another to place them where the tax benefit is greater.
- Deferring tax liability through certain investments and pension plan contributions.
- Structuring your business to obtain a tax deduction for some expenses paid for things that you enjoy (e.g., travel).
- Investing your money to produce income that is exempt from either (or both) federal and state income tax.

This {preparing my tax return} is too difficult for a mathematician. It takes a philosopher.
— Albert Einstein

Preparing Tax Returns •

The three primary methods for preparing tax returns are to do them manually, use a tax software program, or engage the services of an accountant. The two major drawbacks to preparing taxes yourself (either manually or with a software program) are:

- Tax preparation isn't always as straightforward as it seems.
- There are thousands of codes related to deductions that frequently change, although the tax forms list only a few standard deduction categories.

You need to know what expenses are deductible, and they aren't always obvious. For instance, there are options for declaring deductions for business-related food and lodging expenses. Currently, the standard per diem rate in the United States is $99 per day ($60 for lodging, and $39 for meals and incidental expenses). But the rates are higher for certain cities. If you have receipts that are higher than the per diem, you can use those receipts (remember that you can only claim 50 percent of the total meal bill, including tip). The exciting part is that you can take the per diem rate even if it's more than your actual expenses. Loopholes aren't just for the wealthy! Working with a knowledgeable tax professional can ensure that you take advantage of all eligible deductions.

See IRS Publication 1542.

Keep in mind that a tax deduction is what you can deduct, not necessarily what you spent. Sometimes this works in your benefit, as in the above per diem example. The flip side of this is that there are legitimate business expenses for which you can't deduct the full cost (e.g., 50 percent of business entertainment meals) and others for which there are limits (e.g., $25 per person ceiling on gifts).

Pages 292-294

for information on Deductions.

The main problem with using tax software programs is that they aren't designed to handle the complexities of a business. They are great for wage earners who receive W2s. So if you work solely as an employee, then a software program might work well.

Not every practitioner must utilize an accountant, but it's wise to meet with an accountant at least once to determine what deductions you may be overlooking, and to plan for ways to legitimately write off future expenditures.

How to Find the Right Accountant • •

A good accountant looks into ways to save clients money through tax savings, shifting how and where money is spent, increasing revenues and reducing overhead. The problem areas in tax returns are depreciation and "underuse" of eligible deductions. There are hundreds of legitimate tax deductions, and even the best accountant can't spend the time going through each one with you to make sure you're aware of them all.

Find an accountant who takes the time to work with you, not just someone you hand your paperwork and get a tax return to send to the IRS. You also need to feel comfortable with this person. Some accountants take an aggressive approach to tax return preparation while others are conservative. It is also crucial that the two of you can communicate clearly and easily. Your accountant can profoundly affect your business success, so choose wisely.

U.S. Federal Tax Reporting •

The following information provides an overview of federal tax reporting requirements. Check the IRS guidelines to determine filing dates for tax returns. Generally, state tax returns are due at the same time as federal returns. Some states follow the same tax law as the IRS and others don't. Check with your state tax agency to verify requirements.

Employees • •

Check www.irs.gov for current tax information.

Employees receive a Form W-2, Wage and Tax Statement from their employers. They are issued in January for the previous calendar year. Form W-2 combines all wages and reported tips. It lists the amount of taxes withheld and paid throughout the year.

- Form 1040: U.S. Individual Income Tax Return
- Form 1040: ES: Estimated Tax For Individuals (quarterly—if you will owe taxes)
- Form 2106: Employee Business Expenses
- Form 4070: Employee's Report of Tips to Employer (given monthly to your employer)
- Form 4137: Social Security and Medicare Tax on Unreported Tip Income

Employee Business Expenses • • •

According to the IRS regulations, employee expenses are generally listed on Form 2106 and the total amount is carried forward to line 20 of Schedule A (Form 1040) or line 9 of Schedule A (Form 1040NR). This is only applicable if you itemize. Also, don't file Form 2106 if none of your expenses are deductible because of the two percent limit on miscellaneous itemized deductions.

Note: Check to see if the standard deduction amount is greater than your itemized deductions. If so, use the standard deduction.

Gratuities • • •

All tips you receive are income and are subject to federal income tax. You must include in the gross income all tips you receive directly, charged tips paid to you by your employer, and your share of any tips you receive under a tip-splitting or tip-pooling arrangement.

Reporting your tip income correctly is not difficult. You must do three things.

1. Keep a daily tip record.
2. Report tips to your employer.
3. Report all your tips on your income tax return.

You must report tips to your employer so that:

If you are documenting your work and keeping accurate accounts, tax preparation becomes a natural extension of your bookkeeping activities.

- Your employer can withhold federal income tax and Social Security and Medicare taxes.
- Your employer can report the correct amount of your earnings to the Social Security Administration (which affects your benefits when you retire or if you become disabled, or your family's benefits if you die), and
- You can avoid the penalty for not reporting tips to your employer.

If your total tips for any one month from any one job are less than $20, do not report the tips for that month to that employer. Do not report the value of any noncash tips, such as tickets or passes, to your employer. You don't pay Social Security and Medicare taxes on these tips, although their value is supposed to be listed as income and subject to income tax.

If your employer doesn't give you any other way to report your tips, you can use Form 4070, Employee's Report of Tips to Employer. Fill in the information requested on the form, sign and date the form, and give it to your employer.

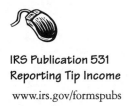

If you do not use Form 4070, give your employer a statement with the following information.

- Your name, address, and Social Security number.
- Your employer's name, address, and business name (if it is different from the employer's name).
- The month (or the dates of any shorter period) in which you received tips.
- The total tips required to be reported for that period.

You must sign and date the statement. You should keep a copy with your personal records.

If you received tips of $20 or more for any month while working for one employer but did not report them to your employer, you must figure and pay Social Security and Medicare taxes on the unreported tips when you file your tax return. If you have unreported tips, you must use Form 1040 and Form 4137 to report them. You may not use Form 1040A or 1040EZ. If you do not report tips to your employer as required, you may be charged a penalty of 50 percent of the Social Security and Medicare taxes due on the unreported tips unless there was reasonable cause for not reporting them.

Sole Proprietors • •

A sole proprietorship is not an independent entity from its owner, so the business does not file a separate tax return. Income or loss is reported on the owner's personal tax return. If you're a sole proprietor you must file:

- Schedule SE: Self-Employment Tax
- Schedule C: Profit or Loss From Business (Sole Proprietorship)
- Form 1040: U.S. Individual Income Tax Return
- Form 1040 ES: Estimated Tax For Individuals (quarterly—if you will owe taxes)

Generally, you must pay estimated tax if you expect to owe (after subtracting your withholding and credits) at least $500 in tax for the current year, and you expect your withholding and credits to be less than:

1. 90 percent of the tax to be shown on current year tax return; or
2. 100 percent of the tax shown on the previous year tax return (given the return covered all 12 months).

The exception to this is if your previous year tax return showed a refund or the tax balance due was less than $500. Plan ahead: If your income level requires you to pay taxes (even if you can avoid making prepayments to the IRS this year), set up a "savings" account for that money.

Page 291
for details on Tips.

IRS Publication 531
Reporting Tip Income
www.irs.gov/formspubs

Partnerships and Limited Liability Corporations (LLCs) • •

Partnerships and LLCs are taxed similarly to sole proprietors. A partnership doesn't pay taxes. Income or loss is reported on the individual partner's tax returns. The partnership must file the following (plus include a copy with their personal tax returns):

- Form 1065: U.S. Partnership Return of Income
- Form 1065 K-1: Partner's Share of Income, Credits, Deductions, etc.

Corporations • •

Corporate annual returns are due by the 15th day of the third month after the close of the corporation's fiscal tax year. Corporations must file the following:

- Form 1120: U.S. Corporation Income Tax Return (or short form version, 1120A)
- Form 8109: Federal Tax Deposit Coupon (estimated tax payment)

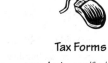

Tax Forms
www.taxadmin.org/fta/
link/forms.html

Employer's Forms • •

As an employer, you're required to file the following:

- Form 941: Employer's Quarterly Federal Tax Return
- Form W-2: Wage and Tax Statement
- Form W-3: Transmittal of Wage and Tax Statements
- Form 940: Employer's Annual Federal Unemployment Tax Return (FUTA)
- Form 1099: Miscellaneous Income (any business that pays more than $600 to a self-employed person must report that payment to the IRS and the sub-contractor)
- Form 1096: Annual Summary and Transmittal of U.S. Information Returns

Tax Credits •

The IRS advises that taxpayers consider claiming eligible tax credits when completing their federal income tax returns. A tax credit is a dollar-for-dollar reduction of taxes owed.

Business Tax Credits • •

Tax credits differ from business deductions in that most tax deductions are the actual costs incurred in running a business and the categories tend to stay the same year after year. Tax credits are government incentives to encourage business owners to take socially responsible actions or to stimulate the economy. The regulations regarding tax credits can frequently change. Historically, business tax credits have included hiring people with disabilities, using renewable energy sources, renovating buildings, purchasing alternative fuel vehicles, operating a business in an empowerment zone or renewal community, and investing in certain types of equipment.

Chapter 5, Pages 96-99
for examples of socially
responsible business practices.

Tax Credit for Handicapped Accessibility • • •

ADA Fact Sheet
www.ada.gov/taxpack.htm

Possible tax credits are available for the purchase of equipment such as hydraulic tables. Practitioners may benefit by Section 44 Disabled Access Credit (Forms 8826 and 3800), which applies to costs incurred by small businesses to comply with the applicable requirements under the Americans with Disabilities Act of 1990. In addition to access expenditures such as ramps, the definition includes, "To acquire or modify equipment or devices for individuals with disabilities." These expenses must meet the standards issued by the Secretary of the Treasury.

To qualify as a small business, the practice must meet the following requirements: the annual gross receipts for the preceding year did not exceed $1 million or had no more than 30 full-time employees during the preceding tax year.

A tax credit is subtracted from your tax liability after you calculate your taxes, while a tax deduction is subtracted from your total income before taxes, to establish your taxable income.

If you work with clients who fit into this category (such as physically challenged or elderly), then you could be eligible for a rebate. Essentially the credit works this way: Take the total expenses, subtract the minimum amount (which is $250 in 2007), and then multiply that amount by 50 percent. For instance, let's say that a table costs $4,000. Deduct the $250 to get a subtotal of $3,750. Multiply that amount by 50 percent, and the total credit available is $1,875. Thus, although the table costs $4,000, the actual out-of-pocket cost for the table is only $2,125. By the way, this $2,125 gets listed as a deductible business expense on your tax return.

The maximum annual purchase limit is $10,250, so the maximum tax credit available is $5,000. This credit can only be applied to reduce an existing tax liability down to zero, but not to the point at which the business would show a loss.

Personal Tax Credits • •

See IRS Publication 970 to determine if you qualify for Education Tax Credits.

Many types of tax credits are available, ranging from the Earned Income Tax Credit (EITC) for certain people who work and have an earned income under certain thresholds, to Child and Dependent Care Credit to Education Credits. Since many of you reading this book are in school or plan to further your education, we've included an overview on education tax credits to help save you some money.

Education Tax Credits • • •

The Hope Credit and Lifetime Learning Credit for "qualified tuition and related expenses" provide potential tax savings on higher education costs incurred by you, your dependents or your spouse. The Hope Credit is for the payment of the first two years of tuition and related expenses for an eligible student. The Lifetime Learning Credit is available for all post-secondary education for an unlimited number of years. A taxpayer cannot claim both credits for the same student in one year.

www.businessmastery.us/ ed-tax.php
for more information on education tax credits.

In the past, educational expenses related to starting a new career were not tax-deductible. Those costs could only be deducted if they were considered to maintain or improve skills related to your current trade or business. This deduction reduces your taxable income, thus lowering the amount of income tax due. The IRS has initiated a program that actually puts money back into your pockets in the form of educational tax credits.

U.S. State Tax Reporting •

In the United States, most states and the District of Columbia require you to file a state return if your income is above some minimum requirement. State tax returns are usually due at the same time as federal returns. Contact your State Department of Revenue or a tax professional to ascertain your state's specific requirements and the way they determine your tax liability.

Sales Tax • •

A taxation area that practitioners sometimes ignore is state sales tax. Unless you live in a state that doesn't levy sales tax, you're required to collect (and remit) sales tax on product sales—regardless of the volume. Some states also tax services. Contact your State Department of Revenue to apply for a Transaction Privilege Tax License. Most states charge a one-time fee of less than $20. Some cities require a separate Transaction Privilege Tax License. The frequency of how often you must submit reports and the collected sales tax varies. Usually you're required to fill out a form on a monthly basis for the first year. If the volume is low, the state might reduce it to quarterly or even annually. Note that while it is called State Sales Tax, the percentages usually vary by the type of taxable activity and the city.

Discuss tax collection requirements with the state, as well as the company from which you buy products for resale (e.g., certain food-based products are not taxed). Also, if you purchase products to resell, you don't need to pay sales tax to the company that sells you the product. The companies from which you purchase products often ask for your Resale Number (which is on the Transaction Privilege Tax License).

The difference between death and taxes is death doesn't get worse every time Congress meets.
— Will Rogers

Canadian Tax Resources •

As in most countries around the world, tax regulations in Canada are complex and change frequently. Regulations and requirements vary among the provinces and territories. To ensure compliance with the most current Canada Revenue Agency (CRA) tax laws, readers are advised to consult with their accountant or financial planner for specific advice prior to making any business decisions.

When it comes to business expenses, some are fully deductible and some are only partially deductible. Any reasonable expense that you incur to earn business income should be treated as a potential deduction. Many expenses can be fully claimed in the year of purchase.

The CRA is responsible for collecting federal, provincial (except Québec) and territorial income taxes. The Canadian tax system is also based on self-assessment. Under the self-assessment system, nonresidents with Canadian income and Canadian residents are responsible for making sure they've paid their taxes according to the Income Tax Act. Income tax rates are set annually. Income and deductions are listed on the Income tax and benefit return so both the tax filer and the CRA can calculate the taxes the tax filer has to pay. Similarly, Canadian corporations and nonresident corporations with Canadian income pay corporate income tax according to the Income Tax Act and provincial and territorial legislation. Corporations file a corporate income tax return.

For those who want to get familiar with the general workings of the Canada Revenue Agency (CRA) tax requirements and tax planning, refer to the Internet websites listed in the margin. They are a good starting point and can help answer many frequently asked questions. The following information is an overview of various tax requirements.

Canada Taxes

www.cra-arc.gc.ca/
menu-e.html

www.sbinfocanada.about.com/
cs/taxinfo/l/bltaxindex.htm

www.canadabusiness.gc.ca/
gol/cbec/site/nsf/en/
index.html

Provincial and Territorial Tax Rates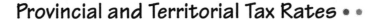

Provincial and territorial tax rates vary. Under the current tax on income method, tax for all provinces (except Quebec) and territories is calculated the same way as federal tax.

Goods and Services Tax (GST) ••

The Goods and Services Tax (GST) was implemented by the Federal Government in January 1992. Some services which had been tax-free became taxable, including wellness services such as massage therapy, chiropractic and acupuncture services. However, not every wellness practitioner has to charge the GST. For sole proprietors, partnerships or corporations with a combined gross business income of $30,000 or less in the last four consecutive calendar quarters or in any single calendar quarter, GST collection is not mandatory. Once the $30,000 mark is surpassed, GST collection becomes mandatory.

Provincial Sales Tax (PST) ••

When you have to charge GST and PST, calculate GST on the price excluding PST. Readers are advised to contact their provincial sales tax offices for more information. Keep in mind that in the participating provinces, HST includes both the federal and provincial parts.

Taxes, after all, are dues that we pay for the privileges of membership in an organized society.
— Franklin D. Roosevelt

Harmonized Sales Tax (HST) ••

Three participating provinces—Nova Scotia, New Brunswick, and Newfoundland and Labrador—harmonized their provincial sales tax with GST to create the Harmonized Sales Tax (HST). For instance, the HST rate in 2007 was 14 percent (6 percent federal part and 8 percent provincial part). HST has the same basic operating rules as GST and is applied at a single rate on the same base of goods and services that are taxable under GST.

• Work Smarter with Barter •

Barter is a cashless exchange of goods and services. This method is not confined to primitive societies. It is the preferred method of managing finances for some, while others use barter only occasionally to enhance their cash flow. Bartering is not a casual activity. According to the International Reciprocal Trade Association (the oldest and largest trade organization representing the reciprocal trade industry), approximately 300,000 companies in North America belong to an organized barter exchange. Those businesses transact approximately $4 billion in sales annually.

Technological advances in electronics (e.g., computers, fax machines, modems and email) have expanded barter from a face-to-face interaction to a global transaction. This enables a small business owner the opportunity to participate in an arena previously dominated by large corporations.

Barter affords you a simple, legal method to conserve cash outlays. If you can trade for something you need, then you can use your cash for other purposes. I've traded for office supplies, printing, advertising and cleaning. You may need your office rewired, your taxes prepared, flowers delivered, or your back adjusted. Bartering is also an excellent method for expanding your client base. Many people who've never received the services of a complementary wellness provider might be more open to scheduling an appointment if they didn't need to pay in cash. I have made several training contracts with companies that probably would not have hired me or anyone else if it meant dipping into their cash reserves. Even though I didn't receive cash, the trade was useful and those clients have referred cash-paying clients to me.

Direct Barter •

Many wellness providers already barter on a direct basis. They identify services and products they need and approach appropriate business owners with a trade proposal. Quite often, too, a client is the one to initiate a barter transaction. These direct trades work best if the items or services are of equal value. You can use gift certificates for trades and get gift certificates or vouchers from the person with whom you're trading. For instance, if you barter chiropractic services with a printer, have the printer give you a voucher for the amount you normally charge for an office visit. Then, when you're ready to do a printing job, you can redeem your vouchers.

Barter is considered taxable income like cash, credit cards and checks.

Here's another example: Let's say a restaurant owner wants to trade you meals for acupuncture treatments. You charge $65 per visit. One method is to have the restaurateur provide you with a $65 voucher for each treatment. Another idea is to transact a trade for a set amount, such as 10 acupuncture certificates for $650 worth of restaurant vouchers (in varying denominations). The beauty of the latter idea is that the certificates and vouchers can be redeemed by anyone. If you don't want to eat $650 worth of food at that restaurant, you can give the vouchers as gifts or use them for trading with someone else. Your client can do the same with the acupuncture certificates you give, which can ultimately bring you additional cash-paying clients.

Two major problems with direct barter arise from inequitable trades and trading for things you don't really need. The following scenario demonstrates the first concern: You want to have someone clean your office. You don't really have the cash to pay for that service so you consider approaching someone to barter. Although you may find an office cleaner, it probably won't work for long. The person is likely to become resentful when five hours of labor (at $10 per hour) equal one hour of your services.

The second problem relates to setting good boundaries. It can be so tempting to accept a barter offer from a potential client, particularly if you feel that the only way the person will utilize your services is if you agree to trade. If this occurs, remind yourself that your time is valuable. If the trade is not for something you want or that you can give to another, then you're essentially giving away your session if you agree to trade. Both of these problems can be eliminated by membership in a barter network.

Developing your own direct barter network takes some thought and a bit of research. Start by listing all the goods and services you need in your business. Then make a second list of the items you would like for personal use. Make a third list of friends, colleagues and clients and the services and goods they offer. Then compare all three lists. You may match a lot of your needs with people you already know. Build your network by telling people that you're interested in bartering—let them know your needs and what you can offer in return.

Barter Exchanges ●

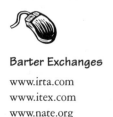

Barter Exchanges
www.irta.com
www.itex.com
www.nate.org

Join a barter exchange if you plan to incorporate more than the occasional barter into your practice. Contact the National Association of Trade Exchanges or the International Reciprocal Trade Association for listings of barter organizations in your city. Approximately 300 barter networks exist in the United States. The International Trade Exchange (ITEX) and International Monetary Systems (IMS) are the two largest exchanges.

Essentially barter organizations work by members selling their goods and services to other members in exchange for trade dollars, which are valued at the equivalent of cash dollars. With each transaction, trade dollars are debited from the buyer's account and credited to the seller's account. The seller can then spend these trade dollars with other exchange members.

Barter exchanges function like a bank. They handle transactions, debit and credit accounts, charge fees and send monthly statements. They may even offer a payment plan or extend a line of credit. You are given either a credit card or checkbook with which to make your transactions. A client getting a treatment from you either charges it and you call it in to the exchange office (a similar procedure to processing bank credit cards) or writes you a barter check which you deposit (just like a bank check). The organization charges 10-15 percent commission (in cash) on the value of the actual trade. Usually the commission is applied against the buyer's account, but some exchanges split the charge between buyer and seller.

Before you join an exchange check how many other people in your specific profession are members. If the total membership of a prospective exchange is under 200, and if five of the same type of practitioners are members, you may want to consider a different group because there might not be a large enough potential client pool.

www.businessmastery.us/
barter-exchange.php
for more tips on how to
work successfully with a
barter exchange.

⁕ Inventory Control ⁕

Practitioners who sell products need to keep track of what has been ordered, how long it takes to receive merchandise, how long it takes to sell merchandise, and what is in stock. You don't want to run out of your best-selling item—particularly if it takes weeks to obtain more. Also it isn't wise to carry too much stock that has a relatively short shelf life—oils that can go rancid or magazines that are published monthly.

If you carry a limited selection of products, daily inventory can be checked visually and a written tally (often referred to as a physical inventory) taken at least twice per year. A more formal approach to inventory is recommended if you stock a wide variety of goods. Most accounting software packages include inventory recordkeeping. These programs keep track of inventory on hand and alert you when stock gets low. Even if you rely on computerized inventory control, do a physical inventory at least twice each year, as posting errors can occur and adjustments need to be made.

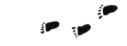

Chapter 13, Pages 263-265
for details on product sales.

Forgetting to place an order can easily happen when you're busy with all the other aspects of running a practice. Charting inventory activities reduces the chances for errors and provides you with a quick overview.

Figure 14.13

Sample Inventory Record							
Item: _____				**Vendor:** _____			
Address: _____				**Phone:** _____			
Date Ordered	Quantity Ordered	Date Received	Quantity Received	Posted on Computer	Quantity Sold	Balance	Date of Physical Inventory

• Selling a Practice •

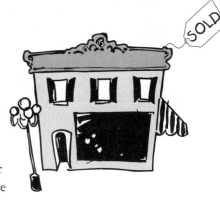

People have many reasons for selling their businesses. The standard ones are burnout, relocation, serious injury or permanent disability, the desire for a career change, death, boredom, disagreement with a business partner, lack of capital, or retirement. Just because you want (or need) a change, selling isn't the only avenue. Many alternatives exist. You can cut back your hours, find partners, incorporate other practitioners, change the business structure, get help, give the business away, sell part of it, franchise or expand.

Chapter 10, Pages 191-194

for information on buying a practice.

The topic of selling a business is fraught with misconceptions—the biggest one being that a buyer will come out of nowhere and make the seller wealthy. Another common fallacy is that selling a business is like selling a house: while everyone needs a place to live, no one needs to buy a business. Also unlike real estate, there are generally no accepted ways to set a selling price, and you can't compare selling prices of other wellness practices. The most frequent assumption is that buyers fully appreciate the years of sacrifice it took you to build your practice; in most instances they don't. Another major misconception is that the less information you give the buyer, the better. Nothing could be further from the truth. Uncertainty is always discounted, and buyers always pay less for less information. Also, legal ramifications can occur if you fail to disclose full information (also known as fraudulent inducement).

Most small business owners either sell or close their business within 20 years. I have no idea what the average is for the various types of wellness practices. Through the mid-1990s, the only practitioners that seemed to sell their practices were primary care providers (mainly medical doctors and dentists). The statistics on other practitioners is still sorely lacking.

With traditional businesses, the majority of sellers hope a family member, employee or associate will buy their business, but in reality only 25 percent of businesses are sold to a family member, and 10 percent are sold to an employee. Over half of the buyers are found through brokers.

Most businesses are bought by individuals. Employees usually don't have the money and competitors usually only want a part of the business. In this field you're most likely to sell your business to another practitioner who is either new to the field, new to the area or wants to expand his target markets. Buyers usually don't fork over the asking price in one cash payment; they want the business to earn more than enough money to make the loan payments. They want a high-return, low-risk, satisfying lifestyle and something that's affordable. Make it easy for them. Help them deal with the uncertainty. Provide understandable information, point out business strengths, answer questions, and help them answer questions they're getting from the significant people in their lives.

I realize this process may seem overwhelming and you may be uncertain if all this work is worthwhile. But if you have built up a thriving business, you owe it to yourself to attempt to sell it and recoup some of your investment of time, energy, money and reputation.

Regardless of where you are in your practice (just starting out or nearing retirement), begin organizing your business now so it is easier to sell at any time. Establish a clear system for documentation of your client files and financial records. Analyze your business using the eight factors highlighted below, and clarify your goals and business vision. Start implementing changes now: capitalize on your strengths and do whatever is necessary to eliminate (or at least abate) your limitations. The effort you invest can only enhance your overall success.

Four Ways to Leave Your Business *

The four most common ways to leave your business are:

- transfer ownership to a family member;
- sell your interest to a co-worker, key employee or all employees;
- sell to a third party, such as a competitor or someone interested in entering your field;
- liquidate by selling off your assets, usually at "fire sale" prices.

Consider the following elements when deciding which method to use: minimizing risk, exercising control, achieving personal objectives, assuring payment, maximizing flexibility in structuring the deal, and fixing value. Your needs in each of these elements determine your best selling strategy.

Transfer ownership to family member * *

The downside to this method is that it simply might not be an option, it could increase family tension, and it might stir resentment from the nonfamily members in your business. The benefits include exercising more control, particularly in terms of setting a monetary value on the business and the repayment schedule.

Sell to a co-worker, key employee or all employees * *

The downside is that you don't have control of the quality of services provided once you leave. Yet this method significantly reduces your risks, and you can increase the likelihood of retaining the same quality and degree of success if you have a staff person buy into your business while you're still active. In effect, you're prequalifying your buyer through on-the-job training and observation. You can even establish a fund within the operation of the business to go toward the eventual purchase price.

Sell to a third party ••

Selling to a third party (e.g., a competitor or someone interested in entering your field) is the preferred method when the business is too valuable to be purchased by anyone other than someone with access to a lot of capital. This is most likely to be your best avenue if you have a sole-practitioner business.

The disadvantages are that the buying party inherently has more bargaining power, you can't be certain if the buyer's style and abilities will fit well with your current clientele and staff, and you may be required to carry some (or even most) of the purchase price, which means you will still be involved in the business for one to three years. The benefits are that you most likely get a good price, and, if you have any staff at all, you will be giving them the opportunity for continued employment.

Liquidation ••

Liquidation or simply closing down your practice should be considered the last resort, although, sadly, it's the most common method chosen by the majority of wellness providers.

The Eight Selling Stages •

The best time to sell your practice is contingent on the readiness of your business and the readiness of the marketplace. Most businesses aren't in a position to be sold because they aren't set up for a smooth transition—particularly in terms of documentation. If most businesses were to attempt to sell, they would not get a good price since owners tend to maximize after-tax cash flow and minimize profitability. They set up their business structure in terms of wages and legitimate perks in a manner which optimizes their lifestyle while doing the best they can to reduce taxes.

Figure 14.14

The Eight-Stage Selling Process

- Review your motives for selling your business and consider the alternatives.
- Analyze your business to determine if you're selling what buyers want.
- Assemble an excellent team of advisors.
- Set a selling price for your business.
- Prepare your business for sale and make it easy to purchase.
- Market the sale of your business.
- Sell the business.
- Transition the business to the new owner.

Selling a business usually takes a lot of work and time. Most businesses take between six months and two years to sell. Using a broker helps to reduce some of your direct time and energy involved, but it doesn't eliminate it.

Review Your Selling Motives and Alternatives • •

Reflect upon the reasons you want to sell your practice and clarify your goals. Determine which methods you will use for selling your business. The following exercise assists you in choosing the best method for you.

Choosing a Method for Selling Your Business

Take out some paper and ask yourself this set of questions for each method:

* Why does this method appeal to me?
* What reasons make this method appropriate?
* What conditions need to be present for this method to be appropriate?
* Why might this method not be appropriate?

Analyze Your Business • •

You need to make sure your business is sellable. Put yourself in the position of a potential buyer. Why would they want to purchase your business? What exactly would they be buying? Can they work with your current clients? Analyze your business point by point to determine its scope and condition. Compile a written analysis which includes the following factors.

Company History: How long has your practice been in existence? What is the growth rate of your client base? What is your educational background?

Staff and Associates: Do you have employees? If so, what are their job descriptions and how long have they worked for you? Do you have associates? If so, what services do they provide, what financial agreements are in place, how long have they been associated with your business and how do they fit in with the overall structure of it?

Description of the Business: Summarize your business in terms of the services offered, equipment, products, supplies, location, resale items, fee structure, client profile, position statement, competition analysis and differential advantage.

Financial Status: Figure out the true profit of your practice. Assemble the appropriate documents such as tax returns, profit and loss statements, accounts payable, accounts receivable and the current year's ledger.

Equipment: If you want to sell your equipment, check its condition. Are the items in good shape? Is it worthwhile to include them in the cost of the sale? Most equipment decreases in value over time, particularly electronics (e.g., telephones and computers). Items such as your table may cost much more to replace at current prices.

Facilities: If the buyer will be utilizing your office space, you need to check the condition of the premises, evaluate the overall appearance, and have options ready for the transfer of real estate.

Overall Risk: This is what buyers use to determine the return they require on their investment and what affects their pricing calculation (see step IV). The risk is evaluated from the point of view of not earning a return on the invested time and money or possibly losing their investment.

Strengths and Limitations: Ironically, this is the last step a seller takes in analyzing the business, yet it's the buyer's first step. After you complete a detailed analysis of your business using the above factors, note which characteristics stand out most clearly. Clarify your opportunities and drawbacks. Think about your strengths as your selling points and your limitations as part of your improvement plan. Keep in mind that your practice may be sellable even if it isn't in shape to be sold right now. Reorganization and improvements can always be made.

Assemble Your Advisory Team ••

Your advisory team saves you a lot of time and eliminates some of the inherent frustration involved in selling your business. Minimally this team includes an accountant and an attorney. Another member to consider is a financial planner. It is also helpful to get feedback from other practitioners who have sold their practices. I highly recommend working with a business broker. Brokers know how to organize the appropriate documentation, set a price and market the sale of your business. You can hire one to handle the total selling process or as a consultant.

Set a Selling Price ••

Many formulae exist for the pricing of a business, although valuing and pricing is hardly an exact science due to the large number of variables. It is extremely difficult to measure certain factors such as goodwill, risk, quality of staff, the ability of the new owner to work well with current clients, and (if your practice is sold to an established wellness provider) the cost savings by eliminating duplication of efforts and reducing potential competition. Unfortunately, very few people sell their wellness practices, so we have limited role models available, and comparisons with other professions or businesses aren't necessarily valid.

Ultimately, the price a buyer pays is a subjective decision which is (hopefully) backed by objective information. The amount you receive depends on the value of the business and its affordability to the buyer. It is important that you distinguish the difference between price, value and affordability.

Price is what someone is willing to pay for it. Value is what something is worth. This figure is derived from what the business owns, what it earns, and its differential advantage. Rarely do businesses sell for what they're "worth," particularly wellness practices. This is mainly due to the high risk involved because of the personal nature of this field and the intangibles which greatly influence the success of a practice, such as the marketing abilities of the owner and the clients' expectations of the types of treatments they receive.

Affordability is what the buyer is capable of paying. You may find a potential buyer who would be ideal to take over your business, agrees to your price, yet still may not purchase your business because of the terms. Thus, in many ways, what the buyer can afford depends on you.

Figure 14.15

The Six Most Common Methods for Pricing a Business

Price Based On:
- Assets
- Capitalized earnings
- Integrating assets and cash flow
- Duplication cost
- Carry back
- Net present value of future earnings

Price based on **assets** is done by determining the market value of the assets being sold and deducting the cost of liabilities to be assumed by the buyer. Assets include furniture, fixtures, equipment, supplies, inventory, client lists, leasehold improvements, accounts receivable, real estate (this isn't limited to owning property, it could include possessing a lease in a prime location) and corporate contracts. This is a fairly straightforward method.

Most service businesses are mainly based on **capitalized earnings**. To obtain this figure, first calculate the adjusted cash flow and deduct a fair wage for the new owner. This is the base figure for this method. Next, determine a fair return that a buyer should receive for investing in this business. Most buyers use a 15-20 percent figure for a low-risk business and a 25 percent or higher for a risky business. Convert this percentage into a multiple by dividing it by 100. Multiply the base figure by the multiple to get a selling price.

If the business has both **assets and cash flow**, the first step is to determine the value of the hard assets. Then calculate the adjusted cash flow. Add those two figures together. If, as the seller, you want a full cash sale, this number is your selling price. If the business is in excellent condition or your selling terms include payments over several years, the amount you can ask for is the hard assets plus up to twice the adjusted cash flow.

Pricing your business on the **duplication cost** is done by taking the market value of assets and combining it with the cost for the number of years it would take a beginning practitioner to reach the same profit level. It can be rather tricky to determine the latter figure, particularly if you didn't market and build your practice on a consistent basis. Also, since the potential buyer is an unknown quantity, he may be excellent or abysmal at marketing.

Carry back is generally appropriate for small businesses. Calculate the adjusted cash flow of the business. Deduct the anticipated wages the buyer would need and the expenses required to run the business for one year. This figure gives you the cash available on which to set the sales amount. If you assume the loan to be a five-year payoff, simply multiply the cash available by five. You can add a reasonable down payment amount to this figure to get a total selling price.

These formulae aren't foolproof. The variables which affect the selling price vary significantly with each business. I highly recommend working with a business broker and an accountant to help you determine which method or combination of methods is best for you.

The **net present value** method is worth considering if you've built a very strong, diversified practice which includes other practitioners, corporate contracts, concessions at a health club or product sales. The technique involves the following steps: Adjust the company statements to show true present profit (e.g., add back in the perks you've taken); develop your business plan and project the growth for the next five years; calculate the profit, investments and returns for the next five years; and then discount the figures to the present using a discount rate which reflects the degree of risk, as well as projected inflation. The major problems with this method are that the projections are purely speculative and the discount rate is totally arbitrary.

Calculate your selling price using all the above methods and see what the results show you. Inherent in all of these methods is the problem that they don't take into account: many practitioners buy an existing practice simply to ensure themselves of a "job." Also, your business may include intangible assets that are difficult to price. These include your credibility, heart, reputation, goodwill and presence in the community. Many clients may stay with the new owner out of their respect and loyalty to you—given that you sell to a practitioner with the same commitment toward quality.

Another idea to consider is incorporating a contingency clause. As a result, you can ask for a higher price since you're minimizing the buyer's risk. After the down payment, the two techniques for contingent payment are: the buyer makes the additional payments only if the business meets certain expectations (e.g., at least 50 percent of the clients stay), or the buyer only has to pay you a set percentage of the fees received from your current clientele.

The bottom line in selling your business revolves around economics—supply and demand: Is your business saleable and are there any buyers?

Buyers will test the desirability of purchasing your business. The first test in buying a small business is how the cost returns and effort required in running the practice measure against investing their money elsewhere. The biggest test is the "justification test." The buyer must be convinced that the business can provide sufficient cash flow to repay the loan, support the business operational expenses, give a reasonable return on the down payment and allow for reasonable wages.

What a buyer can afford and what they are willing to pay more often depends more on the upfront cash required than the selling price. The more favorable the terms of sale (such as no or low cash down, no security deposit, minimal interest, a lengthy repayment schedule or contingency terms), the easier it is for you to find a buyer.

Preparing Your Business For Sale • •

As stated before, the single biggest mistake sellers make is not properly preparing the business for sale. Preparation involves making the requisite improvements in order to enhance the likelihood of your business selling as well as assembling the appropriate documentation. See Figure 14.16 for the items to include in your documentation package.

Figure 14.16

Business Sale Documentation

- Opening Proposal: A one-to-four page overview of the company history, mission statement, brief business description, summary of assets, financial history, reason for sale and pricing terms
- Samples of Promotional Materials
- Detailed Business Description
- Names of All Owners
- Copy of Lease
- Profit and Loss Statements for Past Three Years
- Tax Returns for Past Three Years
- Copies of Current Contracts
- Determination of Value of Leasehold Improvements
- List of Fixtures and Equipment with Replacement Value
- Value of Inventory

Marketing • •

Marketing the sale of your business includes the preparation, pricing, packaging and promotion you do to bring your business and a buyer together. Accurate, organized, appealing documentation is the foundation to the successful sale of your business.

Your presentation package should include your opening proposal, samples of promotional materials and any other documents that highlight your success such as newspaper interviews.

The rest of the documentation should be provided to the prospective buyer only after they've signed a Letter of Intent to Purchase. Granted, this letter doesn't guarantee they will indeed buy your business, but it helps safeguard your business privacy by weeding out the less serious buyers.

The most common marketing methods are advertising, direct mail, telemarketing and networking. Advertising is an effective technique if the potential buyers are numerous and they're easy to reach in print (e.g., through trade journals and newsletters). Direct mail works well if you can identify buyers. It is one of the best for selling a practice because you can target specific practitioners or soon-to-graduate students. Telemarketing is an avenue worth pursuing, particularly if it's done in conjunction with direct mail. Networking is an extremely effective marketing technique. The only problem is that if you do it yourself, you lose confidentiality. Most wellness providers aren't overly concerned about people discovering they're attempting to sell their practices. Although if you don't anticipate selling the business quickly, you may need to proceed cautiously to avoid losing clients. If you desire to keep the sale of your business under wraps until the last possible moment, networking should be done through an intermediary.

2007 Business Reference Guide
www.businessbookpress.com

Buying and Selling a Business
by Robert F. Klueger

*The Complete Guide
to Selling a Business*
by Fred S. Steingold

If you don't match abilities and personalities, the buyer is less likely to retain the client base.

Finding an appropriate buyer is crucial. It is to your benefit (particularly in terms of getting paid) that the buyer can easily take over and work with your clients. This can be difficult if the techniques you utilize are extremely specialized. You need a buyer whose knowledge, training and personality is similar to yours. For instance, if you're a Trager® practitioner, it's wise to sell your practice to another Trager practitioner—not just any touch practitioner. If you incorporate a variety of modalities, find another practitioner with diverse experience.

The Actual Sale • •

Once you have a potential buyer, delineate in writing both parties' expectations regarding the selling process. Keep in mind that most buyers and sellers are inexperienced and don't know what to expect.

The next phase is to qualify the buyer. Find out where he stands financially and his sources of income. You could request a personal financial statement or a copy of the previous three years' tax returns. Realize that, as the seller, you're viewed as the prime source of financing, given that 75-80 percent of businesses are seller-financed, with the seller carrying one-half of the selling price. Another aspect of qualifying a buyer is to find out if there's a good fit between the buyer's goals and needs, and the company as it stands. The last element of qualifying a buyer is obtaining references.

After you've qualified your potential buyer, ask for a *Letter of Intent to Purchase*. This letter contains the names of the buyers and sellers, description of what the buyer intends to purchase, the date of offer, expiration date, price, terms, interest rate, repayment schedule, amount of deposit, closing date and contingencies.

The next stage centers on negotiations and documentation verification. Do not be surprised if the buyer requests you sign a "non-competition" clause stating that you won't set up another practice within certain geographic limits, or requires you to refrain from promoting your business to specific target markets for a reasonable period.

Once the seller accepts the offer, she submits the rest of the documentation. The buyer then performs what is termed "due diligence." This entails examining all of the submitted information to verify its accuracy and confirm that any specified conditions are met. More negotiations may follow and the contract is drawn.

The final stage is the closing. This can be a rather stressful event, so be prepared. To ensure a smooth closing, make sure all parties understand and agree upon the terms of the sale in advance and bring copies of all important documents.

The Post-Sale • •

In most instances, sellers are required to continue involvement in the company for a short time after the official sale. This transition time allows for the new owner to be brought up to speed and provides the seller with the opportunity to introduce the new owner to the clients, suppliers and staff. It may be necessary for the seller to train the new buyer, continue to work in the business for a specified time or provide consulting services to the buyer.

• Retirement Planning •

When you have bills to pay and other priorities demanding your time and money, saving for retirement may seem like a distant goal. No matter the size of your business or your age, it's important to take the first steps toward saving for your retirement and developing an investment plan.

It all starts with the realization that you're not going to work forever—and that you need to save now to pay for future living costs. These concerns require that you act today so you can enjoy a comfortable and worry-free retirement. Whether you're self-employed or an employee, the steps to a successful retirement are simple:

- Develop an effective savings plan: save the right amount; save regularly; save in the right accounts.
- Create an investment strategy: choose the best mix of investments based on your retirement goals and comfort with potential risk.

The first step is to understand what retirement investment options are available. You can either work with a financial planning advisor or spend some time with a good resource book to get the information you need. The next steps are to set retirement goals, estimate what your living expenses will be when you retire, and develop a strategic savings and investment plan to meet your financial goals. Financial experts agree that it's best to treat Social Security retirement income as a supplemental source of retirement income—not the primary source.

Retirement Planning Calculator

http://cgi.money.cnn.com/tools/retirementplanner/retirementplanner.jsp

Prosperity is the fruit of labor. It begins with saving money.
— Abraham Lincoln

Retirement Plan Options •

> Following is a short introduction to retirement planning. We've been given permission by Jan Zobel to excerpt and adapt this information from her book, *Minding Her Own Business: The Self-Employed Woman's Guide to Taxes and Financial Records*. Detailed information can be found at www.businessmastery.us/retire.php.

Tax-deferred retirement plans are valuable because, while saving for your retirement, you delay paying taxes on money you earn and contribute to these plans. Additionally, the interest and dividends earned on the money in the retirement plan are tax deferred. Tax-deferred means that you pay no taxes on the money until it's taken out of your retirement account.

Theoretically, when you take the money out of the account, you're retired or working part time, which puts you in a lower tax bracket than you were in when you invested the money. As a result, the money you contributed and the earned interest or dividends are taxed at a lower rate than they would have been if you hadn't put the money in a tax-deferred account and instead had paid tax on it when it was earned.

Have a set amount of money automatically withdrawn from your checking account on a monthly or biweekly basis and put it into a retirement investment.

Check with the IRS, a pension planning attorney or a financial advisor before implementing a retirement plan to be sure you're optimizing your planning strategy and following IRS regulations. Also, remember that these numbers change.

Due to compounding interest, the earlier in life you begin contributing to a retirement plan, the less total amount you'll need to deposit to accumulate a substantial amount of retirement money. The money you contribute to a retirement plan, however, should be money that you don't expect to need until you're at least 59½ years old. When you take a distribution from your retirement account, you are taxed on that money in the same way as you're taxed on other income. With few exceptions, the IRS also assesses a 10 percent penalty if money is taken out before you're 59½. Your state may have a similar penalty, which means that if you take the money out prior to reaching the minimum age, you may lose nearly 50 percent to federal and state taxes and penalties. No matter how little you contribute, get into the habit of making an annual contribution to your retirement account. Following is a brief overview of retirement plans.

Small Business Retirement Plans • •

Employer Sponsored—Tax-Sheltered or Tax-Deferred Plans and Annuities

> 401(k) Plan
> 403(b) Tax-Sheltered Annuity
> Tax-deferred Annuity Retirement Plan

Contributing to these types of plans gives you an immediate tax deduction and tax-deferred growth on your savings. Deductions are taken from your paycheck and put into your designated retirement account. Many employers offer matching contributions. Plan rules vary.

Self-Employed 401(k) Plan • •

A retirement plan for business owners with no employees.

IRA Details

www.fool.com/money/
allaboutiras/
allaboutiras01.htm

Traditional IRAs • •

IRAs offer huge tax breaks. They can be set up at a bank, brokerage house, mutual fund company or other financial institution.

Roth IRAs: Offers tax-free growth, but does not allow contributions to be tax-deductible.

SEP-IRA Accounts (Simplified Employee Pensions): Available to sole proprietors, partnerships, LLCs and corporations. Contributions are based on a percentage of net employment income. Employers are required to make a contribution on behalf of anyone over age 20 to comply with SEP-IRA account guidelines. Funded by employer contributions.

Keogh Plans: Either a defined contribution plan or defined benefit plan. Rules regarding employee coverage, due dates and maximum contribution limits apply. Funded by employer contributions.

SIMPLE Accounts (Savings Incentive Match Plan for Employees): Enables employees to contribute to a retirement plan. Requires employers to match employee contributions up to a certain percentage according to plan rules. Provides favorable conditions for self-employed small business owners as they may make SIMPLE contributions as both an employer and employee.

Money taken out of an IRA before age 59½ is subject to an early withdrawal penalty. In certain cases the penalty may be waived.

Part VI

Marketing Mastery

Part VI of *Business Mastery* explores how to master the marketing tasks that are essential to your success. Successful practitioners know who they want to work with, understand how to find those potential clients through appropriate marketing techniques, and attract the desired clients by clearly and engagingly describing what they do. They maintain a thriving practice by being client-centered: having an inviting treatment space, using high-quality equipment, conducting thorough treatment plans, following up, and, most importantly, listening and responding to each client's unique needs. What's the best way to begin? Like building a house, it's wise to start with a foundation and build from there.

Chapter 15 provides that foundation by detailing how to identify your target markets, develop a marketing plan, and take action steps to attract new clients and build a thriving practice. The chapter also introduces a virtual toolbox of marketing concepts, such as positioning, branding, and differential advantage, along with valuable insights into how you can put them to work to grow your business.

Chapter 16 provides the framework for a solid house by providing a primer of low-cost marketing techniques that you can use to get your first clients. This chapter is filled with practical information about how to use promotion, advertising, publicity and community relations to build a thriving practice.

Chapter 17 rounds out the house design by focusing on creative ways to retain clients. It explores how exceptional customer service and incentive programs foster long-term client relationships, and how you can put customer service action plans to work to enhance your business success.

Marketing Fundamentals

• Primary Marketing Principles •

The word "marketing" may trigger a wide array of thoughts and feelings ranging from tremendous excitement to fantasies of instant success to studied disinterest to hand-wringing dismay. Although effective marketing is the cornerstone of a flourishing practice, some practitioners shy away from any type of self-promotion as they associate it with pushy sales tactics. This avoidance may also stem from a lack of marketing knowledge or limited resources.

One of the attractions of the wellness field is its dissimilarity with the "typical" business world. But even the wellness profession revolves around sales and marketing. Luckily, we rarely need to rely on traditional methods to promote ourselves. The most effective marketers focus on value-centered marketing: promoting their business in a way that reflects their personality, philosophy and integrity. Within this context, marketing is simply sharing information about yourself and your services with potential and current client so they get a sense of who you are, which allows them to make an informed choice of whether to utilize your services. It isn't about coercion or pretending to be someone you're not.

Simply put, marketing involves identifying your target markets, developing a marketing plan, and taking action steps to attract potential clients and retain current ones. The wide world of marketing includes promotion, advertising, community relations and publicity. Marketing is all about empowering your clientele to value you and your services. Effective marketing involves targeting the appropriate people and informing them about the benefits of your services. The biggest mistake I see people make is overextending themselves; they try to be the practitioner for everyone. One person cannot fulfill all the needs of every client.

Marketing a service can be very different than marketing a product. For example, retailers use mass-marketing techniques such as broad-based advertising campaigns, telemarketing and in-store promotions. Service businesses usually target a well-defined market and use a personal approach. The major portion of marketing a service business is educational in nature.

Quality in a service or product is not what you put into it. It is what the client or customer gets out of it.
— Peter Drucker

Frequently wellness providers leave their marketing to chance. They wait for people to find them—an attitude that's generally counterproductive. (It's okay if you have an alternate source of income.) But consider why you got into this field in the first place. What good is it to desire enhancing people's well-being if they don't know who you are? The key is to create a marketing plan that focuses primarily on low-cost techniques that build relationships.

Very few people can afford the luxury of building their practices solely by word of mouth. If you're very good at what you do, genuinely care about and respect your clients and charge a reasonable rate, you will ultimately develop a strong clientele base. However, most practitioners are interested in accelerating that process, and that requires marketing savvy.

The Essence of Marketing ●

Marketing is about getting yourself known—building a professional reputation. The ulitmate aim is to develop a thriving practice, and that means having a strong and continually growing clientele base.

Everything you do makes a statement about how you feel about yourself, your clients and your practice. Thus, you're always marketing yourself—for better or worse. You may have noticed that marketing concepts and tips appear throughout most of the chapters in this book. This is because marketing isn't just about the outward activities you do, such as advertising and promotions; it also involves the way you relate to your clients, your ethics and your professional demeanor. To attract the right clients and grow your business, your outward image must be consistent with your vision of a successful wellness professional. The more creative and natural your marketing techniques, the more successful they are, mainly because you enjoy doing them. No rule says that you can't have fun while promoting your business!

A popular phrase in this industry (and also the title of a book)[1] is "Do what you love and the money will follow." Unfortunately, most people forget about the verb in the sentence: DO. Having a passion for what you do—and top-notch skills—aren't enough to build a thriving practice. Without a good marketing plan and consistent action steps to reach your marketing goals, it's likely your business and bank account will lag.

Marketing is all about taking the right actions to attract new clients. For instance, if you don't have a full client load, invest that free time in educating people about your work or donate your services (do what you love)—then the money will truly come. Have the courage to do some of the practice building activities that you might not necessarily love, such as public speaking or writing articles.

The Power of Public Opinion ●

Price is what you pay.
Value is what you get.
— Warren Buffett

Before you begin to develop your marketing plan, assess your community's opinions and perceptions about preventive wellness and alternative therapies. Are wellness services such as massage therapy, nutritional counseling and acupuncture viewed as nonessential luxuries (fluff)? Or is your business located in an area where people are open to alternative approaches to wellness and focused on healthy aging? Are there specific target markets within your community that currently work with wellness practitioners on a regular basis?

Understanding the wellness quotient of your community is important, because it's a lot easier to swim with the current than against it. If a high percentage of people are actively seeking alternative therapies and can afford regular preventive wellness services, your odds of success are much greater than in a community that is skeptical of alternative approaches to wellness.

Establish Credibility •

Establishing credibility is essential to the long-term success of your practice and is the foundation of any successful marketing venture. People need to feel that they can trust you and your expertise to assist them in reaching their wellness goals.

Your level of professionalism plays a major role in the status of your credibility. Your actions must echo your words. Don't make promises, either verbally or in printed materials, that you cannot fulfill. Don't make claims that you cannot substantiate. It is better to be conservative in your offerings and exceed them, than to make grandiose proclamations and fall short.

One of the best methods for establishing credibility and increasing visibility is public speaking.

Figure 15.1

Credibility Components

- Length of time in the field
- Hours of education and training
- Appearance and dress
- Demeanor
- Communication skills
- Vocabulary
- Testimonials and success stories
- Pictures
- Guarantees
- Professional affiliations
- Credentials
- Public image

Chapter 5, Pages 90-93 for more on professionalism.

Competition •

A strange paradox of competition versus abundance exists in this career field. There truly are enough potential clients in the world for everyone, and yet not many practitioners have as many clients as they want. Part of the dilemma stems from the fact that the people are "potential" clients. You have to make them aware of you and the benefits of your services. It isn't as though there are limitless numbers of people anxiously waiting for you to let them know you exist; you must create the need.

Understanding how competition impacts your business can help you make wise marketing decisions. Think of competition as a way of distinguishing yourself from other wellness providers. One of the most exciting facets of this industry is that practitioners usually aren't attempting to prove that they're "better" than others—but that they're different. For this reason, marketing is vital to your career. You must sell people on your services and then on you! Don't assume that you're going to attract the people who "know better," take care of themselves and use alternative wellness services. Such people probably already have a network of wellness providers. You may need to attract clients who are exploring new modalities due to a health challenge or life change, and you may need to create new markets, and possibly share an existing market.

Bicyclists race faster against each other than against a clock.
— Norman Triplett

Don't take it for granted that people know what you do because you have a certain title. Define what you do. Explain the benefits of what you offer and what sets you apart from other practitioners in your field. Every practitioner is unique, and brings her experience and personality into play along with whatever techniques are employed. The power of your marketing increases with the level in which YOU are integrated into those marketing strategies.

The other sources of competition are the products and services that your target markets employ to meet their needs. For instance, if you're a nutritionist and one of your target markets is people who suffer from migraines, your competition can include physicians, hypnotherapists, somatic practitioners, meditation instructors, biofeedback practitioners, acupuncturists, herbalists, and pharmaceutical companies. Many factors determine how migraine sufferers choose to address this health concern, such as the severity and frequency of the migraines, the overall cost for care, knowledge of the breadth of care options, attitudes about wellness options, and the perceived value of your type of service.

Some people pay whatever it costs to get the care they need, and they select the method(s) based on their perceived value. Others must choose between options they can afford.

Your Major Competitors ● ●

Rarely is evaluating the competition a straightforward task. You need to do some footwork. It can be easy to ignore this phase since many practitioners aren't willing to challenge their preconceptions about competition. Although your ultimate success depends more on your abilities and communication skills than what your competition does, the more you know about your competition, the easier it is for you to determine the most advantageous manner to market your practice.

The first step is to identify your most direct competition. Begin your research by studying the telephone directory. For example, you look through the directory and discover that 40 other practitioners are listed. Of those 40, perhaps half of them appear to provide similar services as yours. This information tells you that you have at least 20 direct competitors and 20 indirect competitors. First focus on your direct competitors. Start your research by checking out their websites. Look to see what services and products they offer, if they have other practitioners working with them, and their prices. Delve deeper to get a sense of what markets they seem to be targeting by how they describe themselves and their services, the graphics they use and the client testimonials they highlight.

Call them and request brochures, particularly if they don't have websites. Some places to find wellness practitioners' brochures and fliers are bulletin boards at health food stores, offices of other practitioners and bookstores. Also, check out other local publications (you may want to get several months' worth of editions) to discover if your competitors are listed in any of those publications. Ascertain who is doing what and where they're doing it. These local publications and bulletin boards may be your primary source of information about your competitors, since many wellness providers don't advertise in traditional ways.

Finally, use their services. You may discover that only four or five of these people are in direct competition with you, actually offering similar services to the same market at a comparable rate, that is, the same target market.

The best way to evaluate other practitioners is to take notice of what people say about them.

Chapter 10, Pages 185-187

for more tips on scoping out the competition.

Get new clients by purchasing the phone numbers of closed competitors and have the numbers routed to your phone number.

Competition Analysis

Compile a profile on each of your major competitors. Include the following information:

- Name
- Location
- Length of time in business
- Description of services offered
- Manner in which services are provided
- Office hours
- Fee structure
- Clientele description
- Business strengths and limitations
- Differential advantage and market position
- Methods of promotion

Analyze the information you've gathered on your competition. Look for patterns and trends. Compare it to the assessment of your own business.

- How does your business compare to the competition?
- What are the strengths your business has in comparison to the competition?
- What are the challenges your business has in comparison to the competition?
- What are some steps you can take to meet those challenges?
- How can you take your competitors' weaknesses and turn them into unique benefits of your practice?

Cooperation ●

Your marketing ventures can be significantly more successful, enjoyable and less risky if you join with other practitioners in cooperative marketing activities, such as trade shows, advertising or direct mail campaigns. Cooperative marketing is a great way to overcome marketing reluctance. Combining some of your marketing tasks with others saves you time and money. You also generate a powerful synergy as the creative process is significantly enhanced by team effort versus a "solo act." Pooling your resources helps you afford more imaginative, elaborate, expensive and long-term marketing projects.

The benefits of cooperative marketing extend beyond just stretching your marketing budget. Some of the most dreaded aspects of marketing become less of a chore when you don't have to do them alone. For instance, even though public speaking is one of the most effective means of promotion, many people are so uncomfortable being in front of a group, they don't schedule any speaking engagements. Presentations, seminars and demonstrations are much less intimidating and make a greater impact when done by two people. It isn't necessary to do everything by yourself!

As much as most practitioners claim they don't believe in competition, very few actively share in marketing their practices. Many are unwilling to even brainstorm ideas with their colleagues for fear of someone else successfully implementing their plans. We need to alter this scarcity consciousness.

For best results, develop a working relationship with at least three other practitioners:

- A practitioner in your field who targets a different market.
- A practitioner who offers different services to the same target market.
- A practitioner who shares your target market.

Keep in mind that you don't need to limit mutual marketing relationships to other practitioners. You can also work with retail establishments, suppliers and organizations.

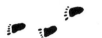

Chapter 10, Page 196

for tips on working in partnership.

One way to ease into working with others is to jointly plan a small scale marketing activity. You can increase the scope of your marketing alliance as you build confidence in yourself, your co-marketers and the process. In essence, you're creating a short-term partnership, so create an alliance proposal that includes the purpose, priorities, goals, financial outlays and interaction expectations.

To give you a picture of how cooperative marketing may work, we look at several examples of marketing alliances and some creative ideas for generating new business.

Same Service—Different Target Market • •

Following are examples of joint marketing ventures among wellness providers who specialize in the same method of wellness care, but work with different target markets:

Any activity becomes creative when the doer cares about doing it right, or better.
—John Updike

Acupuncturists: one mainly works with people in recovery programs, another targets the geriatric population, the third works with people with disabilities.

Nutritionists: one targets construction workers, another works with physical therapy clients, the other works mainly with athletes.

On-site seated chair massage therapists: one works on hair stylists, one targets attorneys, the other works with car salespeople.

Hypnotherapists: one targets other wellness professionals, another works with abuse survivors, the third works with corporate executives.

Marketing Ideas • • •
- Share a booth at conferences, health fairs and expositions. Don't limit your exposure to just the traditional venues; consider participating in home shows, business expos, state and county fairs, and community art festivals.
- Advertise in local publications and also consider radio or television advertising.
- Co-write an article and submit it to your local publications.
- Contact the media to do interviews.
- Give presentations to the general public.

Different Service—Same Target Market ••

Some of the most effective cooperative marketing takes place when providers of different services and products focus on the same market. In this case, let your market determine who is best to join forces with for cooperative marketing. Review your target market profiles to assist you in compiling this list. The following are some examples of matching target markets with a group of allied practitioners.

- Most athletes could use the services of a massage therapist, sports physician, personal trainer and hypnotherapist.
- People active in personal growth might be interested in seeing a massage practitioner, Rolfing® practitioner, hypnotherapist, counselor and aromatherapist.
- Pregnant women might assemble a wellness team consisting of a massage therapist, midwife, gynecologist, Lamaze instructor and nutritionist.

Extend your combined promotional efforts to include other businesses who share the same markets. Some examples are: health food stores, restaurants, educational organizations, hair salons that use natural products, bookstores, specialty clothing shops and cultural groups.

Marketing Ideas • • •

- Design wellness packages for businesses and special interest groups. In addition to the standard wellness providers such as massage therapists, counselors, chiropractors, and physicians, consider including a vendor of ergonomic devices like chairs or pillows, a supplier of relaxation CDs and self-improvement products, a health food restaurant to supply healthy snacks, and a biofeedback specialist for stress management.
- Place cooperative advertisements in local publications. If you're in a professional building or shopping complex, get together with the business owners to do joint advertising to attract new clients to your location. You can also sponsor an open house for the public, advertising free demonstrations, music, munchies and door prizes.
- For those who aren't conveniently located next to one another, consider sharing advertising to promote the benefits of each other's services. This might include wellness providers and related businesses. A recent advertisement in my community paper featured a chiropractic service, a massage therapist and a bookstore.
- Sponsor an event such as a fundraiser for a local charity or a health awareness day. If possible, participate in events such as major races by providing a booth for refreshments or your services.
- Design a special flier that describes the services, products and benefits of the people involved in the cooperative venture. Another possibility is to combine your separate promotional materials into one packet and send a direct mailing to potential clients.
- Co-sponsor seminars on health-related topics. For example, develop a stress management workshop with a counselor, aromatherapist and a bookstore.
- Create packages for celebrations: holidays, birthdays, "thank-goodness-tax-season-is-over" and anniversaries. For example, you could put together a Valentine's Day special that includes dinner, flowers, music and massage for two.
- Place a display with your cards and brochures next to the cash register at a restaurant, and put coupons from the restaurant in your waiting area.

Same Service—Same Target Market • •

The best time to join forces with others in your field who target the same market is when the market is too big for you to handle yourself. For instance, this may occur when you contract to provide services for a large corporation. Depending on the size of the company, you may even need numerous practitioners. Another similar situation arises when you're working with a specialty group such as an athletic team.

Marketing Ideas • • •

- Submit proposals to corporations for your services.
- Send direct mailings to specific groups of people.
- Give in-person or video presentations.
- Volunteer at athletic events.
- Sponsor an athletic or charitable group (e.g., underprivileged children).

Cooperative Marketing

- List at least two people who do similar work as you but target different markets.
- List at least two people in allied fields who share your market.
- List at least two people in totally different businesses who also share your target market.
- List at least three marketing projects that would be a lot more fun to do with others.

Chapter 10, Page 187

for tips on how to gather industry statistics and estimate a community's supply and demand.

Dramatically increase the lifetime value of a client by replacing your typical clients with ideal clients.

The Lifetime Value of a Client •

The lifetime value of a client is the total dollar amount your typical client brings into your business. If you're just starting out, these numbers are guesstimates. Your forecasts can be more accurate if you base them on industry data. The following formula calculates this amount:

1. Determine how much money your average client will spend during the entire client/practitioner relationship in session fees and product sales. For example, let's say that your typical client sees you 10 times a year at $60 per session. This client works with you for four years and purchases $80 in products each year.
   Sessions: $60 x 10 x 4 = $2,400
   Next add the product sales: $80 x 4 = $320
   The total value: = $2,720
2. Calculate the value of client referrals. For example, let's say your average client refers only one new client every year.
   4 x $2,720 = $10,880
   Thus, each client has an overall lifetime value of $13,600.

Understanding the lifetime value of a client puts your marketing time and expenditures into perspective. The cost of actions such as the extra time you occasionally give a client, providing a free or low-cost initial consultation, placing confirmation calls, sending greeting cards and newsletters, and offering special promotions, pales next to the potential return on investment.

Tracking Trends ●

As you work to build a thriving wellness practice, keeping up to date with the latest trends is a vital skill. This requires paying attention to both consumer trends as well as industry trends. Fortunately, plenty of resources are available to help you gain insights into cultural, lifestyle and industry trends. Best of all, it doesn't take a lot of time or money to keep your finger on the pulse of emerging trends.

Trend watching can help identify a unique niche in the marketplace for you and keep you better attuned to the needs of your target markets. In the words of trend-watching guru, Reinier Evers, director of Trendwatching.com, "Knowing where the world of consumerism is heading will give you a point of view—a grip—and from that knowledge, you'll hopefully be able to come up with new goods, services, and experiences that appeal to your customers."

Matching Massage with Societal Trends
www.businessmastery.us/
massage-trends.php

Group Mentality: Exploring Generational Marketing for Spas
www.businessmastery.us/
spa-marketing.php

In short, trend watching can help spark new thinking that results in practical ways to reach new clients and retain existing clients. For instance, time-pressed, busy professional clients highly value convenience and stress reduction, yet they find it difficult to schedule daytime appointments. Based on this insight, you may decide to open your schedule for evening appointments several times a week. You may also decide to implement online scheduling so your clients can schedule appointments 24 hours a day at their convenience.

Tuning into baby boomer trends—such as the avid preoccupation with healthy aging, maintaining a youthful appearance and preventive wellness—may result in a more targeted brochure, a new line of antioxidant nutritional supplements, skin care products or bodywork modalities geared toward satisfying this market's needs.

Other important trends to track from an industry standpoint are legislative activity and educational standards. Knowing where you stand in relation to others in your industry, what certification or continuing education standards may be changing, and how you can best protect your business interests are key to managing your career and professional practice.

The best and simplest way to track consumer trends is to subscribe to the free Trendwatching newsletter. As for industry trends, trade journals often feature insightful articles about consumer perspectives, legal trends and educational standards. Browse a few trade journals and subscribe to one or two that most appeal to you. The information and insights you gain are well worth your investment. Build the habit of trend watching into your professional life by scheduling an hour or two each week to browse the Trendwatching newsletter and trade journals.

Track Trends
www.Trendwatching.com
www.Ubercool.com

Another valuable trend-watching resource is Ubercool, a site that tracks trends worldwide. If you have an extra half hour or so to spare, go to the website and search for "Fountain of Youth," a brief look at baby boomer trends. According to Ubercool, "Born between 1946 and 1964, baby boomers, numbering 450 million in the Western world, are the world's richest generation. Their forever-young attitudes are guaranteed to substantially lift the beauty, wellness and rejuvenation markets. And a youthful spirit is something you can bank on."

No introduction to trend watching would be complete without a look at the work of Faith Popcorn, respected trend watcher and author of *Clicking: 17 Trends That Drive Your Business—And Your Life*.[2] She asserts that for any business to be successful, it needs to click with at least four of the 17 trends. To make it easy for you to evaluate what trends may click with your business, See Figure 15.2 for an overview of the 17 trends.

Figure 15.2

Societal Trends

Cocooning: Consumers are shielding themselves from the harsh, unpredictable realities of the outside world and retreating into safe, cozy "homelike" environments.

Clanning: Consumers seek the comfort and reinforcement of those who share their values and beliefs, or even their interests.

Fantasy Adventure: As an escape from stress and boredom, consumers crave excitement and stimulation in essentially risk-free adventures.

Pleasure Revenge: Tired of being told what's good for them, rebellious consumers are indifferent to rules and regulations. They're cutting loose and publicly savoring forbidden fruits.

Small Indulgences: Busy, stressed-out consumers, seeking quick-hit gratification, are rewarding themselves with affordable luxuries.

Anchoring: Reaching back to their spiritual roots, consumers look for what was comforting, valuable, and spiritually grounded in the past, so they can feel secure in the future.

Egonomics: Feeling unconnected in the depersonalized Information Age, consumers are drawn to customized, individualized products and services.

FemaleThink: The way women think and behave is impacting business, causing a marketing shift away from a hierarchical model toward a relational one.

Mancipation: Rejecting their traditional roles, men are embracing newfound freedom to be whatever they want to be.

99 Lives: Consumers are forced to assume multiple roles to cope with the time pressures produced by ever busier lives.

Cashing Out: Stressed & spent out, consumers are searching for fulfillment in a simpler way of living.

Being Alive: Recognizing the importance of wellness, consumers embrace not only the concept of a longer life but a better overall quality of life.

Down-Aging: Nostalgic for the carefree days of childhood, consumers seek symbols of youth to counterbalance the intensity of their adult lives.

Vigilante Consumer: Frustrated, sometimes angry consumers are manipulating the marketplace through pressure, protest, and politics.

Icon Toppling: Skeptical consumers are ready to bring down the long-accepted monuments of business, government, celebrity, and society.

Save Our Society: Concerned with the fate of the planet, consumers respond to marketers who exhibit a social conscience attuned to ethics, environment, and education.

AtmosFear: Polluted air, contaminated water, and tainted food stir up a storm of consumer doubt and uncertainty.

• Develop a Marketing Plan •

Marketing plans are internal planning documents: they keep you focused and assist you in choosing the most effective ways to build and maintain a thriving practice. Marketing plans answer the following questions: Where are you now? Where do you want to be? How can you meet prospective clients? How can you determine their needs and wants? How can you convey or demonstrate your ability to assist clients in reaching their wellness goals?

An old saying which states, "If you don't know where you're going, what matters the path?" applies to any type of planning—and particularly to marketing. The chart below illustrates the major components of a marketing plan. The subsequent pages contain exercises as well as technical information to assist you in creating an innovative marketing plan that produces solid results.

Figure 15.3

Sample Marketing Plan Outline

I Overview
- Statement of why you're in this business
- Results you intend to create
- Summary of how you will accomplish your goals

II Positioning
- Differential Advantage
- Image

III Target Market Analysis
- Demographics
- Psychographics
- Needs and Goals

IV Marketing Assessment
- Analysis of previous promotional activities
- Recommended changes for future plans
- Overview of competition's marketing

V Strategic Action Plans
- Promotion
- Advertising
- Community Relations
- Publicity
- Timetables
- Budget

Marketing Plan Self-Assessment

- Why are you in this business?
- What is your purpose for marketing?
- What are your priorities for marketing?
- What are your major goals for marketing?
- What are your strategies for developing and implementing your marketing plan?

Positioning

To effectively position your business, you must determine exactly what niche you intend to fill. Prospective clients need an easy way to differentiate you from your competition; your position statement provides that information. Positioning and target markets go hand in hand. It is difficult to explain one without the other. As a matter of fact, if you have more than one target market (which is usually wise), and they're vastly different, you may need a separate position statement for each of those target markets.

Two examples of successful positioning statements are those from Avis® and 7 Up.® Everyone knows that 7 Up's marketing position is: 7 Up, The Uncola.® When Seven-Up was developing its marketing campaign, a soda usually meant Coca-Cola or Pepsi. To counteract that assumption, they promoted their product as something totally "un"like competing soft drinks. Avis had to overcome two problems: another company had a stronghold on the number one position, (can you name it?) and most people find it difficult to differentiate one car rental business from another. Their solution was the slogan: We're Avis. We're Number Two. We Try Harder.™ This position statement made a compelling promise to its potential customers. It was so effective that now Avis' position statement is simply: We try harder.®

Branding Your Image ●●

A brand is a "unique sum of impressions" that can be your business' greatest asset.[3] It is derived from what your clients and the public think and believe about your business. In a marketplace crowded with talented wellness providers and discerning consumers, practitioners that develop a strong brand image have a competitive advantage. Such a brand image is rooted in clarity of purpose—as defined in your mission statement—and is reflected in consistent and concise messages that convey who you are and what you promise to deliver to clients. These messages continually broadcast to your clients what's important to you and what you value. These messages take many shapes, such as marketing programs, promotional materials, logos, business cards, everyday interactions with clients and your office environment.

Wheaties is known as The Breakfast of Champions.® They back up their position statement and reinforce their image by putting pictures of famous athletes on the front of their cereal boxes.

What does a strong brand mean in practical terms? For wellness providers it most often translates into loyal clients and a steady stream of new clients. Whether clients find you through word of mouth or the Internet, your brand is like a trusted friend that creates an emotional connection with clients. In short, a strong brand attracts those who will bond with you and appreciate what you have to offer.

Create Your Brand

- How do your clients and colleagues describe you and your practice?
- Describe the image you wish to portray.
- How do your office environment, client communications, marketing programs, promotional materials and attire align with this image?
- What changes are needed to alter the elements that aren't in sync with your desired image?

The Differential Advantage • •

The next step in developing a position statement is to define your differential advantage, also known as a "unique selling proposition." You must know how to describe what makes you different (unique) from other wellness providers in your field. No two people are exactly alike, even with the identical training.

Reflect upon your practice. Think about what you really do: the intention of your work; your image; the range of skills and techniques you employ; the products you use; the results your clients receive; and what your clients say about you and your work. Your differential advantage may stem from yourself, your specialization, the range of services offered, geographic location, or a combination of factors. Keep in mind that what usually attracts potential clients aren't the features of your practice, but how those features are going to benefit them.

Another way of differentiating yourself from other practitioners is through specialization. You may prefer to work on a particular condition or a specific clientele. Perhaps one of your greatest strengths lies in the actual service you offer. Do you have specialized knowledge? Are you the only one in your area who does a certain type of work? Do you own state-of-the-art equipment? Do you offer a greater range of services and products than most other wellness providers?

One of the most significant yet often overlooked advantages is your actual office location. If you're situated in a large professional building, your appeal is accessibility—people can schedule appointments during breaks, before or after work, and they don't need to drive. If you do on-site work, one of your major benefits is convenience—clients don't have to go anywhere or do anything but enjoy the session. If your office has a particular ambiance (e.g., a fitness motif, a clinic setting or a retreat atmosphere), expound upon those qualities.

In most instances, the strongest factor in your differential advantage is you. What you do and how you do it is greatly influenced by your background, personality, education and philosophy toward the nature of well-being.

To spur your thought process for the next exercise, gather your marketing materials and other practitioners' brochures. Reflect upon the value clients receive from your type of services and remember why you chose this profession for your career.

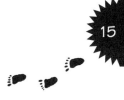

Chapter 5, Pages 90-94
for more information on image and professionalism.

Branding
www.allaboutbranding.com

Stay centered in your enthusiasm about your work and the results it produces. This is what attracts people to want to learn more about who you are and what you do.

Define Your Differential Advantage

- Carefully consider the following questions:
    1. What does your business do?
    2. What needs does your business meet?
    3. What problems does your business solve?
    4. How do your clients benefit psychologically?
    5. How does your business differ from the competition?
- Write a statement that summarizes what makes you unique.
- Summarize why your current clients work with you.
- Describe how potential clients will recognize your differential advantage.

Figure 15.4

Position Statement Examples

The following position statements illustrate the range of differential advantages from types of services, to philosophy, to specific clientele and to location. Position statements are similar to slogans—though not always so catchy.

Services

Some position statements are based solely upon the service(s) provided. This approach is usually taken when a practitioner has specialized knowledge, a unique service, a particularly clever slogan or state-of-the-art equipment.

"On Pins and Needles? Try Acupuncture for Relief"
"We Use the Latest Advances in Dental Technology"
"Trained by the Founder of <insert well-known name here>"

Philosophy

Most wellness providers have strong beliefs about the nature of well-being and their particular approach to wellness. Quite often, this is the major quality that distinguishes one practitioner from another.

"We Treat You as a Whole Person"
"The Beginning of a Healthy Lifestyle"
"The Gentle Approach to Deep Tissue Therapy"
"Combining Ancient Healing Wisdom with State-of-the-Art Technology"

Specialization

Some position statements are based on appealing to a target market. For example, you may prefer to only work with one gender or a specific age group. Maybe your focus is treating a specific condition or part of the body.

"Seniors are Our Specialty"
"Making Your Pregnancy More Comfortable"
"Giving Athletes that Competitive Edge"
"The Specialists in Head and Neck Injuries"

Office Location

Expound upon your location's accessibility, convenience or ambiance.

"Providing All Your Wellness Needs in One Location"
"A Haven from the Hectic Workplace"
"Only Twenty Minutes from Downtown, Yet a World Apart"
"Have Table, Will Travel"

Position Statement Examples

www.businessmastery.us/
position-statements.php

Your Position Statement • •

Some people choose a position statement because it resonates with them. Others create statements to draw a specific clientele. It's best if you can do both.

To prepare for the next exercise, review your responses to the differential advantage questions and highlight the most important facets. Combine those with your image statement to formulate your general position statement. After you finish the next section on target marketing, you may find you need to create additional position statements (for each of the different markets).

Create Your Position Statement

Write your position statement. Evaluate it in terms of the following criteria:

- Does it convey a true benefit?
- Does it differentiate you from your competition?
- Is it unique?

Targeting Markets •

Target markets are groups of people who share similar characteristics. The whole concept of target marketing may seem very scary at first. On the surface, specialization appears to limit the pool of potential clients. Many practitioners fear that by defining a market, they will lose business or choose the wrong one. An additional concern is that other practitioners will take anybody and therefore absorb some of their business.

In most instances, narrowing your field increases your overall number of clients. Target marketing is analogous to archery. In archery, the goal is to get your arrow as close to the center as possible. The outer rings are bigger and easier to hit, but the high score comes from hitting the center. The same goes for attracting clients; you can appeal to the general masses (the outer rings), but it takes more money and time (multiple arrows) to get the same return on your marketing investment than it would be focusing on a target market (hitting the bull's-eye with one arrow).

The purpose of choosing specific target markets is to make your practice more enjoyable, simplify your marketing, and increase the success of your promotional endeavors. The world abounds with opportunities, and it's impossible to pursue them all or attempt to be everything to everyone. You need to decide where to focus your marketing energy and resources. As a side benefit, specialization and having distinct target markets immediately reduce your competition.

Wellness is very intimate work. Think about who you want in your space. Actively seek those types of clients. This doesn't mean you must limit yourself to only working with people in your target markets. While it's fine to work with whomever wanders through the door, invest your marketing time and money toward attracting your desired target markets.

Most successful practitioners have one or two major markets and a couple of minor target markets.

Working with several markets helps to avoid the potential disaster of selecting an unsuitable one. The benefits of not being restricted to only one type of clientele are manifold. In particular, your skills become well rounded by experiencing a variety of people with their own unique issues. Plus, it allows you to balance your altruistic goals with your financial needs. For instance, one of your passions might be working with a specific market that doesn't normally have the funds to pay for your services. If you had another target market that covers your bills, you could work with the former population for free or on a sliding scale. As a side note, consider applying for a grant for working with a needy population.

You may also find that certain aspects of your target markets overlap, such as they all shop at the same health food store. Knowing the commonalities assists you in streamlining your marketing endeavors as you can combine some of your activities, (e.g., conducting demonstrations and posting brochures at the health food store).

Marketing Foundation Exercise

Consider the following questions:

- How would you describe the people who use the kind of services you provide?
- What types of people do you want to reach?
- Which groups do you most relate to or already have clients in?
- What types of services would be the most fulfilling for you to offer?
- What qualities do you want your services to exude?
- What problems, conditions and issues do you want to address in your work?
- What type of environment do you want to work in?

Given your responses to the preceding questions, who would be most easily attracted to working with you?

Check with professional associations to find the client usage statistics for your specific branch of wellness care.

Demographics and Psychographics • •

The more you know about your potential clients, the easier it is to develop an appropriate position statement and design an effective marketing campaign. The two most common means of market analysis are Demographics and Psychographics, which describe a person in terms of objective data and personality attributes.

Figure 15.5

Demographics and Psychographics

Demographics are categorical statistics such as:

- Age
- Income Level
- Occupation
- Gender
- Geographic Location
- Education Level

Psychographics (also known as lifestyle factors) are the major determinants in whether someone becomes a client. They include:

- Special Interest Activities
- Philosophical Beliefs
- Social Factors
- Cultural Involvements
- Wellness Needs
- Wellness Goals

The number of target markets you have depends mainly upon the size of your practice and the scope of your knowledge. Some target markets are more productive than others. You set yourself up for difficulty if you base your target market solely on demographics.

Connecting with the Right Clients • •

Some typical wellness target markets are: high-stress executives, pregnant women, athletes (in general or a specific niche such as triathletes, cyclists, gymnasts), infants, children, people in self-improvement programs, pre- and post-operative recovery, people with disabilities, attorneys, seniors, the entertainment industry, natural disaster casualties, people in addiction recovery programs, patients of other primary care providers, small business owners, crime victims, students, animals, abuse survivors, computer operators, military personnel, restaurateurs, dancers, artists, people with specific issues such as long-term illness or injury rehabilitation, and other wellness providers.

A common misconception in the wellness field is that people with money are a great target market. Affluence isn't a market, it's a demographic statistic only! Just because individuals have the means to easily pay for wellness services doesn't mean they ever avail themselves. If all the people who could afford your type of service attempted to book an appointment, you and your colleagues would have to work 24 hours a day, seven days a week. You need to discover what motivates someone to receive your services.

Still, many wellness providers fall short of their income goals. Obviously, the means isn't a determining factor—the motive is. To grow a successful business you must identify your target markets and clearly communicate the benefits of your services in a way that attracts potential clients' attention and inspires them to schedule a session with you.

People want to feel that their unique needs are understood. So, even though we know just about anyone can benefit from complementary wellness services, we need to find a way to communicate with potential clients in terms and language that appeals to them.

When determining the clients you want to target, ask yourself, "Who do I really enjoy being around?"

We exist to serve the marketplace. The better we do that, the more profits we will make.
— Stephen Martin

Matching Needs and Benefits • •

So far we've explored potential target markets. Now it's time to look at how to analyze those markets. The first two steps are: describing each of your target markets in terms of their general needs, concerns and goals; and connecting specific benefits with each item.

Below are brief descriptions of sample target markets, their concerns, and words or phrases that could address those needs. Use these examples as a springboard for analyzing your target markets. Keep in mind that the more accurately you identify the needs of your target market, the easier it is to determine the appropriate terminology.

The goal is to inspire people to find out more about your services and how those services can benefit them.

Pregnant Women • • •

Pregnancy is a time of great change: physically, hormonally and emotionally. In addition to being concerned about the health of her child, the mother also contends with a changing body image, fluctuating emotions, a possible reduction of activity level, back pain and edema.

When addressing these areas of concern, incorporate phrases such as: reduces edema; increases circulation; eases discomfort; soothes; enhances connection between mother and child; encourages relaxation; promotes a healthier pregnancy; reduces anxiety; relieves muscle tension and stiffness; enhances well-being; increases ease and efficiency of movement; and provides an environment for self-appreciation and nurturing.

Infants • • •

Infants often have difficulty adjusting to being outside of the womb and the birth process itself can be traumatic. They may develop sleeping problems, colic and other ailments that can definitely benefit from complementary health services.

Even though the receiver is the child, the parents are the ones to whom you must market your services. Use terms such as: soothing; nurturing; strengthens immune system; safe; gentle; fosters easier and deeper breathing; encourages sound sleep; and promotes healthy development.

Seniors • • •

As people age they become more concerned about their overall health, mobility and mental acuity. They may be experiencing stiffness, pain and a lack of touch. Emphasize your benefits with terms such as these: increases blood and lymph circulation; tonifies; promotes healthier, better nourished skin; improves digestion; optimizes joint flexibility; increases range of motion; offers caring and nurturing touch; maintains health; improves posture; reduces blood pressure; heightens capacity for clearer thinking; reduces stress; and relieves muscle tension and stiffness.

Athletes • • •

Athletes are concerned with avoiding injuries, improving performance and reducing downtime due to pain or injury.

Accentuate benefits such as: increases circulation, flexibility, and mobility; relieves muscle soreness and chronic pain; improves endurance; lessens recovery time; tonifies; achieve peak performance; reduces risk of injuries; and enhances concentration.

Entrepreneurs • • •

Your typical entrepreneur is on the go, experiences a lot of stress, must make decisions quickly, has numerous responsibilities and "job titles," and keeps a tight schedule.

To appeal to this market, focus on the results and convenience. Use phrases such as: increases stamina; rejuvenates; relieves stress and tension; improves concentration and creativity; alleviates headaches; enhances sense of well-being; convenient; accessible; increases productivity; promotes deep relaxation; and provides an easy, affordable way to take care of yourself.

Wellness Providers • • •

Caregivers often ignore their own well-being. In addition to the actual physical stress of their jobs, they often experience fatigue and burnout.

To best reach this market, remind them that they know the importance of taking care of themselves. Use phrases like: take time for yourself; relieves tension and stiffness; balances chi; relaxed state of alertness; increases stamina; reduces injury; improves posture; enhances self-image; increases career longevity; and provides care for the caregiver.

Personal Growth • • •

People who are actively involved in their personal growth experience this clearing physically, spiritually and emotionally. Their self-image tends to undergo major shifts.

In approaching this group, use phrases such as: tonify your body as well as your soul; soothing; reduces stress and tension; "natural adjunct" to current personal growth techniques; greater ease of emotional expression; increases self-esteem; strengthens immune system; promotes deep relaxation; encourages peak performance; and evokes a heightened awareness of the mind-body connection.

Target Market Profiles • •

A target market profile is a statement that defines your market in terms of their needs, how your services address those needs, who else caters to the target market and where they can be found. Once you've determined those components, you can choose effective marketing methods. At this point you may be wondering how you could possibly know this information, particularly if you're just beginning your practice or are branching out into new directions. Start by conducting research. Read books and articles about your target market. Get feedback from wellness practitioners as well as other businesses that cater to your desired market. Research trends online. Discover information by contacting organizations that deal with your target market and by conversing with people who train practitioners to work with that specific population. Talk with those who are in the know—members of your target market.

15

I cannot give you the formula for success, but I can give you the formula for failure—which is: Try to please everybody.
— Herbert B. Swope

Most of the information gathered in a target market analysis applies to the majority of the members of the given target market. For instance, factors such as trends, basic needs and goals, types of group they belong to and national publications they read are the same for cyclists regardless of where they live. The details that vary include the specific local publications, stores, practitioners, groups and events.

After you've completed a target market analysis, you're ready to create a target market profile. Start with the general known facts about your target population and adjust them according to your own findings and feedback from others. If you're in practice, review your client files and integrate that data with the research results. The whole purpose of creating a profile is to assist you in developing an effective, natural marketing plan.

Figure 15.6

Target Market Analysis

- Target market group title
- Applicable Demographics
  Age, income level, occupation, gender, geographic location, education level
- Target's physical, emotional and personal needs and goals
- Features your practice offers*
- Benefits your services provide*
- Places to find members of this market
  Stores where they shop, places where they socialize, online newsgroups
- Publications they read
  Local and national magazines, print and online newsletters
- Groups they belong to
  Support groups, civic organizations, professional associations, social clubs
- Special events and important dates
  Specific awareness days, races (for athletes), seasonal stresses (e.g., January - April for accountants)
- Companies and wellness providers who service this market
- Trends that will most likely affect this market
- Where they look for help
  Online resources, telephone book, bulletin boards, friends, organizations
- Needs that aren't being met by traditional services and products
  This could range from physical relief from current condition to emotional components such as compassion and understanding
- Target's philosophical beliefs about wellness
- Target's perceived value of your services
- Primary reasons the target does or would use your services
- Average number of sessions per client per year
- Session intervals
  Daily, weekly, biweekly, monthly, bimonthly, occasionally

*Whenever possible, match these to the Needs and Goals

Sample Target Market Profiles • •

The following fictitious examples include client analyses, profiles and ideas for reaching those populations. Additional in-depth marketing techniques are explored in the next chapter.

Massage Therapy Prenatal Clients • • •

Figure 15.7

Massage Therapy Prenatal Client Analysis and Profile:

- Thirty percent are referred by childbirth educators, midwives and health centers.
- Twenty percent are referred by friends.
- Twenty percent were clients before they became pregnant.
- Thirty percent are referred from direct promotional endeavors.
- The average age range is between 28-35 years.
- The majority experience discomfort.
- They are under the care of a physician.
- Seventy percent take health-related classes like Lamaze and exercise.
- Fifty percent never had a professional massage before their pregnancy.
- Seventy percent shop at The Bouncing Baby Boutique.
- The majority read the local Entertainment Guide.
- Sixty percent are professionals or teachers.
- The combined family income level is between $45,000 and $80,000.
- Seventy percent attend at least two cultural events per year.
- Sixty-five percent are interested in nutrition and shop at health food stores.
- Seventy percent receive massage once per month.
- Ten percent receive massage once per week.
- Fifteen percent receive massage twice per month.
- The majority are more motivated to receive massage in their last trimester.

By compiling this information, you could create this profile:

"My typical prenatal client is 32 years old. She has been married at least three years and already has one child. She is under the care of a physician, keeps a healthy diet, goes to Lamaze classes, exercises regularly and gets a massage once per month. She attends cultural events such as theater or concerts at least two times per year and dines out at least once per week. She shops at The Bouncing Baby Boutique, buys books on child care at The Basic Book Store, frequents Nature's Haven Health Food Store, reads the local weekly Entertainment Guide and subscribes to Parents magazine. Her combined family income is greater than $50,000. She holds an administrative position and works through her eighth month of pregnancy. She is a strong believer in the healing arts. Her major reasons for getting massage are to have an easy, healthy pregnancy and to feel better about herself—relieve her lower back pain, increase her stamina, decrease edema, improve her body image, reduce stress and enhance the overall well-being of herself and her baby."

Reaching the Prenatal Market • • • •

The prenatal market can be approached in many different ways. Before investing any time or money into a promotional endeavor, check your profile to evaluate the likelihood of success. Let's say someone approaches you with an opportunity to place a listing in a promotional piece that is being mailed to "working women" within a three-mile radius of your office. You need to obtain much more information before determining if it's worth the risk. Keeping in mind that no promotion is ever guaranteed to be successful, compare their proposed demographic and psychographic statistics with your target market profiles to see how well they match.

In developing your marketing plan, prepare for potential obstacles— especially with a target market such as pregnant women. Many other people such as a partner, physician or even a mother may influence whether or not a woman receives massage. Your promotional efforts, particularly your print media such as brochures and cards, need to reassure the significant people in the pregnant woman's life. The following ideas are a starting point for reaching this market.

Design attractive promotional materials. In addition to business cards and brochures, consider creating one-sided fliers that are good for tacking on bulletin boards and making informational handouts on different topics of concern to pregnant women. Print these on your letterhead or include your name, title, address and phone number at the bottom of the page. Place your promotional materials wherever pregnant women tend to frequent: obstetricians' offices, Lamaze classes, fitness centers, health food stores, maternity shops, bookstores, childbirth centers, and offices of other allied wellness professionals.

Establish your credibility and build up contacts by volunteering your services (massage or other) at organizations that serve pregnant women, such as wellness clinics, the La Leche League and Planned Parenthood. Write articles on topics of interest to pregnant women and those around them, such as prenatal well-being care or the benefits of massage during pregnancy, and submit them to your local publications. Also post your articles on a variety of e-zine sites.

Regularly update your website with your articles and include a tips section on wellness care for the expectant mother, new moms and babies. Also, link with online sites that provide support or products to this market. Put client testimonials on your website. Also include photos of some of your happy, pregnant clients. Keep people returning to your site by including weekly health tips, announcements and special offers. Be sure to also list your practice on other sites which this market is likely to visit.

Give an instructional program that teaches birthing partners how to use basic Swedish massage strokes such as effleurage and kneading the back, legs and arms on their pregnant partners. Arrange speaking engagements by contacting pregnancy-related organizations, Lamaze classes, birthing centers and midwifery associations, as well as business networking groups such as Entrepreneurial Mothers. You could even get another business to sponsor a more extensive program—and handle the promotion and cover the expenses.

Establish a strong referral network of allied professionals such as obstetricians, midwives, nutritionists, other wellness providers and childbirth educators. List your name and a concise, engaging description of your practice in appropriate print and online publications. Be sure to put these listings under the heading of "Pregnancy" or "Prenatal Care" in addition to "Massage." Some recommended publications are telephone directories, local wellness publications, newsletters directed toward pregnant women, and special editions of the newspaper, such as an annual health and fitness guide.

Increase your visibility by participating in joint promotions. Some techniques are: include your brochures in mailings with other businesses that cater to pregnant women (e.g., maternity shops and baby stores); set up a booth at expositions such as baby shows, fitness fairs, and anyplace else that attracts your target market; and donate a few sessions as prizes at a major fundraising event. The list goes on....

Acupuncture Senior Clients • • •

Figure 15.8

Acupuncture Senior Client Analysis and Profile:

- Seventy-five percent are retired.
- Eighty percent are on a fixed annual income of $20,000 to $30,000.
- The average age range is between 65-90 years.
- Sixty-five percent are women.
- The majority eat dinner before 6 p.m.
- Sixty percent regularly volunteer for charities.
- Sixty-five percent are on a modified exercise routine: walking, swimming, golfing.
- Twenty percent live in a "retirement" community.
- Seventy percent own their own homes.
- Fifty percent listen to classical music.
- Forty percent regularly listen to a radio station that plays music from the 1940s and 1950s.
- Thirty-five percent belong to the American Association for Retired Persons.
- The majority are concerned about their longevity and quality of life.
- Sixty percent are on a nutritional program.
- Sixty-five percent read the local *Senior World Monthly* publication.
- The majority have a lot of free time.
- Fifty-five percent attend community theater.
- The majority experience pain, stiffness and some restriction of movement.
- Sixty percent have more than one chronic medical condition.
- Seventy percent see a doctor at least once per quarter.

Given this information, the senior client profile could resemble this:

"My typical senior client is a retired 70-year-old woman. She leads a semi-active lifestyle—walks two miles at least four times per week and swims in the summer months. She is on a fixed annual income of less than $24,000 and dines out only once or twice per month. She is a member of at least one senior's club and attends four to five cultural events per year. She frequents museums, libraries and historical sites, does at least three hours of volunteer work each week and takes one class per year at the community college. She reads the local Senior World Monthly, *gets massaged every six weeks, receives an acupuncture treatment every three weeks, occasionally shops at Nature's Haven Health Food Store and takes three vacations per year. While she does work with a few wellness practitioners, she mainly uses conventional medicine for her healthcare. This client's major reasons for getting acupuncture are to feel better and be more energetic: enhance mobility, reduce joint inflammation, increase circulation and relieve pain and stiffness."*

Reaching the Senior Market ● ● ● ●

The senior market is best reached through education. Create a promotional packet that contains your brochure, and be sure it incorporates appropriate terminology and is printed in an easy-to-read, large-sized typeface. Also create cards, informational handouts and reprints of articles on the benefits of acupuncture and Traditional Chinese Medicine for seniors.

By the way, this packet is also useful to send with your letter of introduction to allied professionals. Place your promotional material on bulletin boards at senior centers, golf courses, wellness centers, medical supply outlets, Elderhostels, community centers, libraries, gerontologists' offices, the Department of Parks and Recreation, pharmacies, bingo halls, volunteer centers, fitness clubs and offices of allied wellness providers.

Establish your credibility and build contacts by volunteering your services at a local nursing home, a seniors' rights advocacy association or even a senior center. Get your name in print by publishing an article on the benefits of acupuncture or by being interviewed by the press. You can also promote goodwill and gain publicity by donating treatments to major fundraising events.

Give presentations at wellness centers, community colleges, senior centers, nursing homes and other groups like civic organizations that seniors tend to join. Choose the organizations you want to develop an affiliation with and mail them your promotional packet that includes a cover letter expressing your interest in presenting a lecture or demonstration.

Also, consider teaching an extended weekly class on geriatric wellness at one of the centers or colleges. Many cities have a community cable channel. Find out if they broadcast a program designed for seniors, and get yourself booked to appear on that show.

Take out listings in appropriate print and online publications. Again, be certain to also put your name under the headings of "Senior Wellness" or "Geriatric Care" in addition to "Acupuncture." Some suggested publications are telephone directories, your local seniors' publication, newsletters directed toward seniors, and special "senior sections" in the newspapers.

Put client testimonials on your website. Also include photos of some of your senior clients doing activities, such as stretching or playing golf. Each season post information on the suggested changes in diet, herbs and activities. Keep people returning to your site by including weekly health tips, announcements and special offers. Be sure to also list your practice on other sites which seniors are likely to visit.

Another effective promotional technique is setting up a booth at events that attract seniors, such as golf tournaments, garden shows and health fairs.

You can be very creative in reaching the senior market. For example, many restaurants offer senior discounts on early dinners. You could join forces with one of those restaurants and have your cards (with or without a discount of your own) displayed on the tables at the restaurant, and, in return, you distribute the restaurant's coupons to your senior clients.

These examples are only a small segment of available options to reach the senior market. Whatever methods you choose to increase your clientele, take the time to establish credibility, allay concerns and build rapport.

If a window of opportunity appears, don't pull down the shade.
— Tom Peters

Target Market Exercise

Describe Your Current Clientele

Define your current client base and ascertain the specific markets you currently have. Start by completing a target market analysis. Then look for traits that your clients share and see if you find patterns. Next, write a descriptive profile for each of your target markets.

Identify New Markets

Select at least two target markets and complete a target market analysis and profile for each one.

Evaluate Your Markets

Examine the data from your current and desired target markets. Highlight areas of commonality. Evaluate your position statement (from the exercise on page 339): Does it appeal to your target markets? Do you need to change it or create additional position statements? If so, rewrite it now.

Marketing Assessment •

The next phase in developing your marketing plan is to assess your previous promotional endeavors and those of your competitors. If you're just starting out in practice, skip this exercise and proceed to the next section. I recommend you do this assessment exercise at least once per quarter.

Marketing Assessment

- List the marketing venues you currently employ.
- How is your business perceived by your clients, colleagues and prospective clients?
- If you offer more than one service, have you promoted each one? Yes No If no, why not?
- Have you been satisfied with the quality of your marketing efforts? Yes No If no, why not?
- What have been the results of your promotional activities so far?
- What changes would you like to see happen?

Strategic Action Plans ●

The final portion of the marketing plan is the design of your marketing campaign. Refer to the next two chapters for specific marketing techniques. Keep in mind all important dates such as holidays, clients' meaningful occasions and seasonal events. Plan your campaigns thoroughly. Be aware that you may need separate promotional strategies for each target market.

Figure 15.9

Successful marketing is based on having a clear vision for your business, defining your target markets, clarifying your differential advantage, determining your position statement, and designing a marketing plan that utilizes creative and effective strategies which reflect your values.

> ## Marketing Strategy Questionnaire
>
> For each marketing strategy, ask yourself the following questions:
>
> - Is the strategy realistic?
> - Does this strategy fit into your budget?
> - What are the ramifications of spending money on this strategy?
> - Is this strategy unique?
> - Is the market large enough to return a profit from this strategy?
> - Does this strategy relate to your other strategies?
> - Does this strategy accent your strengths and differences?
> - Does this strategy appeal to your target markets?
> - Is this strategy directed toward your target markets?
> - Are people likely to respond to this strategy? If yes, why?

If your answer to any of these questions is no, alter your strategy. If your answers are all yes, it's time to put your marketing plan into action.

Implementing your marketing plan of action begins by setting up a schedule. Establish a timeline and specific deadlines for all the steps—and stay on schedule. Setting realistic deadlines and integrating your goals into the timelines so they follow a logical order enables you to stay within your time frame.

The next phase is to evaluate the results. If things are going as anticipated, review the rest of the plan to see if you can make any changes to further enhance the results. If you appear to be off target, identify the problems by asking yourself the following questions: Were the goals realistic? Was the timeline too ambitious? Did you need to rely upon too many outside factors? Did you expect more of a percentage increase than occurred? Were there any errors in your plan? Did you incorrectly add any of the numbers? Was any of your data inaccurate? Did you choose an inappropriate target market?

Once you've identified the obstacles, some possibilities for alleviating them are to change the basic goals, alter the timeline, correct the mistakes or possibly even modify the overall strategy.

In summary, developing a top-notch marketing campaign requires creativity, clarity and insightful analysis to design strategies, determine an annual marketing budget and assess how well the various parts of the plan complement each other. Be sure to allot time to evaluate the effectiveness of your campaign during each phase. Track what works and what doesn't—and make adjustments as needed to ensure outstanding results.

Marketing Mastery

www.sohnen-moe.com/ marketingmastery.php This free subscription service includes a full-year marketing plan, followed by monthly goals and weekly activity reminders.

Marketing in Action

• Marketing Techniques Primer •

Now that you've clearly defined your target markets and gained a solid understanding of marketing basics, we take a look at how to put marketing techniques to work to grow a thriving practice. These techniques can be divided into four major components: promotion, publicity, advertising and community relations.

Promotion involves the activities and materials you produce to gain visibility. The money invested is indirect (e.g., it costs money to print business cards; it costs nothing to distribute them), and the activities are often free of cost. *Publicity* involves building media awareness about you or your business, often in connection with a special event or milestone. *Advertising* differs from publicity and promotions in that you must pay directly for your exposure. *Community relations* are goodwill activities that create a positive public image for you and your business. (See Figure 16.1.)

In marketing I've seen only one strategy that can't miss, and that's to market to your best customers first, your best prospects second and the rest of the world last.
— John Romero

Marketing Mix •

Successful practitioners include a good mix of promotion, advertising, publicity and community relations in their marketing plans. Marketing your business takes time and creativity—particularly with a small practice. Don't always rely on previously used methods (even if they seemed to work), especially if you're approaching the same target group. People like and respond to variety. They tire of seeing or hearing the same thing over and over again. The other reason for altering your marketing modes is to reach potential clients who may have been uninspired by your earlier endeavors. Use an assortment of approaches in an ongoing, consistent manner. Marketing never ends; it's an integral component of your business. Plan on investing at least 15 percent of your time in marketing to maintain your practice and more to expand it. If you're just starting out, you may need to increase it to more than 50 percent.

The methods available for marketing your practice are vast (unless your specific profession has distinct precepts). You don't have to be a genius to develop a sound marketing plan, you don't have to go the traditional route, and it isn't necessary to spend a lot of money (although it's so easy to do).

The crucial factor for selecting a marketing venue is: Does it appeal to your target market? Many years ago I heard a speaker talk about the need to learn how to broadcast on station WIIFM (What's In It For Me?). This is particularly true in marketing. Your marketing endeavors need to convey to the recipients exactly how your company is going to help them.

This chapter contains valuable tips on how to use promotion, advertising, publicity and community relations to attract new clients. It also takes a look at how to jumpstart your practice and choose the right graphic artist. The chapter closes with a list of more than 100 creative marketing ideas and a sample marketing action plan.

Figure 16.1

The Bicycle Story

A massage therapist wants to build her sports massage practice. She places an advertisement on a bus stop bench outside the most popular cycling shop in town. That's **advertising**.

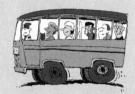

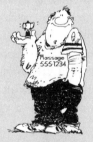
She decides to sponsor a cycling team (offers team members discounts on her services and free pre- and post-race mini-sessions for major local events). She prints T-shirts with her name and number for the cyclists to wear. They wear the T-shirts while riding through town carrying a banner announcing their next big race. That's **promotion** (for both the therapist and the cyclists in this latter instance).

In their excitement, the cyclists topple three elderly gentlemen while riding through the park. A newspaper reporter just happens to be there and reports it. That's **publicity** (although not the best kind).
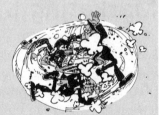

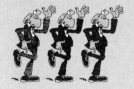
The therapist gives each gentleman a 15-minute massage. They are no longer in pain and harbor no bad feelings toward "her" cycling team. The gentlemen come to the race to cheer on the team. That's mastering **community relations**.

• Getting Your First Clients •

I am often asked, "What is the best way to market my practice?" Alas, as much as I would love to give a concrete answer to that question, it's impossible. No one-size-fits-all formula works. The marketing venues you choose are best determined by your target markets. The trick to marketing success is to determine what's most important to your potential clients and communicate how you can meet their needs and goals.

When starting out, talk with everyone about your profession: family, friends, neighbors, and people in line at the grocery store, movies and department of motor vehicles.... Share your enthusiasm for your work and the results it produces. Excitement is contagious!

Decide how many sessions you want to work each week and do it. It doesn't matter if you have to give free sessions in the beginning. You need to establish your credibility and build relationships. The way to do that is to work with as many people as possible. Actually, many companies use the stratagem of giving things away to obtain long-term customers. Think about all the book, music and DVD clubs. They lose money on their initial sales, yet they know that the lifetime value of the customer is worth it. Other large corporations bank on the reliability of this type of promotion and give away samples of their products. They are confident that once people experience the products, they'll continue to use them.

Chapter 15, Page 332
to calculate the Lifetime
Value of a client.

The concept of "giving to get" also holds true for wellness services. For example, if you give away 40 sessions in one month and only 10 of those people become regular clients (or refer you regular clients), then those 40 hours of work will bring you $136,000 over the next four years. Not a bad investment at all!

Estimate how much money you want to make and how many clients it takes to reach that goal. Program your mind to expect a set number of sessions, and soon you will find that those sessions are all filled with paying clients. Having said that, it's best if those free sessions are given to people who are likely to become clients or actively generate word-of-mouth referrals.

Chapter 10, Page 213
for a Time/Income Factor
Analysis.

Building a practice requires consistent marketing, business acumen, perseverance and optimism. Many practitioners give up too soon because they don't receive enough positive feedback and rewards don't come as quickly as desired. While exceptions do exist, it takes most people two to three years to build a thriving practice. You might need to take a part-time job in the beginning to augment your income. The caveat is to make sure that at the outset of your career, you set specific parameters for when you will take the plunge into full-time practice (e.g., number of clients, amount of money saved). Otherwise, you may never make that transition.

Almost No-Cost Start-up ●

All you need to start out are business cards and a telephone. These may be the only tools you need if you want to work part time or reside in a community where you're the only practitioner of your kind.

Marketing a wellness practice is based on education and relationships. Make emotional connections with people. Do whatever you can to increase your visibility in your community. Attend networking meetings, take classes, write articles, hold open houses, deliver talks and give demonstrations. Wear logo clothing with your profession or slogan emblazoned on it. Always carry your business cards with you. Volunteer in your community and get interviewed by the media. Post your business cards and brochures wherever your target markets are likely to see them.

Moving Forward ●

Once you have your first clients, it's time to take the steps to fill your appointment book. Marketing your practice can oftentimes appear overwhelming and arduous, yet no rule says you can't have fun while promoting your business. You can incorporate creative approaches to building your clientele. Keep in mind that the most effective means of marketing wellness services is through a personal approach. Given that the majority of people become your clients out of an experience with you, it's vital that your marketing plan include informal ways for people to get to know you and your work.

● Promotion: Person-to-Person ●

Promotion techniques and tools attract the attention of potential and current clients, as well as keep you and your services favorably positioned. Some of the most effective promotional techniques are: networking, generating word-of-mouth referrals, holding open houses, presenting workshops and demonstrations; and writing articles about your services or general well-being for local newspapers, magazines and newsletters.

Other promotional activities include: booths at community events, health expos and state fairs; sending direct mail pieces and newsletters; providing your services at conventions, store openings, sporting events and at malls during the holidays; obtaining referrals; and offering specials and incentives. Key promotional tools include professional brochures, business cards and an Internet website. Personalized items, such as pens embossed with your name and logo, also fall under the category of promotion even though they're commonly referred to as specialty advertising.

Specialty clothing

www.4imprint.com
www.cafepress.com
www.insideoutbodywear.com

**Companies that
Market for You**

www.businessmastery.us/
market-company.php

*Without promotion something
terrible happens… Nothing!*
— P.T. Barnum

Word-of-Mouth Referrals ●

People prefer to receive wellness care from someone they know. The second best option is working with a professional who has been highly recommended by a friend or family member. Many claim that wellness is a word-of-mouth industry, yet few know how to foster referrals. They think that offering an excellent service at a fair price is enough.

Most clients have a natural inclination to share their experiences with family, friends and colleagues, yet they can be reluctant to be forthcoming about their wellness care. Unfortunately, satisfied clients don't necessarily talk about you—at least not usually enough to fill your appointment book with new clients. Actually, people are more likely to talk about your business when they're unhappy. However, there are many things you can do to encourage positive word-of-mouth referrals.

The most effective way to build word-of-mouth referrals is to cultivate relationships. Developing a solid reputation and fostering goodwill is pivotal, and it's even more crucial if you reside in a small town.

Natural vs. Planned Word of Mouth ●●

Most practitioners rely on the natural word of mouth that results from doing good work, genuinely caring about clients and having a solid reputation. You can increase referrals by incorporating the tips in Chapter 17 on excellent customer service. Still, unless you have a strong network of supporters, this approach could take a long time. While you cannot control how and when you get referrals, there are many ways to generate a positive buzz about your practice.

Figure 16.2

Chapter 5, Page 95
for tips on enhancing goodwill.

Word of Mouth Marketing Association
http://www.womma.org

Word of Mouth Marketing: How Smart Companies Get People Talking
by Andy Sernovitz

> ### Top 10 Tips to Generate Buzz
>
> - Cultivate relationships with centers of influence.
> - Recruit cheerleaders.
> - Make it easy for people to share about you (e.g., brochures, cards, newsletters, websites, open houses).
> - Be interesting and innovative.
> - Cultivate an attitude of gratitude—thank your clients in writing or in a brief telephone call.
> - Develop a referral incentive program for current clients.
> - Send regular communications (e.g., greeting cards, newsletters, wellness tips).
> - Be a source of knowledge (e.g., give presentations and demonstrations, write articles).
> - Establish a presence in your community (network, volunteer, send press releases, get interviewed).
> - Refer clients to appropriate colleagues.
> - Do a good job and pay attention to "the little things."

The Direct Referral Process • •

Directly asking for referrals is a common and accepted form of building any service business. If you don't tell your clients you would like their assistance, they might assume you're fully booked and aren't accepting new clients. The direct referral process consists of four major stages: request the referral, repeat the request, reward the referral and reciprocate the referral.

Request the Referral • • •

Pages 372-373
for details on developing a dynamic introduction.

Talk with your most satisfied clients and enlist their support. Ask them to tell their colleagues and friends about you. Supply them with business cards, brochures, and perhaps even some discount coupons for a percentage off an initial session (see Figure 16.3).

You can also email each client a brief description of yourself and a personalized statement of how your services assisted that specific client in achieving her wellness goals. Request that the client make any desired adaptations and send the note to people who might be interested in your services.

Repeat the Request • • •

The next time you talk with your clients, repeat the request. People don't always hear things the first time. They may have been preoccupied (or if it was right after a session, they may have been too relaxed for the request to sink in). Find out if they need more promotional materials, and ask them how you can make it easier for them to promote your practice. Also, send them a thank-you note even if you haven't received any referrals.

Sample Referral Note Card
www.businessmastery.us/ referral-card.php

Recognize them for their intentions and support. They could be sharing information about you and passing out your cards, but you might never know it. They don't have control over whether or not the people they talk to call you to set up an appointment. Everyone likes to be acknowledged, and knowing that you appreciate their efforts can inspire them to continue referring people to you.

Reward the Referral • • •

When you do get a referral, immediately send a thank-you note. Reward the referral with something tangible such as a free session, a product sample, a plant or flowers.

Reciprocate the Referral • • •

The last stage in the referral process is reciprocation. Whenever someone refers a client to you, go out of your way to either refer another client or customer back, use his services and products yourself, or supply the person with some type of desired information.

Figure 16.3 Client Referral Card

Client Referral Card

To: _____

From: _____

Give this card to a friend for $10 off their first appointment... and you get $10 off your next visit too!

Mia Lan Acupuncture
518 Broadway, Suite 3, Anytown, NJ 08413   207-555-3271
www.mialan.com

Generating Indirect Referrals • •

Another option to cultivate referrals is to compile a list of referral sources (e.g., all former and current clients, colleagues, friends and family members) who value your work. Ask them to write down the names, addresses and phone numbers of people whom they think could benefit from your services. Send those prospects a personalized letter of introduction, your brochure and include a discount coupon or referral card. Keep track of which people respond to your letter. Call the rest within a month. Inquire if they received the letter and ask if they would like additional information (such as articles or pamphlets), invite them to an open house or workshop, offer a free consultation or perhaps even book a session.

Developing a solid referral process is great for augmenting your practice as long as you don't depend on it as your major source for new clients. Ultimately, when it comes to establishing a thriving practice, you're the only one who can do it. The key is to design and implement a sound customer service plan. When it comes to word-of-mouth promotion, the most important mouth is your own!

Networking •

Establishing a strong network is fundamental for success in the wellness field. Since so much of our business comes from word-of-mouth (referrals from clients, friends and other networking associates), it's crucial to begin fostering these associations immediately!

Networking is essentially a group of interconnected or cooperating individuals who develop and share contacts, information and support. An effective network is composed of many different types of people: individuals from whom you get information; experts whose services you utilize and can refer to others; people who keep you informed of events and opportunities; role models; those who are genuinely concerned about you, listen to you and support you; mentors; people who actively refer potential clients to you; and centers of influence.

Networking is a perfect example of the adage, "The more you give, the more you receive."

Centers of influence can have a dramatic impact on your practice. These are individuals who are well known and highly respected by your target markets. Just one word from them could inspire droves of people to flock to your roost.

You can network informally by sharing resources with the people you contact or formally by joining a networking group. The most successful networkers are those who actively support others in making connections. Networking is a perfect example of the adage: the more you give, the more you receive.

Work Your Network • •

Become visible in your community by attending business, civic and social events, and joining professional and networking associations. Take seminars and classes. Attend various types of functions so you can widen the scope of people you meet.

Chapter 12, Page 243
for contact management ideas.

Enhance your networking abilities by recognizing the vast potential for making connections for yourself and others. Whenever you meet someone, jot a few notes about them: where and when you met, who introduced you, what line of business they're in, what their interests are and what types of resources they have. Think about the other people you know to see if it would be beneficial for them to meet each other. Even if you're unable to make any connections right away, you may do so in the future. You never know when a contact will come in handy.

Follow up on leads and information with a phone call or note. Take the initiative. Always thank people that help you (either by giving you their time, support, advice, leads or contacts), even if you don't use their help or if the leads don't work out. When you're given a recommendation to utilize someone's services, tell the person who referred you. When you give out referrals, make note of who you referred to whom. Find out if the referral was successful.

You can make more friends in two months by becoming interested in other people than you can in two years by trying to get people interested in you.
— Dale Carnegie

Maintain contact with people in your network and stay up-to-date with what's happening. People's lives are constantly changing and so are their networking needs. Given natural attrition, add at least two people per month to your active network to keep it thriving. The most fundamental element in effective networking is to follow through on your commitments.

Choosing a Networking Group • •

It is essential for your professional and personal well-being to belong to at least one networking organization. Numerous types of networking groups exist from monthly social clubs, to community groups such as the Chamber of Commerce, to weekly "needs and leads" business associations. Participate in functions at which you meet people to develop mutually beneficial relationships.

Determine which organization is best for you by assessing your needs and clarifying your purpose and goals for networking in general. Ascertain the types of contacts you desire and appraise the assets you have to offer others. Delineate your purpose and goals for each specific group you're considering joining. You may want to become a member of one group mainly as a means for getting clients and join another association because you strongly support their goals and activities. You may decide to become part of an organization for the educational and informational opportunities or join a club to make new friends and have fun. Sometimes one organization can meet several of your criteria.

Attend one or two meetings as a guest. Get a feel for the group. Notice whether or not you share any common interests and goals. Ask to see their bylaws and mission statement. If they don't have anything written, talk to several members and get feedback on their impressions of the group's purpose and philosophy. Find out the types of businesses and professions represented by the membership. Many organizations have a substantial membership fee, so it's wise to do some research before joining to determine if it's the right group for you.

Effective networking can be exciting as well as financially rewarding! Become active in at least one business association, and invest time in building your network of contacts and refining your networking skills.

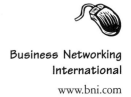

Business Networking International

www.bni.com

16

Figure 16.4

Networking Tips

- Wear clothes with pockets when attending networking events; one pocket holds your business cards, the other for cards you collect. Also, keep your hands as free as possible—it's extremely difficult to shake hands when you're balancing a beverage, plate of food and purse or briefcase.
- Clearly state what you do. After a brief conversation, people are more apt to remember an occupation than a name.
- Periodically reassess your needs, priorities and contacts.
- Have a professional address book, computerized contact manager, PDA or Rolodex.® Keep it current.
- Collect business cards. On the back of the card write the date, where you met the person, who introduced you and any other specific information you want to remember.
- When you give out referrals, make note of who you referred to whom. Then find out if the referral was successful.
- Follow up initial meetings with a phone call or a note. Take the initiative. Everyone likes to know that people are interested in them.
- Maintain contact with people in your network. Know what is happening.
- Add at least two people per month to your active network.
- Join professional associations.
- Develop your own personal, professional or educational support groups.
- Attend workshops.
- Always take plenty of business cards to networking events and keep them in an easily accessible spot.
- Share your resources and contacts.
- Attend community functions.
- Thank people who help you (either by giving you their time, support, advice, leads or contacts). Be a giver and a receiver.
- Follow through on your commitments.
- Actively cultivate your current network and begin increasing it today.

Figure 16.5

Contact/Referral Record

www.businessmastery.us/
forms.php#busman

Decide to Network Poem

www.businessmastery.us/
network-poem.php

Networking Group Checklist

Assess Your Needs and Goals
❏ Identify the types of support you need.
❏ Determine the type(s) of groups that would be in alignment.

Research Potential Groups
❏ What is the group's purpose (mission statement)?
❏ What year was it established?
❏ When does it meet, duration and location?
❏ What are the dues and fees?
❏ How many total members?
❏ How many active members?
❏ What is the number of members in your field?
❏ What types of businesses and professions are represented?

Attend at Least Two Meetings
❏ Determine the group's philosophy.
❏ See if you share any common interests and goals.
❏ Decide if you're comfortable referring business to the members.

Building an Effective Network

An effective network is composed of many different types of people. List the names or titles of the people who fit into each category (some names may be repeated since people often have more than one role in your life).

- Who are your sources of business- and practice-related information?
- List the people who could be centers of influence.
- Who are the people who actively refer potential clients to you?
- List the experts whose services you use and can refer to others.
- Who keeps you informed of events and opportunities?
- List the people who genuinely care about you, listen to you and support you.
- Who are your mentors?
- List your role models.

Now that you have specified the people in your current network, review the lists. Do one or two people perform most of the roles? Are there any areas that are lacking names? Are most of the people the same "type"? How do you feel about your network?

- List the kinds of support you would like to have right now.
- What additional types of support do you need over the next year?
- Who would you like to add to your network?
- List at least 10 goals for improving your network.

Building Professional Alliances ●

Every day the wellness field becomes more integrated. Providers from all realms are working together—blending philosophies, as well as actual client care. You can guide the direction this takes by developing affiliations with other wellness providers. Cultivating strong professional alliances provides value for you personally, as well as for your clients.

One of the most important benefits is having a diverse referral base to properly support your clients' well-being. Working with other practitioners provides you with a means to get away from working alone. These associations can also supply you with new clients and offer you the opportunity to participate in case management.

Professional alliances take time and commitment. They can be best developed with a two-tiered approach. The first level is built on increasing awareness of the benefits of your specific services. The second level involves forming direct affiliations with other practitioners. It is crucial to always be working on both levels.

Increasing Public Awareness ● ●

Increasing public awareness can be accomplished in many ways—from distributing educational materials to hosting elaborate media events. One of the most effective techniques is public speaking: offer to do presentations and demonstrations for professional, business, civic and special interest organizations (such as fibromyalgia support groups). Host exhibits at health fairs and expositions. Write articles for local publications. Get interviewed by the newspaper, radio and television. Be a guest on local health-related talk shows. Find out if and when your local paper publishes a special health supplement and arrange for your interview to appear in that section.

To see power as the ability to enhance others' lives expands society's narrow understanding of more traditional concepts of power.
— Pythia S. Peay

Although these activities are geared toward increasing public awareness about the benefits of your services, they also increase your credibility and visibility. Additionally, the exposure serves to establish you as an expert.

Developing Direct Affiliations ● ●

Build your network of professional wellness alliances through establishing credibility, initiating contact, forging relationships and maintaining connections. Determine your purpose, priorities and goals for developing these alliances, and create an action plan. Consider how much time you want to invest, the types of professions (and how many) you want to include in your network, and the levels of interaction you desire.

Foster Professional Alliances

- List the types of service providers that could assist your clients in achieving their well-being goals.
- Match those categories with names of providers whom you currently know.
- Note which categories are lacking names, and set goals to meet those types of practitioners.

The first step in developing professional relationships is to establish credibility. Many allied providers (particularly physicians) are required to obtain layers of licensure and certification. This leads them to judge competency by the number and types of certificates hanging on a wall—so some type of professional certification is helpful. Yet pieces of paper aren't the only badges of credibility.

You can enhance your visibility and credibility by getting involved in the activities described in the previous section on increasing public awareness. In addition to those activities, you could attend meetings at which there are other practitioners, join a local wellness organization (usually sponsored by a hospital), or volunteer your services for a charitable organization.

An interesting synergy often occurs in developing affiliations. Once the first connection is made, others occur more easily.

If you aren't well versed in the language of professional healthcare providers, learn to speak it now: be aware of their philosophy, approach and terminology. While it's fine to refer to your lower leg as a "calf" when talking to the general public, you're less credible if you aren't more technical while addressing other practitioners (in those instances, reference the "gastrocnemius"). Keep in mind that not everyone shares your particular approach to wellness care. While many practitioners believe in and specialize in prevention, others (e.g., physical therapists, general physicians, surgeons) spend most of their time working with people on the remedial side of healthcare.

Initiating Contact • •

Some people prefer the front-door approach while others feel more comfortable with the side-door or even back-door method of developing affiliations. You might consider using a combination of these approaches discussed below.

Introduction Letter

www.businessmastery.us/
intro-letter.php

Front-Door Approach • • •

The three most common front-door approaches are the telephone, the mail or in person. Some people feel very comfortable just walking in and introducing themselves. This is a lot easier if your office is located close to other providers. In general, though, people prefer to initiate contact with a letter or telephone call. When you know the practitioner, a phone call usually suffices.

An effective technique for generating prospective alliance partners is to send a mailing to targeted wellness professionals. Direct the emphasis of your letter to the benefits of the reader. First introduce yourself and say what you do, including your abilities and qualifications. Focus on how you can help them, their practices and their clients. Create a separate letter for each type of practitioner you contact. For each type of provider you contact, include examples of how your services address their specific needs. (See Sample Introduction Letter, Figure 16.7.)

For instance, chiropractors see people who suffer from arthritis, back pain, fibromyalgia, migraines, injuries from sports activities, job injuries and automobile accidents. Psychiatrists work with people experiencing pain, stress disorders and migraines, as well as support people in personal growth and well-being. Obstetricians work with women experiencing back pain, edema, hormonal fluctuations and body image issues, as well as support general mother/child well-being. Touch therapists work with people of all ages, providing services ranging from relaxation to injury rehabilitation.

Highlight the mutual benefits of your association. Reassure your prospective colleagues that your intent is to support and complement each other's practice, not compete for clientele. Close the letter by telling them how to contact you, and that if you don't hear from them within the next two weeks, you will contact them.

Enclose your promotional material and an article that lends credence to your claim for potential benefits. You can also include a stamped, pre-printed return postcard that allows the practitioner to respond directly. (See Figure 16.6, Sample Reply Postcard.) After the letter has been sent, you must follow up.

Remember that a man's name is, to him, the sweetest and most important sound in any language.
— Dale Carnegie

Figure 16.6 Sample Reply Postcard

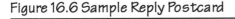
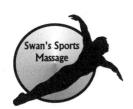

Swan's Sports Massage

Sports Massage Clinic
3197 Bender Creek Circle
Burlington, VT 43579
802-555-5555
ginny@sportsmassageclinic.com
www.sportsmassageclinic.com

Yes, I am interested in pursuing a possible alliance.

❏ Please send me more information.
❏ Please call me to set up a meeting to discuss our possible alliance.
❏ Please call me to schedule my complimentary session.
     The best time to reach me is:
     My phone number is:
❏ I'm not interested in developing a professional alliance at this time.

Chapter 12, Pages 246-249
for HIPAA guidelines.

Side-Door Approach • • •

The side-door approach is usually taken with the practitioner who keeps a buffer person—a nurse, assistant or office manager—between herself and the public. This mainly occurs with medical doctors, chiropractors, dentists and other clinicians. Always treat these gatekeepers courteously because they're the ones who will get you in the door to meet the practitioner (and encourage client referrals once a relationship is established). Be direct. Inform the office staff that you're interested in developing alliances with other providers.

If you're unable to make an appointment with the practitioner, ask when would be a good time to drop off your brochure. When you deliver your brochure, ask the office manager if she has any questions about your services or background, and offer to demonstrate your work, for example, by teaching a five-minute self-massage routine. Give free sessions to the provider and the staff. This is time well invested, because if you have the opportunity to demonstrate your services, and the recipient is impressed with the benefits, that person is likely to be interested in building an alliance with you. Give a certificate for the session(s), and if possible, book the appointment(s) before you leave.

Another way to build alliances through the side door involves your current clients. When conducting intake interviews, ask your clients if they're working with other wellness providers. If so, get their permission to send a note to those providers. This could range from a simple letter of introduction informing each practitioner that you're working with their client, to a more in-depth report with a brief description of your assessment, treatment plan and progress notes. (Note: Be sure to follow HIPAA guidelines, and also include your promotional literature and extra business cards.)

Back-Door Approach • • •

The back-door approach can appear to be the least threatening entrance to developing professional relationships. There are various ways to enter through the back door. You can get to know other practitioners by sponsoring a talk show on radio or cable on which you bring wellness providers as guests. You can also encounter practitioners by attending networking events, social engagements, professional society meetings, special interest group meetings, professional development seminars and civic functions. Research these groups to determine which ones are most likely to attract the types of practitioners you wish to meet.

An example of attending events to develop professional alliances and clients happened when I did a seminar tour in Australia. One of the participants in my workshop in Brisbane was a business coach. She attended my seminar for a dual purpose: to learn new information, but mainly to get new clients. Here was a perfect opportunity: she could spend two days getting to know many people who were obviously interested in their professional development—with the knowledge that I wouldn't be there to work with them on an ongoing basis.

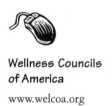

**Wellness Councils
of America**

www.welcoa.org

*No road is long with
good company.*
— Turkish Proverb

Forging Relationships ● ●

Your first official meeting with a wellness provider sets the tone for the relationship. Be punctual and look professional. Ideally you will also be giving a session, so your clothing can be a little more casual. Business attire is appropriate if you aren't giving a session. Greet the practitioner with a handshake and smile.

Briefly share information about yourself and encourage the provider to share information about her practice. Discuss ways in which you could be of mutual benefit (including reducing the demands on her time and energy), and set goals. Confer about approaches to different situations, and determine how you would like to work together. Be certain to cover the preferred methods of future communication about shared clients. Some people favor written correspondence only, while others like to discuss cases and proactively work together to enhance clients' well-being.

While it isn't imperative that the practitioner experience your work, I strongly advise you make it happen. If she claims she is too busy, offer to do a modified session at her convenience. Also give a free session to the staff (see the previous section on initiating contact). Be upfront: tell her that it's important to experience your work firsthand to ethically feel good about making referrals to you. The converse is also true. For you to refer clients to her, you need to experience her work—or in the very least get a sense of her methodology and style, which can be done by assessing the person's demeanor, office environment and written materials (such as intake forms and information pamphlets).

When you give her a treatment, do an intake interview (modify it if time is limited), take notes, and submit a sample of your records. This is of particular importance if you aren't a primary care provider, because it demonstrates your ability to do charting and follow-up. Before you leave this meeting schedule the next one—whether it's a telephone conversation, another session or a more formal face-to-face meeting. Sometimes the steps to forging a relationship take several meetings to accomplish.

Maintaining Connections ● ●

Maintain connections by employing customer service principles. For example: send a thank-you note after your first meeting; if they haven't used your certificate within three weeks, remind them, and ask them when they would like to book the session; acknowledge all referrals; regularly submit typed progress reports (check with client first); call about dramatic results; schedule a brief meeting at least twice per year; reciprocate by sending them clients; leave an ample supply of your brochures and business cards for display in the office and distribution to clients/patients; obtain a plentiful stock of their cards and brochures; and place monthly check-in calls (instead of asking if they've run out of brochures or cards, assume that they have, and ask how many you can bring by).

You want to make it as easy as possible for allied health providers to make referrals to you. In addition to stocking your promotional material, consider printing referral pads with your contact information to give to the providers and their office staff.

Sample Prescription Pad
www.businessmastery.us/
dr-pad.php

16

Figure 16.7 Sample Introduction Letter

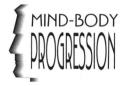

October 15, 2020

Ben Casey, Ph.D.
123 North Swan Road
Sea City, CA 90000

Dear Dr. Casey,

I was intrigued by your advertisement in the Yellow Pages under "Psychotherapy." You appear dedicated to the health of the whole person. As a licensed acupuncturist and Traditional Chinese Medicine (TCM) practitioner I, too, see the mind-body as so interwoven that addressing the health of one area while excluding the other is an incomplete process.

I am interested in developing an alliance between us for mutual referrals to better serve our clients. I provide a complete range of services that include general wellness, stress reduction, pain relief, injury rehabilitation, and illness intervention. Many of these were listed in your advertisement as well. I am also a master herbologist and have worked with people of varying ages.

Acupuncture and TCM, as a complement to psychological counseling, can support optimal well-being in powerful and beneficial ways. As an adjunct to your therapy, clients utilizing my services may find a decreased need for medication, thus lowering the possibilities of medication interactions.

As we tend to approach holistic health from different angles, I believe many of our clients could benefit from our combined services. For example, I see clients who experience emotional releases during sessions and who would benefit from professional counseling. Likewise, I'm sure you have clients who could benefit from acupuncture and TCM.

I look forward to meeting with you personally to discuss the possibilities. Feel free to call my office at 555-5555. Otherwise, I'll contact you within the next two weeks to schedule a time to meet.

Sincerely,

James Kildare

Enclosures

721 N. Somerset Place ❖ Arcadia, CA 91077 ❖ 415-555-5555
jkildare@mind-bodyprogression.com
www.mind-bodyprogression.com

Show and Tell •

Remember "show and tell" from grade school? This was your opportunity to share something wonderful that happened to you or to show off a favorite possession with your fellow students. Most kids look forward to show and tell. I hated it at first. My family never went anywhere exciting, and I didn't have any exotic toys. But that's when I discovered the two keys to grabbing people's attention: exude enthusiasm, and demonstrate uniqueness and benefits. Both elements are crucial. Who would have known back then that I was learning how to be a good public speaker? For most of us, show and tell was our first experience at public speaking—only it wasn't called that. It was simply sharing, and usually it was fun.

As the school years progressed, most of us had to get up in front of a class to give reports, recite poems, make speeches and engage in debates. Often the topics were imposed on us, and it was difficult to muster much enthusiasm. It is no wonder that, as adults, most people dread public speaking. In fact, surveys show the majority of people are more afraid of public speaking than they are of death.

Public speaking isn't just about getting up in front of 25 (or even 2,500) people and giving a formal presentation. It is about the ways you share information with others. These activities range from casual encounters, such as talking with people while waiting in lines and networking at social and business functions, to informal events, such as holding open houses and giving parties, to more formal examples, such as providing free talks at civic, professional and business meetings, doing demonstrations at public events (e.g., fairs and health expositions), facilitating workshops and giving keynote speeches.

As in show and tell, public speaking is easy as long as you share something that excites you and can make a difference in the audience's lives. As wellness providers you've got it covered—you frequently witness profound changes in your clients! How can you NOT be enthusiastic about your work? When I was in practice, I was always talking with people about massage—whether or not I initiated the conversation. Granted, I didn't corner people in elevators (well, hardly ever), but I wanted the world to know how wonderful massage was and how it could change people's lives. It isn't necessary to become a zealot— just be open. I suggest that every day before leaving your house you remind yourself of all the benefits of your services, and recall at least two instances when you or one of your clients experienced a significant change. This puts your work in your conscious awareness so that you're more cognizant of appropriate instances in which to share it.

One of the most successful ways to do "public speaking" is to talk with people whenever you're waiting in a line: share information about your services; recommend stretches; tell them about the latest product you've discovered; and offer to show them something to alleviate their pain. It may sound hokey, but if you're enthusiastic and sincere, it's the best form of education and marketing.

16

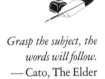

Grasp the subject, the words will follow.
— Cato, The Elder

Educating people about your field is vital to the growth of your profession, as well as building your own practice. Start where you're most comfortable (typically casual encounters or informal events). Commit to sharing information about your services at least five times weekly. Once you've increased your level of comfort and confidence, you can move on to more formal presentations and demonstrations.

Formal presentations can be fun. They aren't limited to traditional platform speaking. Plus, you don't have to do them alone. You can ease your discomfort and make the presentation more appealing by co-leading or holding panel discussions. Actually, in this industry, the most effective presentations are informal in nature and include demonstrations and group participation.

The Public Speaking Circuit ● ●

Many wellness providers contend that the major catalyst for growing their practices is giving "free" talks. Even though you don't get paid for these presentations, they're a superb training ground and a great way to attract new clients. I recommend approaching public speaking from two points: general education and marketing. General education public speaking involves talking to anyone who will listen. While the audience might not be likely candidates for your services, you raise the consciousness level—which benefits the profession as a whole.

As a marketing tool, public speaking requires finding out which groups are most likely to include your target markets as members. Utilize your public speaking time wisely by making certain that at least one-half of your formal presentations are to groups with members in your target markets. The following list contains examples of several target markets and places where they could be found (and likely sponsors of your presentations).

Figure 16.8

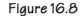

> ### Target Markets for Giving Presentations
>
> - Specific Health Concerns: Support groups, clinics, bookstores, wellness provider's offices and health food stores.
> - People in Recovery: Counseling offices, treatment centers and specialty bookstores.
> - Animals: Veterinary clinics, pet stores, grooming centers, 4-H clubs, dog obedience classes and county fairs.
> - Seniors: Volunteer organizations, senior centers, civic groups and parks.
> - Pregnant Women: Lamaze classes, the La Leche League, baby boutiques and Ob/Gyn offices.
> - Athletes: Sporting events, health fairs, sporting goods stores, sports medicine facilities and health food stores.
> - Attorneys: Bar association meetings, law library and legal aid department.

How to Prepare, Stage and Deliver Winning Presentations
by Thomas Leech

Present Yourself Powerfully
by Cherie Sohnen-Moe

You can speak well if your tongue can deliver the message of your heart.
—John Ford

Getting on the public speaking circuit is easy. Contact civic clubs, professional societies, business groups and networking associations. These organizations are always on the lookout for speakers. Their members enjoy learning specific techniques that improve the quality of their lives. Indeed, any topic relating to well-being or stress reduction is in demand. Even bookstores sponsor talks regularly. The most common duration of these presentations is 20 minutes, but they can range up to one hour.

Successful Presentations ● ●

The key to successful presentations is planning. Investing the time in planning can make the difference between a powerful, flowing, fun presentation and one that's stilted and ineffective. Planning includes understanding the audience, assessing their needs and objectives, determining the presentation purpose, researching the topic, designing the presentation, and matching facilities to program requirements. It's important to evaluate and update your information and audio-visual materials before each presentation—regardless of whether you're preparing a talk from scratch or if you're delivering the same topic for the fiftieth time.

Research Studies
www6.miami.edu/
touch-research/

www.massagetherapy
foundation.org

www.acubriefs.com

Sample Topics ● ● ●

Some general ideas for wellness presentations are: Stress Management Techniques, Self-Massage, Stretches and Exercises People Can Do at Their Desks, Self-Hypnosis to Gain the Competitive Edge, Couples Massage, Acupressure, Peak Performance Through Proper Nutrition, Preventive Wellness, Infant Massage, Hydrotherapy, Nutrition, Movement, Dream Analysis, Aromatherapy, Healthy Baby Care, Common Use of Herbs, Personal Growth and Fitness. You can also give talks on other subjects in which you have experience or training. Some of the most enjoyable "talks" are when you demonstrate your services. You could create numerous different presentations for every example given above. You can also tie in your presentation with holidays or major events and title them accordingly. Two examples are: "Stress Deduction" during tax time; and "The Gift of Touch" for the pre-holiday buying season.

A Physician's Guide to Therapeutic Massage
by John Yates, Ph.D.

Alternative Medicine: What Works
by A. Fugh-Berman, M.D.

Resources ● ● ●

Vast resources are available for ideas on presentation topics, products to sell and handouts. Peruse your personal library and search the Internet. Check your books and magazines for topics of interest. Go to health food stores and bookstores. Research information about your specific industry, and then look at general topics such as health, wellness, fitness, stress and alternative health.

Figure 16.9

Presentation Design

I	Presentation Purpose	Decide whether the focus is informative, persuasive or a bit of both. Think about what you want your audience to take away from the presentation.
II	Audience Analysis	Attempt to find out ahead of time what types of people will be attending, their interests and special needs.
III	Presentation Opening	In addition to your personal introduction, customary openings are stating a central idea, asking a question or previewing the presentation.
IV	Presentation Body	This section typically focuses on a single point with information or evidence to support the premise. Incorporate a mixture of experiential activities and audio-visual materials. Allow time for questions.
V	Presentation Conclusion	Summarize key points, restate the central idea, answer the opening question, or call the audience to action. Thank the audience and your host, and remind them how they can contact you.

Delivery ● ● ●

It's all right to have butterflies in your stomach. Just get them to fly in formation.
— Dr. Ron Gilbert

In any presentation, how you say something is just as important as what you say. Approximately 55 percent of your presentation impact comes from your nonverbal communications, 35 percent from your voice, and 10 percent from the actual content. Being unaware of these numbers, most people spend the majority of their preparation on the content. Power and presence are established through the mastery of body language, while the energy in your voice conveys your sincerity. The methods used to communicate information often determine whether or not the information is fully received.

Incorporate activities that involve the major senses of sight, sound and touch. If you work with aromatherapy, also include smell. People like to feel as though they're being talked with directly—even if they're part of a large group. Some creative techniques for involving your audience are: have the audience participate in an activity such as stretching; lead a visualization exercise; ask questions, and have the group raise their hands or stand up in response (e.g., How many of you get headaches? How many of you have ever received an acupuncture treatment? How many receive acupuncture regularly?); make specific reference to a participant or the group (e.g., "Since everyone here today either suffers from fibromyalgia or is close to someone who does, you know how debilitating pain can be."); request feedback; facilitate a question-and-answer format; and give a demonstration.

The more experiential the activity, the better. When talking about touch therapies, show the group how to do some simple techniques on themselves or each other. If the group members know each other well and aren't dressed in business suits, you can organize a massage circle. If you're including information on aromatherapy, bring some essential oils for the audience to smell.

The activities need not be elaborate to be fun and effective. For instance, you can demonstrate stretches that the audience can do with you while sitting in their chairs. You can lead activities based on popular games, such as crossword puzzles and Scrabble,® and even design a wellness edition of Trivial Pursuit® or Jeopardy® that includes facts about your specific industry.

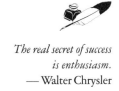

16

Overcoming Nervousness • • •

Some people are fortunate in that they're naturally good speakers; they feel comfortable being in front of a group, easily relate to their audiences, and can think while on their feet. Most people must develop these speaking skills. The first step is to assess your attitude. Many people are hesitant to do any type of public speaking for fear of appearing inept. The beauty of doing presentations about health and well-being is that you intrinsically know the benefits of this work. Granted, you might not know everything about a specific topic or have an answer for every question—but no audience expects that.

The second step is to increase your knowledge and experience of public speaking. Take classes (through your local community college, university or a private company), read books, or join a public speaking group such as Toastmasters International.

The final step is to practice. By joining a group such as Toastmasters, you get weekly practice in public speaking. You can always devise ways to weave information about your services into your topics. Another practice option is to create a support group; members can meet to coach each other on presentations and do public speaking engagements together.

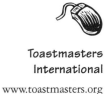

Toastmasters International
www.toastmasters.org

Everyone gets nervous. The difference between a good presenter and a poor one is that the good presenter knows how to manage her fears. Use the adrenaline that's pumping through your system to keep you alert and sustain a high energy level.

Figure 16.10

Top 10 Tips to Alleviate Nervousness

- Before your presentation, visualize yourself having a fabulous time; being dynamic, energetic and connecting with the audience.
- Take a few deep breaths and relax your body.
- Get a touch therapy treatment prior to speaking.
- Avoid eating a heavy meal before speaking.
- Drink warm noncaffeinated liquids (e.g., lemon tea).
- Maintain good posture: unlock your knees and stand with equal weight on both feet.
- Organize your notes and audio-visuals.
- Wear comfortable clothes.
- Find a friendly face to look at when discomfort arises.
- Practice, practice, practice.

Develop a Dynamic Introduction •

No matter what you do in life, your ability to introduce yourself well greatly impacts your success. Because this business thrives on word-of-mouth promotion, you must inspire others by the way you introduce yourself.

Actually, it's wise to have several exciting introductions down pat. The advantage is this: you may want to vary what you say and how you say it depending on the time parameters and the audience. Your introduction will differ if you're talking directly with one person rather than a group. Most likely you'll use different terminology when you're talking to a group of your peers rather than a business group, or even a mixed group.

In most networking groups, you're only allotted 30 seconds or less to introduce yourself. Without a prepared introduction, you probably will only say a small portion of what you wish to convey. Yet 20 seconds is ample time if your basic introduction is clear, concise and engaging.

I recommend creating a memorized 20-second and 30-second introduction. It is also wise to design a one-minute and a five-minute presentation in which you memorize your opening and closing lines, and have a clear outline of key points you wish to cover. Conversely, I highly discourage memorizing any presentation that's more than 30 seconds in length, since this puts too much emphasis on the words and not the relationship between you and your audience. Another problem with a memorized speech is that if you forget a word, or someone asks you a question, you may get totally thrown off track and not gracefully recover.

Figure 16.11

Simple Yet Effective 20-30 Second Introductions

"How would you like to make your pregnancy—or that of a friend's—much more enjoyable and comfortable? This can be achieved by receiving regular massages. I am Mary Smith, and I'm a licensed massage therapist, specializing in prenatal massage. The work I do with pregnant women assists them in increasing circulation, reducing edema, improving muscle tone, and easing tension and fatigue. Please feel free to talk with me after the meeting. I have cards, brochures and gift certificates available at the back table."

"Hello, I am Kerry Billings, and I am a chiropractor. I've been in practice since 1995 and have recently moved to Sunny Hills. My focus is on well-being and preventive care. I have an extensive background in Oriental philosophy and incorporate that into my approach. Please call me if you're interested in more information. I don't charge for an initial consultation. I look forward to meeting with you and assisting you in achieving optimal health."

"Do you experience a lot of stress? Is your life filled with activities—career, family and friends? Are you involved in a fitness program? If you answered yes to any of these questions, you probably experience some form of physical discomfort —be it muscular aches and pain, fatigue, or even tension headaches. Yoga can help reduce stress, improve circulation, ease tension and improve muscle tone. I am Randy Harris, and I am a certified yoga practitioner. If you would like more information on how yoga can enhance your well-being, please talk with me after the meeting."

Designing your introduction needn't be a grueling experience. You can generate and refine several introductions in several hours. Make it fun by getting together with several friends to work on your introductions. As a side benefit, the material you develop for your introduction(s) can be used to create other promotional material, such as brochures and press releases.

Introduction Design

- Begin your adventure by collecting descriptive material: informational packets on your services, magazine articles, brochures from other practitioners and promotional pieces on yourself. Go through this information and highlight the words and phrases that appeal to you.
- Write a detailed statement of what you do. Be certain to distinguish the features from the benefits. Features are the descriptive characteristics about your service and your background, including experience and education in this profession. Benefits are the results that a client receives by utilizing your services.
- Review your differential advantage statement (i.e., what makes your services unique).
- Write your introduction. Choose a specific audience and a time frame (e.g., a business networking meeting and 30-second general introduction). Look over all of the material you have—the highlights from your sample promotional pieces, your business description, and your differential advantage statement. Combine these to formulate your written introduction; review it, replacing any passive words or phrases with dynamic, active, present tense terms. Avoid well-worn language patterns and vocabulary by using a thesaurus to discover different words (terms, jargon, expressions). If you do this exercise with colleagues, read your introductions to each other and get feedback. Repeat this process for each introduction you decide to prepare.
- Refine your introduction. The best way to do this is to practice it in front of friends who will be honest with you. Get their input on the content and your delivery. If this isn't feasible, practice out loud, standing tall in front of a mirror. Use a tape recorder (videotape if available), and critique the results. "All the world's a stage," and these are your lines. Remember, the more comfortable you are in dynamically introducing yourself, the greater your impact. And in this profession, first impressions have a significant influence on your success.

Parties •

A party is a fun and creative way to market your services. The best way to hold this event is to have a current client sponsor a casual in-home or in-office gathering. This approach has proven extremely effective with products such as vitamins, cosmetics, designer clothing, and, of course, the most famous, Tupperware.®

This marketing strategy works because the guests feel comfortable. They are in a safe environment, the atmosphere is festive, and they can experience the services or products firsthand. I know a Rolfing® practitioner who dramatically increased her clientele through these types of parties.

You may be wondering how a party differs from an introductory demonstration given at your office. The major differences are in the sponsorship and the tone of the event. These parties tend to be small and intimate—five to 10 friends or colleagues of the sponsor.

People attend the party not only to find out more about what you have to offer, but also because their friend invited them. These people are usually more open to your presentation and more likely to become clients than strangers who come to an introductory demonstration they saw announced in the newspaper. Also, guests at the party expect to have fun and receive more personalized attention than if they were at a more formal demonstration.

Party Setup • •

Design the party in such a way that the atmosphere is lively and promotes involvement. The sponsor usually provides refreshments, and the first portion of the party is spent casually getting to know each other.

When you begin your presentation, give a brief overview of who you are, your training and your philosophy toward your work and health. Describe your work and do a formal demonstration on a model (preferably the client who is the sponsor). Position your table, chair or mat so that the guests can easily gather around to see you in action. Encourage people to ask you and the model questions.

If you're a touch therapist, allow every participant the opportunity to experience your technique after you've finished the demonstration. This could be anything from a five-minute neck session to a three-minute hand massage—and you can do it while talking and answering questions.

If the group is playful, include health-oriented games. Offer prizes for correct answers to general health questions, such as how much water the average person should drink each day, or to the first person to correctly identify a specific muscle.

Product Sales • •

Depending upon the type of work you do, you may also want to display products at the party. Be sure to describe the products, their benefits and how to use them. Do a product demonstration. If possible, use the products while working on your model.

If you intend to sell products at the party, you must be clear on your focus, and the guests should be told ahead of time so they bring their checkbooks. Realize that most people have never seen some of the wonderful accouterments available for their wellness and relaxation, and they will enjoy the opportunity to see and test these products.

The income generated by the product sales gives you immediate compensation for your time, whereas the long-term benefits are achieved by the new clients you generate from the party. As long as you keep perspective and concentrate the majority of your presentation on hands-on work, product sales can be a profitable adjunct.

Far better it is to dare mighty things, to win glorious triumphs even though checkered by failure, than to rank with those poor spirits who neither enjoy nor suffer much because they live in the gray twilight that knows neither victory nor defeat.
— Theodore Roosevelt

Some examples of suitable products to display are: books; relaxation tools and implements (e.g., percussion instruments, massage pads); audio cassettes and CDs; hot and cold packs; ice pillows; lotions and oils; support pillows and similar ergonomic devices; stretching bands and balls; herbs; supplements; remedies; essences (such as aromatherapy) and the equipment to use with them; and self-health videos.

Choosing a Sponsor ● ●

The first step to organizing a party is to choose an appropriate sponsor. Review your client list and pick several possibilities. The most important characteristics are that the client values your work, is fairly outgoing, is reliable and knows a lot of people.

Talk with your potential sponsors. Most clients eagerly agree to sponsor a party if you offer them some form of compensation either in services or products. I recommend giving the client one treatment just for organizing the party, and one treatment for every three to four attendees. You can also give a bonus of one session for every person who becomes a client. Be certain to tell the sponsor to limit the number of guests to approximately 15. If too many participate, the informal nature becomes disrupted, and you lose the power of intimacy.

The secret of success is to be ready for opportunity when it comes.
— Benjamin Disraeli

Even though your sponsors may be enthusiastic about the party, it doesn't necessarily follow that they can coordinate well. Play an active role in the party's preparation and promotion. Once a client has decided to be a sponsor, set aside at least one hour to plan the event. Choose a date and select the format. Factors that influence the choice of format include the number of prospective guests, their background, the time allotted, and the time of year the party is scheduled to take place.

For instance, if five people attend, you could include more hands-on time with them than if 15 people show up. Also, if the guests are conversant with your type of services, there's no need to spend much time covering the basics—you can focus on the specific benefits of your techniques. If the party is slated for three hours, you must prepare more information and activities than if the party lasts an hour.

Party Preparations ● ●

After the date has been chosen and the format selected, the sponsor creates a guest list and sends out invitations that include RSVPs. The next stages of preparation include scripting the party and rehearsing, creating appropriate handouts, assembling supplies, and supporting your sponsor.

Create a Theme ● ● ●

Be creative by incorporating the time of year into your presentation. Make it a theme party. For example, if the party takes place close to St. Patrick's Day, you can use green paper for your handouts, and decorate accordingly. If the party occurs close to Thanksgiving, include an exercise or discussion about the things for which everyone is thankful—particularly regarding their health, and discuss ways to ensure continued good health.

Party Script • • •

When you script the party, designate time parameters for each segment. A sample party outline might look like this: 15 minutes informal talking; five minutes self-introduction; 10 minutes discussion on benefits of your services and description of your work; 10 minutes group activity; 10 minutes break; 15 minutes demonstration on model; 20 minutes questions and demonstrations on guests; 10 minutes break; 15 minutes additional questions and demonstrations on guests; and 10 minutes wrap-up. Your script would include more details of the actual content to be covered in each section. After designing the outline, rehearse the presentation several times, making any necessary adjustments to the script.

Handouts • • •

Handouts are an integral part of any successful presentation. Most people are visually oriented, so it's important to give the guests something to look at and hold. Design one or more handouts that are tailored to the specific presentation or to the group. For instance, let's say the guests are all co-workers at a computer data entry company. You could create a handout that shows self-care techniques for alleviating eye strain and avoiding repetitive stress syndrome. However you design your handouts, include your name, phone number and website.

Supplies • • •

The basic supplies needed for any presentation are: promotional materials (e.g., cards, brochures, gift certificates, appointment book); personal items (e.g., throat lozenges); and general purpose supplies such as facial tissue, name tags, markers, transparent tape, scissors, masking tape, glue, an extension cord, trash bags, a clock, writing implements, paper and a receipt book. I always keep a small, lidded carrying box stocked with these items. Also, bring any specialized equipment or supplies needed for your specific presentation, such as handouts, table, sheets, lubricant, music system, music, props and charts.

Sponsor Support • • •

The final element in pre-party preparation involves supporting your sponsor. Keep in contact with this person. Check in regularly to get updates on the responses to the invitations and offer any assistance in follow-up or organization of the event. Call your sponsor to find out if there are any last-minute hitches. Arrive at the party at least one hour ahead of time to help with any logistical needs, arrange your equipment and supplies, display your promotional materials and products, and prepare yourself. You want to be organized and centered when the guests arrive so you can concentrate on building rapport and getting to know them.

Party Follow-up • •

The final activity to ensure positive results from the party is follow-up. Send a thank-you letter to your sponsor, mail notes to all guests thanking them for attending, and confirm any appointments made.

Open Houses •

Hosting open houses is an excellent stage for promoting your practice. Open houses provide low stress, relatively inexpensive opportunities to meet your neighbors, network with allied practitioners, introduce potential clients to your services and products, and inspire current clients to increase the amount or type of treatments they receive.

People often avoid hosting open houses for fear that no one will attend. The following steps help ensure a successful event.

Figure 16.12

10 Steps to A Great Open House

1. Decide the purpose, priorities and goals of each open house. Incorporate an educational element, such as a presentation (e.g., stress reduction techniques, nutrition, self-massage, or stretching), or a demonstration of a specific technique, product, or piece of equipment. Make sure that the educational segment's duration is under 10 minutes and perform it several times throughout the event.
2. Envision the event and outline the flow of activities. If possible, create a theme, such as "Spring Rejuvenation."
3. Compile a guest list, including general categories such as all the allied health practitioners in a half-mile radius or people with fibromyalgia.
4. Pick a good date and time. "Good" depends on your office location and the flexibility of your intended audience. For instance, if your office is surrounded by other professional practices, and your main purpose is to network with your neighbors, perhaps an open house during lunchtime or one that takes place midweek from 4:00 to 6:00 p.m. might be most appropriate.
5. Design attractive fliers. Use an attention-grabbing headline, describe the planned activities, and highlight the benefits of attending. Always offer some type of freebie that everyone receives (e.g., "All guests receive a sample of XYZ product."), and offer at least one major door prize such as a free session. Also boost attendance by mentioning that refreshments are served.
6. Distribute fliers. Personally deliver them to the nearby offices. This is also a great opportunity to introduce yourself and network. Post them in places where your intended guests are likely to see them, such as bulletin boards in specialty stores. Mail fliers to potential guests (e.g., your current client list).
7. Send personal invitations to key guests and place follow-up phone calls.
8. Post an announcement on your website.
9. Send press releases to the local media.
10. Place reminder calls to key guests several hours before the open house.

Booths •

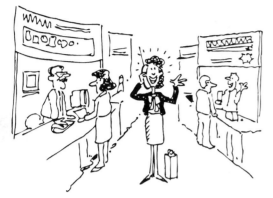

Another effective method for gaining visibility is to set up a booth at conferences, conventions, expositions and trade shows. You can meet a lot of people at these events. Choose shows that attract your target markets. Be creative in your choices. For instance, if one of your target markets is infants, take a booth at a baby fair or even a bridal trade show. A wellness booth will stand out amongst the plethora of product vendors. Establish your community presence by being part of wellness and health expositions. Other factors to consider when selecting shows are: the targeted attendees, the cost in terms of time and money, the other companies exhibiting, and the show's past success.

Trade Show Displays

www.tradeshowdisplayzone.com
www.exhibitoronline.com

Find out which shows are happening in your community by contacting your convention bureau, the Chamber of Commerce and the sales directors at major hotels. Check specific trade journals, local business publications, and the Internet.

Make sure your booth design fits your image. You can create your own or purchase a portable display. The following tips assist in making this a productive experience.

Figure 16.13

Making the Most of Your Booth

- Send out invitations to prospects to attend the show and pick up a free product at your booth.
- Be sure to have ample promotional materials available. You may want to print special fliers (much less expensive than brochures) for these events.
- Display your promotional materials in such a way that people will take them. This enables you to engage in a conversation with someone and not be concerned about missing potential clients.
- Although it's great to have an elaborate booth, don't let the lack of one be a deterrent. Do the best that you can within your budget. Just be sure to personalize it somehow with plants, photographs or flowers.
- Grab potential clients' attention with an eye-catching sign. If you're unable to hang it up, put it on an easel. Make sure the graphics and words are easily viewed from all sight lines.
- Provide ongoing hands-on demonstrations.
- Give away product samples.
- Set out a bowl or basket to collect business cards. Put a sign in front of the bowl stating, "Enter here for a free drawing of...." If possible, donate your services or products. If that isn't appropriate, then give a prize, such as a book, a basket of healthy goodies, or a gift certificate from a local store.
- Play a DVD that either demonstrates your services or gives interesting information (in an entertaining format). Be sure the program is less than six minutes long and looped (so it plays continuously).
- Bring necessary supplies. In addition to your promotional materials, make sure you have plenty of logistical supplies (e.g., equipment, masking tape, extension cords, pencils, paper, tissues), refreshments and clothing (in case you get cold, sweaty or spill something on yourself).
- Bring a friendly, knowledgeable person to help staff your booth. You need to take breaks. You must walk around and check out the other booths. Some of the best networking takes place between booth owners.

• Promotion: The Written Word •

The written word is a powerful tool. Like a magnet, clearly written and compelling promotional materials can attract the interest of potential clients actively looking for a wellness practitioner. Equally important is developing a "voice" in your writing that communicates your unique personality, philosophy and talents in a way that differentiates you from your competitors. Promotional writing can take the shape of articles for magazines, "quick tips" to distribute at speaking engagements, or a post on your website, a paper-based or online newsletter, and special reports that offer solutions to your clients' health concerns.

Articles •

There are more than 100,000 newspapers, magazines, journals and association newsletters published regularly in North America. They welcome information that is beneficial to their readership. Many of these publications are quite receptive to freelance article submissions. Sometimes they even pay you for the articles—but even if they don't, it's great exposure!

Writing Articles

List five topics you feel comfortable writing about. For each of the topics:

- Locate at least two publications that might be interested in the topic.
- Obtain copies of the publications to find out their format, average word count and style.
- Request submission guidelines (usually available online).
- Send a one-page query letter that describes your article idea and why you think it will benefit the publication's readers. Also include a brief biography that lists your credentials.

The Article Writing Process • •

Write articles on general wellness, the value of your particular area of expertise, or the latest innovations in your field. If you're at a loss for topics, think about the types of questions your clients frequently ask you. The steps to writing an article are similar to those when preparing for a presentation. Begin by writing a summary of what you want the readers to learn and what actions you want them to take. Next create an outline. Then write the article.

Regardless of whether your articles get published, use them as promotional tools. Send them to current clients, and make them available to prospective clients.

Figure 16.14

Article Development

I	Title	Construct a catchy title. Some people recommend starting off with a title, although I've found that oftentimes, the title doesn't come to me until the article is completed.
II	Opening	Write an opening paragraph that grabs the readers. Briefly review the topic and explain the benefits the readers will receive by reading the article. Remember WIIFM! (What's In It For Me.)
III	Body	Use this section to elaborate on the subject matter. Include facts, research findings, anecdotes, quotes from experts and testimonials. Keep the paragraphs relatively short and include subheads.
IV	Conclusion	End your article with a strong conclusion. Summarize key points, tell the readers how they can apply the information in the article to enhance their wellness, and provide a call to action.
V	Author's Box	Write a very brief biography that lists your credentials, expertise, other published articles or books, and contact information.

Article Submission Websites

www.goarticles.com
www.ezinearticles.com
www.naturalhealthweb.com

Don't worry about whether your article is written perfectly. After you've completed the article, set it aside for a couple of days. Then reread it and make any edits. Enlist editing assistance from friends, colleagues and a member of the target market the article addresses. While you want to submit a clearly written article, it's ultimately the editor's job to finesse it. Another option is to hire a professional journalist to write an article for or about you.

Reports

A free report is another way to build a relationship with a new client. Reports range from a one-page handout to a multipage bound booklet. Give these reports to clients, and distribute them at other wellness professionals' offices, centers where your target markets congregate, health food stores, health expositions, and places where you give presentations.

Create reports on a variety of topics that address your target markets concerns. For example, you could give new clients a report on "What to Expect After Your First [ ] Session." Think about your client's concerns and write reports to address them (very similar to writing articles).

If you don't want to create this type of educational material, you can purchase preprinted pamphlets that address various wellness topics.

Newsletters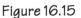

Newsletters are used by all kinds of organizations and businesses as an effective informational marketing tool. Newsletters provide a forum to communicate with your current and potential clients. Readers tend to pay more attention to a newsletter than an advertisement—and it's less likely to get tossed out as junk mail.

Good newsletters pique the interest of the reader. They balance promotional content with specific information that benefits the reader. The language tends to be more conversational in tone than a typical advertising piece or technical publication.

Most wellness providers are multitalented, and oftentimes clients are unaware of the scope of services they have available. A newsletter gives you an ideal opportunity to educate your clients about your other areas of expertise.

Newsletters don't need to be an elaborate production to be effective. You can even create a simple one-page newsletter on your letterhead. Many people also publish their newsletters on their websites. Before you decide upon the appropriate length, style, format and content of your newsletter, you must first clarify your purpose and goals for your newsletter and determine how to make it attractive to your target markets.

Ready-Made Newsletters
www.acupuncturemediaworks.com
www.massagemarketing.com
www.info4people.com

16

Figure 16.15

Newsletter Benefits

- Educate readers on the benefits your services offer.
- Attract new clients.
- Encourage current clients to come in more often.
- Bring back lost clients.
- Inspire clients to try different services.
- Promote products.
- Provide information.
- Build client loyalty and improve client retention.
- Enhance credibility and improve your image.
- Increase referrals and gift certificate sales.

Ready-Made Newsletters ● ●

Several companies produce newsletters specifically for wellness providers to purchase and distribute to their clients. The advantages of buying a ready-made newsletter over designing your own are a lower overall cost and time savings. The disadvantages are that ready-made newsletters lack your personal touch and you have no control over the content or layout. If the newsletter templates aren't sold in a kit, you have to hope the publisher gets them out in a timely manner. Also the information may be inaccurate or dated. Most of these companies now offer online versions of their newsletters that can be customized.

Pages 401-409
for more details on
Internet marketing.

Two ways to personalize a ready-made newsletter to maximize the benefits are: write a column for a pre-existing newsletter; or purchase a ready-made newsletter and insert a note or personalized page. If you decide to insert a page, be sure that it matches graphically in terms of overall style and typefaces. Some newsletter publishers place a blank section on the template for personalization.

Cooperative Newsletters • •

Creating a printed newsletter from scratch can seem overwhelming and financially prohibitive. To ease the burden, consider teaming with wellness providers and people who provide products or services to the same target market. Thoroughly analyze your target market so you can determine who to consider as a co-producer of your newsletter.

For example, let's say that one of your target markets is infants. Many other professionals and companies service this market: pediatricians; baby food companies; specialty stores (clothing, toys); baby seat manufacturers; bookstores; massage therapists; and educational companies that publish information for the parents of infants.

If anything is worth trying at all, it's worth trying at least 10 times.
— Art Linkletter

Another market with a multitude of attending providers is personal growth. People in this category often utilize the services of psychotherapists, counselors and other wellness providers such as touch therapists, nutritionists, holistic physicians, homeopaths, acupuncturists, chiropractors, herbalists and estheticians. They may attend workshops and 12-Step meetings. They read books on personal development and spirituality. They often shop at health food stores and natural clothing shops. And they're probably involved in some type of physical fitness program, such as exercise and yoga.

Don't limit yourself to the obvious. Sometimes the more unique the pairing, the more effective. For example, an on-site massage therapist and a "quick-print" copy shop might co-produce a newsletter. They could utilize a slogan such as, "For people who don't have an extra hour." Also, your co-sponsors can be located in a different city. For example, you could team up with a baby food company or a home exercise equipment manufacturer from another locale.

Newsletters often center on a theme, particularly when they're a cooperative venture. Several possibilities are: a "generic" well-being newsletter that appeals to a specific market such as athletes, pregnant women or stressed executives; or a newsletter that addresses specific health issues like arthritis, aging or carpal tunnel syndrome.

e-Newsletters • •

Pages 407-408 for e-Newsletter tips.

Publishing an e-newsletter is a good option, since the majority of people have access to email and the Internet. Online newsletters are eco-friendly, save you postage, and get delivered immediately. Plus you can easily update them, and add brilliant colors and pictures.

You can send newsletters to subscribers and post them on your website. Create a separate subscribers' email address book so that you can easily send out your newsletters to your list. Make sure you get permission from people before sending them your e-newsletters.

Newsletter Content • •

In terms of content, your newsletter can encompass new services, changes in hours, how-to's for stretches, relaxation exercises, specific tips on self-care, technical information regarding new research, survey results and product reviews, a detailed description of one of your services, websites and toll-free numbers of interest, articles, new products, success stories about your clients (get written permission first), book reviews, cartoons, advertisements, specialty columns such as a question-and-answer column, a section on different wellness modalities and their specific benefits, a "what's new in..." column, poems, articles written by clients, puzzles, contests, quotes, interviews, anecdotes, letters to the editor and discount coupons.

Gather information for your newsletter from newspapers, magazines, books, radio and television programs, documentaries, workshops, other wellness providers and your clients. It is fairly easy to obtain reprint rights of articles from existing publications. These are usually available at low or no cost. They provide variety for your readers and ease the load of material you personally have to generate. After you have located appropriate articles, contact the editor of each publication to ascertain their reprint policies.

There are also many online services that allow you to reprint articles. Search for articles by subject, such as "massage" or "stress" or "nutrition" or by your target market's concerns, such as arthritis. If your newsletter is targeted to a specific market, contact the public relations department of other organizations that cater to that market. Those organizations might have articles of interest and most likely will gladly give them to you free of charge. If you're unable to get reprint rights for material that you want to include, you can directly quote a sentence or two under "fair use" regulations. Be sure to attribute the source. Getting other professionals that serve your target markets to write a regular column for your newsletter is another source of material.

Newsletter Design • •

The personal computer has allowed desktop publishing to flourish. Most people who use newsletters to promote their practices either buy pre-printed ones or create them on their computer. But even if you don't own a computer, many graphic designers and print shops can produce your newsletter for you. If you plan to self-publish a newsletter on a regular basis, I highly recommend that you invest in a quality page-layout program such as PageMaker®, InDesign® or QuarkXPress.® Using word processors is generally not a good idea.

Sources for visuals include clip art images (either computer-generated or cut-and-paste), original drawings and photographs. If you're producing the newsletter on your computer, you can purchase various clip art packages that allow you reproduction rights. If you have a picture or piece of artwork (that you created or own the rights to), you can scan it into your computer and incorporate it into your newsletter. If you don't own a scanner, a service bureau can scan in the art, clean it up and give it back to you on a disk. Also, a print shop can place the art (reducing the size if necessary) directly on the layout sheets.

16

Free articles
www.misterarticle.com
www.articledashboard.com

Popular newsletter sections are industry news, wellness tips, editorials, cartoons, product and service reviews, success stories and announcements.

Be certain the newsletter style and colors match your image, as well as appeal to your target markets. To start off, consider keeping your newsletter to two pages. Either use your letterhead or some fun stationery. If you decide to publish a newsletter that is four or more pages long, I recommend you hire a professional graphic artist to create a template (a reusable design form) to use for each issue. Of course, if you're artistically inclined and possess the appropriate software and artwork packages, you can do it yourself. If you aren't certain about the look you want or the number of pages, you can purchase pre-designed laser-printer newsletter paper from companies such as Paper Direct. These sheets are usually on a high-quality 11" x 17" paper, printed on both sides with a pre-set layout for columns and announcements. Most are printed in full color. The major drawback to using this paper is adjusting your content to fit in their layout. But then again, that could also simplify things for you.

Avoid staples. Use clear or color-coordinated tabs.

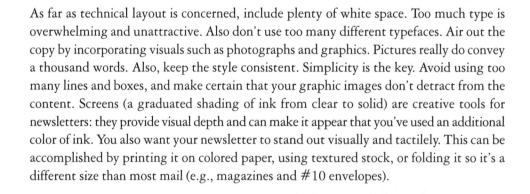

We produce a school newsletter totally in-house. We hired a graphic artist to design the basic layout so we could simply place the new information within the template. We usually add a different clip art graphic for the cover page of each issue that reflects the subject matter or season. We change the color of the paper with each issue. At first we printed them on our own copier; now that we produce more than 2,000 at a time, it's more cost-effective to take them to a printer. If you're reproducing 200 copies or less, it may be advantageous to print them on your laser printer or copier. Keep in mind that your newsletter will continue to evolve, so don't worry about it being perfect from the start.

Quick and Easy Newsletters
by Elaine Floyd

As far as technical layout is concerned, include plenty of white space. Too much type is overwhelming and unattractive. Also don't use too many different typefaces. Air out the copy by incorporating visuals such as photographs and graphics. Pictures really do convey a thousand words. Also, keep the style consistent. Simplicity is the key. Avoid using too many lines and boxes, and make certain that your graphic images don't detract from the content. Screens (a graduated shading of ink from clear to solid) are creative tools for newsletters: they provide visual depth and can make it appear that you've used an additional color of ink. You also want your newsletter to stand out visually and tactilely. This can be accomplished by printing it on colored paper, using textured stock, or folding it so it's a different size than most mail (e.g., magazines and #10 envelopes).

Be Seasonal!

Change the paper color to reflect the seasons, (e.g., orange in autumn). Use graphic images, such as snowflakes for winter or flowers for spring.

Entice your potential readers to open your newsletter immediately by prominently displaying your company name and logo. If you're unsure that readers would recognize your name, highlight the newsletter's purpose or slogan. Then list the contents or use some type of teaser. Let your potential readers know why they should read your newsletter right now!

Keep your newsletter length to six pages or less. You want to provide enough information to inspire someone to read it, but you don't want it so filled with material that it requires a significant block of time to read it. The idea is to create a newsletter that grabs your potential readers' attention so they pick it up and read it immediately, and to furnish readers with just the right balance of graphically appealing and interesting material so they read it from cover to cover in one sitting.

Also, leave your readers anticipating your next issue by giving them a preview. For example, say "In the next issue we describe six techniques for alleviating headaches," or "Next issue includes an interview with Alexa Swift, a local track star who shares how she reduced her sprint time by 10 percent."

Newsletters can be published on a set schedule (e.g., monthly, quarterly, biannually) or you can simply produce them whenever it's appropriate. Oftentimes a business owner generates a newsletter when a change occurs in the company or something major happens within the industry.

Keep your newsletter straightforward and personal. Remember, it isn't a magazine or a newspaper—it's a personal communication to keep you in touch with your current clients, educate the public and promote your practice. Newsletters keep you and your clients connected.

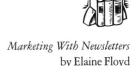

Marketing With Newsletters
by Elaine Floyd

16

Figure 16.16

> ## Marketing with Newsletters
> ### by Jon Lumsden of Massage Marketing
>
> A newsletter works in 10 different ways. You can get a lot more mileage from each issue than by just mailing copies to your existing clients. You have an effective marketing tool at your disposal, so make the most of it:
>
> 1. Mail or email your newsletter to potential clients.
> 2. Encourage your clients to share their issues with others.
> 3. Generate new business by mailing to selected professionals with a cover letter introducing your services.
> 4. Use it as a handout at health fairs and public presentations.
> 5. Leave copies with willing merchants, such as health food stores and chiropractors.
> 6. Use as inserts in community newspapers.
> 7. Mail to nearby residents.
> 8. Use with a cover letter and mail to new neighbors with a first-visit discount.
> 9. Provide issues to services like Welcome Wagon.
> 10. Use in place of business cards.

**Newsletter and
Mailing List Software**

www.raizlabs.com
www.comdevweb.com
www.interspire.com

• Promotion: Marketing Materials •

High-quality printed marketing materials such as business cards, letterhead, envelopes, brochures, gift certificates, newsletters (covered in the previous section), client information sheets, postcards, greeting cards and fliers are essential to generate a professional image. Your visual promotional pieces reflect the character of your business. The ultimate design of your materials depends on your target market(s) and the image you wish to portray. These items don't all have to look identical (actually that isn't a good idea), but the colors, designs and overall look should blend well. For your visual promotional materials to be effective, they must appeal to the clients you want to attract—which might not be the layout that you personally like the best.

Desktop Publishing Paper

www.PaperDirect.com
www.desktopsupplies.com

Although most of your printed materials are given out by you, your friends, colleagues and clients, it's still worthwhile to post your materials in appropriate locations. Place them in health clubs, wellness centers, medical care supply shops, health food stores, offices of other wellness practitioners, bookstores and places that the people in your target markets frequent. Your print materials should tastefully stand out (through design, ink color or paper color) when floating in a sea of other wellness practitioners' marketing pieces.

Select an email address that ties into the name of your business or the type of work you do. Catchy and clever nicknames have their place, but not on your business cards.

The first time you contact the owners or managers at these establishments, do it in person. This gives you an opportunity to introduce yourself and build rapport. Show them your materials so they can easily recognize them and hopefully point them out to their customers. After a relationship is built, it isn't necessary for you to hand-deliver the materials each time; you can mail them or have a service distribute them. It's wise to visit these establishments at least twice a year to maintain connections and deliver an appropriate gift (e.g., healthy treats or a plant) once a year.

The three major choices for most of your basic marketing materials are: work with a graphic artist to design your marketing materials; purchase preprinted materials that you can personalize by affixing an address label or inserting a panel with specific information about yourself; order semi-customizable, pre-formatted materials.

Pages 431-432

for tips on working with graphic artists.

My own experience in preparing my printed materials leads me to recommend leaving it to the experts by hiring a graphic artist to do the job. If cost is a concern, find an artist who is willing to barter services. Be very cautious about adopting a logo. Avoid using one unless you're certain that you want to live with that symbol for a very long time. People tend to remember logos and associate you with your logo even if you no longer use that particular symbol. It's much easier to change a business name or image and alter the design or style of stationery if it's without a logo. Wait until you're certain it's what you want. Also, check to see if anyone else has the same or similar one. Contact your Secretary of State for requisite forms to trademark your logo.

Chapter 10, Pages 199-200

for more information on trademarking.

You can create attractive stationery on a computer, particularly if you purchase paper products that are specifically designed for desktop publishing. You can find hundreds of full-color brochure paper complete with matching business card stock, letterhead, envelopes, postcards and even labels. These companies also provide specialty papers to be used for newsletters, certificates, greeting cards, note cards, fliers and signs. These paper products provide an opportunity for you to experiment without a huge outlay of money.

Figure 16.17

Marketing Materials Checklist

Basic
- ❏ Business Cards
- ❏ Appointment Cards
- ❏ Brochures
- ❏ Stationery: letterhead and envelopes
- ❏ Greeting Cards
- ❏ Gift Certificates
- ❏ Coupons
- ❏ Educational Pamphlets and Handouts
- ❏ Client Forms
- ❏ Newsletters
- ❏ Website

Optional
- ❏ Displays
- ❏ Signage
- ❏ Posters
- ❏ Referral Cards
- ❏ Personalized gift items
- ❏ Doorhangers
- ❏ Fliers
- ❏ Direct Mail Letters
- ❏ Articles
- ❏ Informational Videos/DVDs
- ❏ Comment Cards

16

Business Cards ●

The business card can be your most effective, least costly marketing tool. Choose a card that reflects who you are and captures the essence of your practice. Always carry lots of business cards wherever you go. Keep extra cards in your car or alternate method of transportation. Be generous with your promotional materials. The whole purpose is to circulate them, not hoard them. Whenever you pass out your cards, always hand out at least three per person.

Remember that when it comes to cards, the beauty is in simplicity. A lot of controversy surrounds the amount and type of information to include on your card. Some people attempt to turn their business card into a brochure. In designing your cards, keep in mind that they aren't meant for you; they must appeal to your target market!

Effective business cards convey the major benefits you offer in a quick glance. They should grab attention, but not be so jam-packed with information that potential clients don't feel the need to ask you questions.

The first step in designing your cards is to look at the business cards you've collected over the years (including your competitors' cards) and identify what you like and dislike. Determine the content (refer to your differential advantage exercise) using as few words as possible. Choose an appropriate image for your target market(s) that matches your other print materials. Add color whenever possible. Print them on high-quality card stock and consider using the back of your card for additional copy or as an appointment reminder.

Be sure to include the basics: name, address, phone number, cell phone number, email address and your website information. I'm amazed at the number of cards without phone numbers or area codes. *Always proofread carefully!*

The two major *faux pas* with business cards are not having them when you need them (which is *always*), and correcting information by hand.

Sample Business Cards

www.businessmastery.us/
biz-cards.php

Business Cards

www.vistaprint.com
www.watercolorscards.com
www.printbusinesscards.com
www.info4people.com

Figure 16.18 Sample Business Cards

Deep Tissue • Neuromuscular Therapy • Swedish

Total Health Through Massage
Relieve stress, decrease pain, increase flexibility and enhance your well-being.

Leslie R. Vandruff, L.M.T.
3692 Horndell Lane, Suite 120
South Williams, NE 84207

394~555~3692
www.thtm.com

Client Bonus Session Card
Buy 10, get the 11th session free!

 1 ☐   2 ☐   3 ☐   4 ☐   5 ☐

 6 ☐   7 ☐   8 ☐ 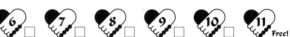 9 ☐  10 ☐ 11 Free!

Create Balance
Between Your
Personal and
Professional
Endeavors

Laura Fonds, Ph.D.
Certified Personal and
Professional Coach

- Career Counselling
- Stress Management
- Relationship Counselling
- Personal Adjustment Counselling

www.laurathecoach.com ▪ **231-555-9734**
3001 N. Walton Drive, Suite 210 ▪ Mountain, WV 26441

Has an appointment on

_____

Day   Month   Date

At _____ a.m. _____ p.m.

Please give 24 hours notice of appointment changes

Mia Lan Acupuncture

*allergies • sleeplessness • arthritis
headaches • stress • body aches*

Mia Lan, L.Ac.
Practicing Since 1971
Under Master Lee Wong

518 Broadway, Suite 3
Anytown, NJ 08413

394~555~3692
www.mia_lan_acupuncture.com

Monica Everett, M.D.
Holistic Practitioner

In Service for the Totality of Your Being

520-555-1125

Holladay Medical Centre
1871 Wells Drive, Suite 142 • Hollistown, AZ 85791
www.monicaeverett.com

Hair Design • Manicures/Pedicures • Cosmetics • Permanent Make-up

Godiva Salon and Minispa

for rejuvenating and toning the body

In Service Since 1979
Open Wednesday-Sunday
196 E. Maine Terrace #129
Landtown, MO 94162

624~555~9721
www.godivaminispa.com

Body and Facial Waxing • Hydrotherapy • Customized European Facials

---

Jon Darbey, D.C.
Doctor of Chiropractic

Cortwell Chiropractic Center
for gentle, fast, effective pain relief

406-555-3216 • 139 Mordnar Street, Big Sky, MT 84139
www.cortwellcenter.com

---

388 • Marketing Mastery

Brochures

Your brochure is often the hub of your printed marketing materials. The purpose of a brochure is to inspire prospective clients to call you. When developing your brochure, remember that you must establish credibility and focus on the benefits a client derives from using your services. Techniques for establishing credibility in printed materials include providing credentials, numbers, lists, specific details, research findings, testimonials, success stories, pictures and guarantees.

With unfortunate frequency, we describe ourselves (and our businesses) in terms of our features. A feature isn't what attracts clients. They want to know how your services will make a difference in their wellness. A *feature* is a description of your service or product, (i.e., how the product was made, the training you received, and the background of the practitioner and the company).

A *benefit* is a description of how the client profits from using the services and product, how the service or product solves the client's problem, the differential advantage you provide, and the results that the client can expect.

One of the key elements of an effective brochure is to include at least one photograph of yourself—preferably one in which you're working with a contented client. The old cliche is true, "A picture says a thousand words."

Brochure design can be a bit complicated. As with business cards, collect other practitioners' brochures to determine what appeals to you. Ask for input from current and prospective clients. It is usually unwise to spend a lot of money on your first brochure since, invariably, you will want to alter it somehow. You may discover that the type style doesn't work well with the paper stock, someone points out an error, the perfect way to express yourself finally dawns on you, or you find something you don't like. If you plan on creating your own brochure, purchase a book on effective brochure design.

Many wellness providers utilize preprinted brochures. The bright side is that someone other than you has invested the time and money to design an effective, attractive, informational marketing tool. Often the cost is significantly less than if you were to design and print your own. The problem is that they aren't personalized. You are the most important aspect of your practice, and your marketing materials need to reflect that. One of the best ways to overcome the impersonal nature of preprinted brochures is to insert a panel with your specific information.

Here is how a massage therapist in Tucson did it. When she purchased the preprinted brochures, she asked for the following details: the type of paper; font names; and the actual ink color name and number used for the fonts and major graphic image. She also obtained permission to duplicate the graphic image on her insert. The insert included her picture, information about her background and philosophy, as well as the specific features and benefits of her practice. It was printed on the same paper as the brochure, with matching fonts, ink colors and the graphic image—it was classy.

Save money, trees and energy by utilizing the Internet to send promotional materials such as announcements and newsletters.

Whatever you do with preprinted brochures, don't handwrite your name, address and phone number on the back—it looks tacky! Ideally, run the brochures through a laser printer (some companies offer that option when you order their brochures), so it looks like you created the brochure. If that isn't an option, print labels on a complementary colored stock and affix them to the back of the brochures.

You can usually obtain preprinted brochures through your professional association or independent vendors.

Figure 16.19

Brochure Design Criteria

- Does it easily distinguish who it's for?
- Does it identify with the target client's problem?
- Does it provide a solution to the problem?
- Does it appeal to the target client's needs?
- Does it have an interesting teaser?
- Are the main benefits listed first?
- Is it believable?
- Is it attractive?
- Is it easy to read? Does it flow?
- Does it have sufficient white space?
- Are the type sizes and styles easy to read?
- Does it have appropriate photographs?
- Is it written in common language?
- Does it establish credibility?
- Is your address included?
- Does it include a map of your location?
- Does it include contact names and numbers?
- Does it include a website and email address?
- Does it provide a call for action?

Most practitioners design their basic brochures and purchase preprinted brochures that describe in detail the adjunct services they offer or the history of their profession.

Ready Made Brochures

info4people.com
HemingwayMassageProducts.com
bluepoppy.com
acupuncturemediaworks.com

Figure 16.20 Sample Brochure

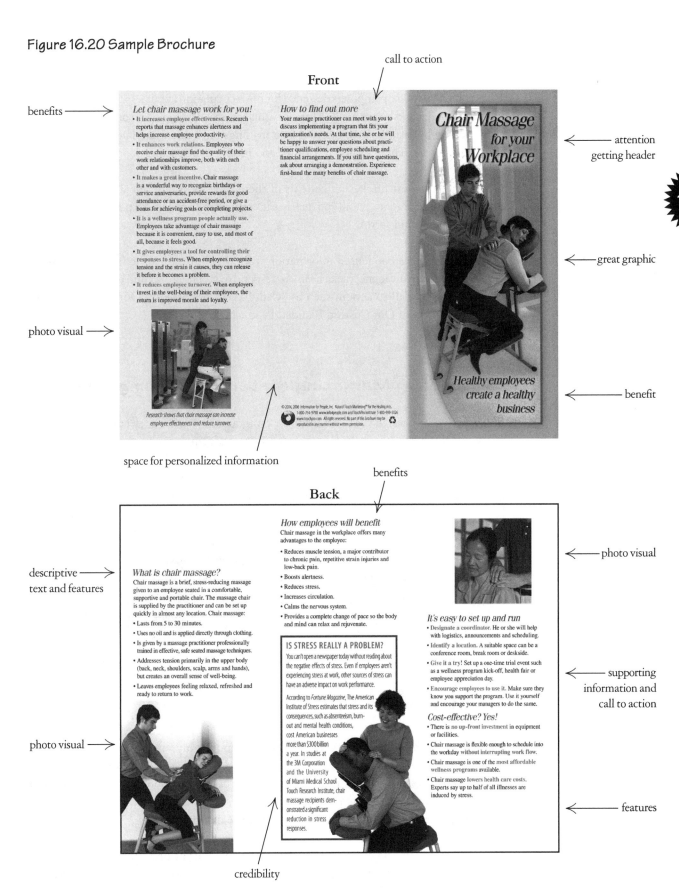

Front

call to action

benefits →

Let chair massage work for you!
- **It increases employee effectiveness.** Research reports that massage enhances alertness and helps increase employee productivity.
- **It enhances work relations.** Employees who receive chair massage find the quality of their work relationships improve, both with each other and with customers.
- **It makes a great incentive.** Chair massage is a wonderful way to recognize birthdays or service anniversaries, provide rewards for good attendance or an accident-free period, or give a bonus for achieving goals or completing projects.
- **It is a wellness program people actually use.** Employees take advantage of chair massage because it is convenient, easy to use, and most of all, because it feels good.
- **It gives employees a tool for controlling their responses to stress.** When employees recognize tension and the strain it causes, they can release it before it becomes a problem.
- **It reduces employee turnover.** When employers invest in the well-being of their employees, the return is improved morale and loyalty.

How to find out more
Your massage practitioner can meet with you to discuss implementing a program that fits your organization's needs. At that time, she or he will be happy to answer your questions about practitioner qualifications, employee scheduling and financial arrangements. If you still have questions, ask about arranging a demonstration. Experience first-hand the many benefits of chair massage.

← attention getting header

Chair Massage for your Workplace

← great graphic

photo visual →

Research shows that chair massage can increase employee effectiveness and reduce turnover.

© 2004, 2006 Information for People, Inc. Natural Touch Marketing™ for the Healing Arts. 1-800-754-9790 www.info4people.com and TouchPro Institute 1-800-999-5026 www.touchpro.com. All rights reserved. No part of this brochure may be reproduced in any manner without written permission.

Healthy employees create a healthy business

← benefit

space for personalized information

benefits

Back

descriptive text and features →

What is chair massage?
Chair massage is a brief, stress-reducing massage given to an employee seated in a comfortable, supportive and portable chair. The massage chair is supplied by the practitioner and can be set up quickly in almost any location. Chair massage:
- Lasts from 5 to 30 minutes.
- Uses no oil and is applied directly through clothing.
- Is given by a massage practitioner professionally trained in effective, safe seated massage techniques.
- Addresses tension primarily in the upper body (back, neck, shoulders, scalp, arms and hands), but creates an overall sense of well-being.
- Leaves employees feeling relaxed, refreshed and ready to return to work.

How employees will benefit
Chair massage in the workplace offers many advantages to the employee:
- Reduces muscle tension, a major contributor to chronic pain, repetitive strain injuries and low-back pain.
- Boosts alertness.
- Reduces stress.
- Increases circulation.
- Calms the nervous system.
- Provides a complete change of pace so the body and mind can relax and rejuvenate.

IS STRESS REALLY A PROBLEM?
You can't open a newspaper today without reading about the negative effects of stress. Even if employees aren't experiencing stress at work, other sources of stress can have an adverse impact on work performance.

According to *Fortune Magazine*, The American Institute of Stress estimates that stress and its consequences, such as absenteeism, burnout and mental health conditions, cost American businesses more than $300 billion a year. In studies at the 3M Corporation and the University of Miami Medical School Touch Research Institute, chair massage recipients demonstrated a significant reduction in stress responses.

← photo visual

It's easy to set up and run
- **Designate a coordinator.** He or she will help with logistics, announcements and scheduling.
- **Identify a location.** A suitable space can be a conference room, break room or deskside.
- **Give it a try!** Set up a one-time trial event such as a wellness program kick-off, health fair or employee appreciation day.
- **Encourage employees to use it.** Make sure they know you support the program. Use it yourself and encourage your managers to do the same.

Cost-effective? Yes!
- There is no up-front investment in equipment or facilities.
- Chair massage is flexible enough to schedule into the workday without interrupting work flow.
- Chair massage is one of the most affordable wellness programs available.
- Chair massage lowers health care costs. Experts say up to half of all illnesses are induced by stress.

← supporting information and call to action

← features

photo visual →

credibility

The sample brochure is used for illustrative purposes only with permission by Information For People. Please honor the company's copyright.

Fliers and Circulars •

Fliers and circulars are pamphlets designed for mass circulation about a specific event such as an open house, workshop or a sale. They are usually printed or copied on one side so they can be posted on bulletin boards, inserted into mailings, and distributed at your colleagues' places of business. They can also be printed specifically to be used as door hangers.

One of the strongest marketing benefits of these types of promotional tools is that you determine your target (e.g., all the dentists in a three-mile radius, or people who shop at the local health food store).

Sample Flier
www.businessmastery.us/
flier.php

Design tips include condensed information from brochures plus the following: Use an attention-grabbing headline, make it easy to respond (e.g., phone, fax and toll-free numbers), and close with a call to action, such as "Call Today," or "Stop by Our Open House to Receive a Sample of Our Custom Blended Products."

Figure 16.21

Reducing Marketing Materials Printing Costs

Whether you design your own printed promotional materials or elect to utilize the services of a graphic artist, follow these tips for reducing your print media costs:

- Work with interns from local colleges.
- Barter for services.
- Get at least three bids.
- Use standard size and weight paper.
- Use a photocopier for short print runs.
- Print samples before using expensive paper and ink.
- Use the printing services of trade and vocational schools.
- Reuse effective material (as long as it isn't being sent to the same people).
- Purchase customizable business cards, brochures & postcards from online vendors.

Direct Mail •

Direct mail promotions are simple, inexpensive and highly effective marketing tools. They are great for introducing yourself to potential clients, as well as keeping in touch with current ones. They range from a formal letter of introduction to announcements to surveys. (See Figure 16.22 for a sample survey.) These materials are personalized, and you can address specific needs in a friendly, low-pressure manner.

Many local printers and online companies, such as VistaPrint print and mail your direct mail pieces. Some companies even have templates to help you design your marketing materials and others offer design services.

Postcards ● ●

Postcards are a fast, easy and inexpensive method of reminding clients of follow-ups and appointments, sending announcements or just saying hello. They are also a good technique for generating new clients. Postcards can be sent one at a time or in a mass mailing. They encourage people to take action quickly and are most effective when the action required is free (e.g., "Visit our website for the top 10 things you can do to improve your health today," "Call for a free wellness update today"), or includes an upgrade in services, such as "Book your next private yoga appointment by March 31st and receive a pass for two free group classes."

Design, print, address and mail your postcards
www.postcardmania.com

16

Greeting Cards ● ●

Greeting Cards are an excellent tool for connecting with clients, networking associates and referring professionals. They can be used to wish people good tidings, as well as encourage client retention. Keep a variety of cards on hand so that you can quickly send one when it's appropriate. If you have to make a special effort to buy a card, then you might not do it. Here are some ideas for when to send a greeting card:

- Reaffirm the professional relationship. After a client's first visit, state that you look forward to working with her to achieve her wellness goals.
- Thank-you for referrals.
- Keeping in touch.
- Special occasions, such as birthdays and anniversaries of their first appointment with you.
- Milestones reached in their work with you, their profession or personal achievements.
- Inspire clients to return.

Greeting Cards
www.koglecards.com
www.watercolorscards.com
www.info4people.com

Wellness Surveys ● ●

Sending a wellness survey to potential clients can attract interest in your services and open the door to new business. It also works well to invite potential clients to educational events in connection with a survey. This can be a very effective way to introduce the benefits of your service, build trust and foster new client relationships. Be sure to offer a free gift or discount as an incentive and send a thank-you for participating in the survey (see Figure 16.22).

Figure 16.22 Prospecting Survey

Westside Wellness Center

6000 N. Windy Way • Fairbanks, AK 99710

907-555-5555 • www.westsidewellness.com

Susan Izensnow
1900 Frostbite Circle
Fairbanks, AK 99711

Dear Ms. Izensnow,

We realize that your well-being is a high priority. Your opinion of chiropractic care is important to us, and finding out what how you feel assists us in meeting your expectations. Please return this survey and we will send you a free booklet titled, *Ten Things You Can Do Today to Increase Your Vitality and Longevity.*

Are you currently under chiropractic care? ❏ Yes ❏ No

If yes, how often?	❏ On a regular schedule	❏ On an as-needed basis
❏ Weekly	❏ Biweekly	❏ Monthly
❏ 6 times a year	❏ 4 times a year	❏ Less than 2 times a year

If you're currently under chiropractic care, please describe what you like best about it:

_____

_____

What you like least about it: _____

_____

If you don't receive chiropractic care, please check which of these reasons apply:

❏ Too expensive	❏ My insurance doesn't cover it
❏ My insurance limit is up	❏ I don't have the time
❏ My course of treatment has concluded	❏ I'm not certain of the benefits
❏ Not a convenient location	❏ Hours not convenient
❏ Other _____	

If you were to utilize chiropractic care, which of these features would be most important to you?

❏ Working with the same physician each time
❏ Flexible office hours, including evenings and Saturdays
❏ Honoring insurance claims
❏ A guarantee of satisfaction
❏ Other _____

Thank you very much for your time in filling out this form. Return this survey today and receive your free booklet.

Sincerely,

Thomas Moore

Thomas Morre, D.C.

P.S. If we receive your survey in the next 10 days, we will also send you a complimentary registration for one of our upcoming seminars.

Sales Letters • •

Make sure your sales letter is typed and kept to one page. As most people's mailboxes are overflowing with form letters and marketing pitches, tailor each letter to a specific individual within a target market. Do your homework and find out as much specific information as possible. Add your special touch. Consider signing your letter in an ink that's a different color than the type (I like to use a teal-colored felt pen).

Research shows that sales letters garner a response rate of up to 80 percent higher than other types of mailers. The key elements to success are a great design, an excellent mailing list and follow-up.

Figure 16.23

Design Tips

- Use an eye-catching headline.
- Highlight the benefits immediately.
- Use your prospect's name.
- Clarify why you have selected the recipient to receive your letter.
- Build rapport and develop credibility.
- Keep it short.
- Use sincere, friendly language.
- Include powerful words such as "new," "free," "save," and "now."
- Provide a guarantee.
- Offer incentives.
- Include testimonials. Always use a full name. If possible, include a company name, title and location.
- Include a time limit or expiration date.
- State your offer in clear, simple terms.
- Provide step-by-step instructions so your readers know how to respond.
- Close with a call to action.
- Use a postscript (P.S.) at the end of the letter—next to the headline, it's the most-often read part of any letter.
- Compose the letter on a computer.
- Use bold type to emphasize key points.
- Print the letter on high-quality paper.
- Enclose a response card or an invitation.

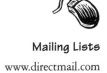

Mailing Lists
www.directmail.com
www.listsareus.com

Envelopes • •

Your envelope needs to motivate readers to open it and see what's inside. Printing teaser copy or an illustration on the outside helps. Also, a large or irregularly shaped envelope stands out from regular mail. If you're sending letters to general consumers (current and prospective clients), use a first-class stamp instead of metered or bulk mail to increase the odds of your letter getting opened. (See Figure 16.24)

Figure 16.24 Direct Mail Envelope

Stress Reduction Clinic
971 Montrose Canyon Way
Cleveland, OH 44114

Look Inside for
5 Easy Ideas to
Reduce Stress
by 50%!

Miriam Webster
129 Miracle Highway
Cleveland, OH 44114

Mailing Lists ● ●

You can develop your own internal mailing list or purchase lists through a broker. The fees for mailing lists range from $45 to $200 per 1,000 names. The major problems with purchasing brokered lists are that it's difficult to get a list of qualified prospects and the list itself may be of poor quality (outdated or contains incomplete information). Another option for mailing lists is to contact organizations and associations that serve your target markets. They often share their lists for a nominal charge or free. Sometimes you can obtain the addresses of new residents for free through the utility companies.

Generating Responses ● ●

Some incentives that inspire people to respond to direct mail are: free merchandise or service; free demonstration; free literature such as a newsletter, catalog or handout; technical assistance; discount coupon; free training; and a free consultation.

Generate an internal mailing list. Collect business cards at networking events and your public speaking functions. Combine the information with your client list.

Response cards are very effective for generating leads and come in two major categories: Business Reply Cards (postpaid) and Courtesy Reply Cards (not postpaid). Postpaid cards get the best response (free is usually better). Keep the information clear, concise and engaging. Restate your offer, and include an incentive for a quick reply. Use check-off boxes with different options—the less amount of time and energy the recipient has to expend, the more likely you're to get a response. Perhaps include "Maybe" along with "Yes" and "No" options. Put your name, address, phone number and website on the bottom. If possible, print the recipient's name on the top of the card.

An alternative to mass mailing is to send out one letter each day to prospective clients and other wellness providers with whom you wish to develop alliances.

Follow-up is crucial. You can increase your direct mail letter response up to 800 percent by following up the mailing with a telephone call.

Gift Certificates ●

Gift certificates provide a surge of income into your practice and offer an easy way for clients to share your services with their family, friends and colleagues. They can also be both a marketing tool to generate new clients and a goodwill promotion when given as presents or donated to charities.

Gift certificates are a tool to increase your client base, so it's in your best interest that they get redeemed. Each person who uses a gift certificate can become a regular client. Thus the initial certificate (whether purchased or given as a promotion) can launch a wonderful business relationship and bring in thousands of dollars in fees.

In today's time-pressed and hectic world, gift certificates for wellness services are growing in popularity. Many clients appreciate the convenience of this gift-giving option, and are enthusiastic about this unique and thoughtful way to support others' well-being.

Expiration Date Debate ● ●

Many states have strict regulations concerning gift certificates: some don't allow expiration dates, some dictate how far they may be postdated, and several require that if the certificates aren't redeemed within a certain period of time, then the money must be deposited with the state. You can put an expiration date on gift certificates when they're used as promotions (no money has been exchanged), such as donating certificates to a charity auction.

Some people advocate increasing one's revenue stream by aggressively selling gift certificates with very short expiration terms. Often the majority of certificates expire before being redeemed, and the practitioner receives the income without having to perform any services. While this scam might appear tempting, consider the long-term consequences of this and the ill will that this might generate.

For most people, a gift certificate is a significant investment. Your gift certificate sales will dramatically increase if you develop a system that allays concerns about purchasing something that might not be used. People feel more comfortable purchasing certificates that either have a flexible expiration date or no expiration date. Another approach is for the certificate to revert to the purchaser if not used by the expiration date.

Some practitioners put a reasonably short expiration date on their gift certificates (such as three or six months) to encourage people to come in soon, yet always extend the date upon request. Others charge a token reactivation fee to extend the expiration.

> In one of my workshops, a massage therapist shared the following method for successfully integrating gift certificate sales: Whenever he sells a gift certificate, he posts who bought the certificate and the name and phone number of the intended recipient (if this is unknown at the time the certificate is bought, he checks back with the purchaser in a month or so). His gift certificates include a six-month expiration. One month prior to the expiration, he calls the recipient to give notice that a session needs to be booked before the certificate expires. After six months elapse without redemption and he cannot contact the recipient or the recipient doesn't schedule an appointment, he contacts the original purchaser and tells her that the gift certificate reverts to her use. He sells a lot of gift certificates and has a redemption rate in the high 90th percentile! His clients feel comfortable about purchasing gift certificates from him because they don't have to worry about the certificates (and their money) going to waste.

Chapter 14, Page 290

for tips on managing gift certificate finances.

Stocking Up • •

You can purchase ready-made gift certificates or design and print your own. The three major benefits of purchasing ready-made certificates are a lower initial investment of time and money and the variety of design options. Most of these certificates are printed in full color on high-quality paper and are available in a wide range of styles (some generic and others for specific events, such as birthdays).

If you're in a solo practice and sell a large quantity of certificates, then you might consider printing your own. You can customize the certificates with your contact information (e.g., name, address, phone number and a listing of your services). If you choose this route, the certificate design can match the style and color palette of your letterhead, business cards and brochures. There are some very attractive gift certificates printed on card stock and bordered in foil (silver, gold, or copper) with a matching foil-lined envelope. Regardless of whether you purchase certificates or make your own, be sure they convey your desired image.

Key information to include on a gift certificate is the recipient's name, the giver's name, and a description of the services to be provided. Other useful items to add are the certificate number, date of issue, the name of the practitioner who issued the certificate (particularly for a multipractitioner office), and (if you insist) an expiration date. If you custom-print your certificates, include your contact information. If you purchase ready-made certificates, put your business card in the envelope or attach it to the certificate (some certificates are slit so you can easily attach your card).

Early Redemption • •

The sooner your gift certificates get redeemed, the better. Print an encouraging phrase on the bottom of the certificate to assist in early redemption, such as:

- Take Time Out for Yourself Today
- Enhance Your Well-Being Right Now
- Relax and Revitalize Today

Another idea is to offer incentives for early redemption, such as:

- Book your appointment within two weeks and receive a free paraffin dip for your hands
- Use this gift certificate within one month and receive an extra 15 minutes
- Redeem this certificate within one month and receive a 15 percent discount on all self-care supplies

Marketing Gift Certificates • •

Some work settings lend themselves to a high volume of gift certificate sales. Upscale salons and day spas are a prime example, since gift certificates for services and products are commonplace in these settings. Yet relatively few practicing wellness practitioners actively promote gift certificate sales—they typically make them available only to current clients. The certificates are an afterthought. Usually the only action a practitioner takes is a special holiday promotion, reminding clients that they can give the gift of touch. Don't be limited to seasonal sales; gift certificate sales can be an integral part of a year-round marketing program.

At the very least, insert a sample gift certificate in your welcome kit and prominently display one in your waiting area (framed and either on a stand or hung on the wall). Mention your gift certificates in all your promotional materials, particularly brochures, fliers, website and advertisements. If you distribute a newsletter, print a notice about gift certificate sales in every issue. Tactful, tasteful reminders about gift certificate availability are always appreciated.

Always keep a stack of gift certificates handy (and be certain to display a sample one) whenever you're involved in an activity associated with your practice, such as a public speaking event, open houses and exposition booths.

Also, sell your certificates to businesses to use as incentives or rewards. Many companies regularly reward customers, clients, and employees with substantial gifts. For example, real estate agencies and title companies usually give gifts to their clients upon closing. Purchasing a home can be extremely stressful, so wellness care makes an excellent gift alternative to the customary houseplant or kitchen accessory.

While gift certificate sales are excellent tools for increasing revenue, keep in mind that the true profit is generated not from the sale of the certificate but from the subsequent sessions that the new client books.

Another option to increase your gift certificate sales is to offer free gift certificates (for services or products) to cross-promoting partners to use as incentives. They can make a similar offer for their customers who purchase gift certificates (or some other incentive program). A bookstore could be a great barter partner. You could offer a $10 book gift certificate for every two wellness certificates purchased. The bookstore could offer a 15-minute mini-service certificate for every $75 worth of book certificates purchased. The certificates don't need to be of equal value as long as the total exchange is equitable. For instance, you could give the bookstore 10 certificates for mini-sessions (let's say at a value of $30 each) or five full-session certificates to be used in whatever type of promotion the bookstore chooses, and, in return, the bookstore would give you thirty $10 book gift certificates.

Coupons •

Coupons encourage people to try new services and products. They help generate new clients and prompt current clients to return. Some people don't use them because they think they're somehow demeaning. The bottom line is that they're extremely effective when used correctly. While free is always best in the consumer's eye, it isn't the only option. Still, the discount needs to be enough to provide impetus. For instance, $5 dollars off a $75 session most likely won't produce a huge influx of new clients (although it would certainly make current clients happy).

Another option that works for many practitioners is to offer a short session for free (e.g., a 30-minute massage) that can be upgraded for a fee to a full session. Coupons can also be used to promote ancillary services or products. For instance, a coupon could state, "Bring this coupon to your next session and get a FREE six-ounce container of The World's Best Aloe Vera Ointment."

Coupons are easily printed from your computer, so they can be customized. If you don't have a color printer, use a jazzy paper or purchase special laser printer stock that's designed to be used as coupons or mini-certificates. This paper is usually heavier, has borders and is perforated. When you print coupons in small batches, you can include a short expiration date. Unlike gift certificates, coupons can have an expiration date without any legal concerns since the client doesn't purchase the coupon.

Personalized Gift Items •

Personalized gift items—also known as premiums and specialty advertising—provide a daily reminder of your business while either being passed around from person to person, landing on a refrigerator or being seen on handy items. Some typical gift items in this category are erasers, magnets, pens, pencils, note pads, letter openers, stress balls, bookmarks, bumper stickers, calendars, mugs, visors, nail files, aromatherapy eye pillows, sports bottles and T-shirts. You can distribute these as gifts at special events or whenever a new client comes in for an initial visit. Include them in your mailings or hand them out whenever you're so inclined.

Premiums can be worthwhile in any business. They are fun promotional tools and often quite inexpensive. For wellness providers, the main focus of premiums is to develop relationships with prospective or current clients. In most instances, the perceived monetary value of the item isn't as important as its use, so select items that the recipients want or need.

Gift items can also be used as incentives (e.g., offer a free tote bag with every $50 spent on products). In addition to the national catalogs listed in the margin, check your local yellow pages for names of advertising specialty companies. Call them and request a catalog. The variety of these items is amazing. You can get almost anything personalized with your company name or logo! Choose items that either directly remind your clients of you (or your specific services) or are of definite interest (or benefit) to the people in your target markets. The key elements to print on these items are your company's name, phone number and website.

An inexpensive idea for a beneficial personalized gift item is to print labels and affix them to water bottles. You can purchase bottled water by the case (they usually come in eight to 24-ounce bottles). Most print shops have specialty labels in different colors, shapes and designs (e.g., golf balls, hearts, stars) that you can imprint with your name, phone number, address and website. Every time your clients come in for an appointment, greet them with a smile, a handshake and a water bottle. If they drink all the water before they leave, offer to refill it from your water cooler.

Premium Sales
www.bestimpressions.com
www.4imprint.com
www.amsterdamprinting.com

16

Sites to List Yourself
www.FindHealer.com
www.holistichealersnetwork.com
www.massagesoup.com
www.massagenetwork.com
www.acufinder.com

• Promotion: Internet •

The Internet offers a wealth of resources for growing your business. Some marketing experts refer to the Web as the hub of "keep-in-touch marketing," marketing that builds strong, lasting relationships. From websites to blogs, from email newsletters to online discussion groups, these web-based marketing tools make it easy to connect with thousands of people with a minimum investment. Best of all, these tools can boost your income in a big way by attracting new clients. According to Michael Port, author of *Book Yourself Solid*, "If you're not online, you're out of line."[1]

As the landscape of Internet marketing is vast, this section provides valuable insights and resources to help you understand the toolbox known as online marketing. It also gives you the practical know-how to evaluate what online tools are best suited to your business. For a more in-depth orientation, plan to read several of the recommended books and online sources, or attend a seminar with a local Internet marketing expert.

Page 409
for Internet Advertising ideas.

Website Savvy •

A website is one of the most powerful marketing tools ever invented. It increases your visibility and credibility, and gives instant access to information about you and your services. Think of it as an electronic brochure. A website makes it possible for existing clients to refer people to you more easily. You can also enhance your "convenience quotient" by adding an online scheduling component to your site. An e-newsletter archive with news, health tips and special promotions also adds interest and value to your site.

If those aren't enough reasons to spark your interest in a website, talk to any wellness practitioner with a website and you'll hear rave reviews about online coupons. These easy-to-use promotional tools—which can be printed from your site and redeemed for introductory visits or special promotions—are proven business builders. Online coupons are one of the most effective ways to attract new clients and build loyalty with existing clients.

A website can also make it easy for time-pressed clients to purchase gift certificates and package deals. In short, you want a website that educates new clients and persuades them to make an appointment with you, and that strengthens your relationship with existing clients.

For those unfamiliar with Internet terminology, here are a few basic definitions:

- Home page: The first page of your website.
- Website: A collection of web pages.
- Internet Service Provider (ISP): A private or public entity that provides high-speed or dial-up access to the Internet.
- Uniform Resource Locator (URL): The website's address (e.g., www.sohnen-moe.com).

The speed of the Internet lends itself well to communicating the latest news to your clients via your website. For instance, if you have activities and announcements about classes, open houses, discounts, promotions and product specials, you can make changes to your website in minutes at little or no cost—in comparison to the expense of reprinting brochures.

Website Design •

The most common methods for wellness providers to develop a web presence are to create a website on their own, work with a company that specializes in template designs, work with a web designer to create a customized site, or rent a home page on another site, usually as part of a professional association or a "health mall."

Although it may be a breeze for some tech savvy practitioners to get a website up and running, the learning curve is too steep for most practitioners to create a professional looking website. Working with a professional designer to launch a website can cost anywhere from $500 to $2,500 or more. A less costly approach is to work with an intern at a local university or design college, or find someone who will barter all or part of the cost of producing a website.

How to Use the Internet to Advertise, Promote and Market Your Business or Website with Little or No Money
by Bruce C. Brown

Internet Marketing for Less Than $500/Year
by Marcia Yudkin

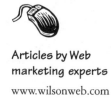

Articles by Web marketing experts
www.wilsonweb.com

Companies that specialize in website "template" designs for wellness practitioners can help you get a site up and running in a short amount of time. By standardizing design elements and simplifying site maintenance, they keep costs affordable. You can choose from several "looks," and some packages include email systems and newsletter services. Most charge a one-time setup fee along with a standard monthly fee.

Whatever route you choose, some basic rules apply to site design, content development and navigation. The most talented website designers possess a combination of marketing, design and technical know-how. Ideally, you want to work with someone who has a good balance of all of these skills. Sometimes a designer can lean heavily toward the technical and lack a solid marketing sense, in which case the end result may be less than optimal. A traditional graphic artist might not be the best choice.

If you hire a graphic designer to create the visuals for your website, make sure that person knows how to translate the graphic design to the website or also hire a website developer. In addition to the site looking good, it needs to be created in such a way that it's simple to update, looks the same on a variety of systems, is friendly for people who are visually or movement impaired, and the search engines can easily find it.

Plan and develop your site's content, layout, color scheme and "look" before turning your website project over to a designer. The best way to jump-start this process is to search the Internet for websites that you like—ideally those of other wellness practitioners in your field. Print out copies of five of these sites and keep them in a file folder. When you interview various website designers, use this file to identify what design elements and content features you want to incorporate into your website. Likewise, ask to see a designer's portfolio of websites to get a sense of whether she is the right fit for your project.

If you want to keep things simple on your website, plan to include three essential pages: a home page; a biography page; and a page that outlines your services, prices and contact information.

16

Template companies
www.yourwebpro.com
www.holisticalliance.com

Writing for the Web
by Crawford Kilian

The Non-Designer's Web Book
by Robin Williams

Figure 16.25

Elements of Website Design

Good
- Eye appeal, pleasing color scheme
- Clear and easy-to-use navigation
- High information value
- Quick-loading graphics
- Easy-to-find contact information
- Balance of content and white space
- Simple graphics

Poor
- Clutter
- Poor navigation
- Lack of contrast
- Flash or animated graphics
- Ugly background images
- Sound files
- Slow-to-load pages
- Black background color

The next step in website design is to create a rough draft of your website content using your brochure and other existing marketing materials as a starting point. Reference your sample websites and develop your content pages according to the various categories of information, such as home page, biography or credentials, about us, services, philosophy, gift certificates, online scheduling, special promotions, maps or directions, links, contact us, what's new, e-newsletter archives, frequently asked questions and testimonials. Plan to include photos to add a personal touch.

Figure 16.26

Free Clipart
www.123clipart.com

Web Design Tips
www.thebodyworker.com/
websitetips.htm

www.webpagesthatsuck.com

Website Design Tips

These tips and techniques make your website more search engine friendly (easier to find) and more appealing to clients.

- Use headings that catch the interest of your reader.
- Use appropriate meta-description and meta-keyword tags on each page.
- Don't try any "tricks" to get higher placement in search engines. Learn about what search engines are looking for, and work within that framework.
- The Page Title must match the page's main heading.
- Your main keywords should comprise about two to five percent of the page content and are most effective in the title, filename, and near the top of the document.
- You have five seconds to show something that will keep a visitor on your site.
- Your homepage is the first page a visitors sees, so it should load quickly, grab his attention, and provide a clear roadmap to where he can find what he wants. The more you stuff into it beyond this, the less effective it becomes.

Website Hosting Services ●

A webhost provides the online "space" and resources to operate your website. You can work through your Internet Service Provider or other company for these services. Choosing the right web hosting company ensures the smooth sailing of your website, and avoids unexpected bouts of downtime that may result in clients perceiving you as unreliable or unresponsive. A good starting point is to ask people you know who have websites for their recommendations.

Website hosting services generally cost from $5 to $50 per month. Annual contracts may offer a reduced fee. The difference in fees depends on the additional services you select, such as server side scripting, databases, online "storefronts," and the number of different websites and email accounts you require. Multiple email accounts are normal for a website: "Webmaster," "service," "sales," and "info" are common generic accounts. Other factors that impact cost are uptime guarantees (i.e., how often the service becomes unavailable), site development assistance, levels of technical support, secure hosting services, and site backup services.

Search Engine Listings •

Regardless of where your site is technically located, you need to let people know how to find you. Notify the Internet search engines (e.g., Google, Yahoo) and directories, as well as other sites related to your specific field and your target market's interests. It is becoming more commonplace for search engines to require a listing fee. Otherwise it may take three to six months before your site has a presence in the search engine.

Many cities have websites that list local businesses and even provide direct links. Contact these sites to arrange listings. Also advise people on your mailing list of your newly launched website by sending them an announcement or publishing the address in your newsletter.

List your URL
www.scrubtheweb.com/addurl.html

www.google.com/addurl/

16

Figure 16.27

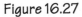

> ## Make Your Site Inviting
>
> - Create a section for electronic news releases and media materials (e.g., include announcements about workshops, open houses and special promotions).
> - Include a web page that highlights new developments and research findings in your field and of general interest in the holistic health field.
> - Include links to websites of holistic wellness professionals and organizations.
> - Post success stories and testimonials (be sure and obtain clients' permission).
> - Offer discount incentives for online purchase of products and gift certificates.
> - Promote online appointment scheduling by offering package deals.
> - Provide a way for visitors to give you feedback (e.g., a "Contact Me" form, direct email link, or a survey).
> - Purchase a digital camera so you can take pictures at events and upload them to your site.

Search Engine Details
www.searchenginewatch.com

Online Marketing Tips
www.webpromote.com
www.whatsnextonline.com
www.website101.com

Figure 16.28

> ## Website Marketing Tips
>
> - Print your website address on all your promotional materials (e.g., business cards, brochures, fliers, newsletters).
> - List your website on professional directories for your field (e.g., acufinder.com).
> - Send press releases to local media about your website.
> - Notify your Chamber of Commerce and Visitor's Bureau about your special events.
> - Post your address with regional website directories and city sites (usually the listing is free but a charge is assessed if you want a direct link to your site).
> - Link your site to other wellness practitioners' websites (contact the Webmaster or site manager to determine if linking is an option).
> - Crosslink your site with affiliated sites (i.e., provide reciprocal links). For example, if you specialize in working with fibromyalgia, link up with some of the online fibromyalgia support groups and resource organizations).
> - Visit www.ineedhits.com/free/popularity/ to find out which sites on the Internet are linking to your site.
> - Purchase advertising on sites that you feel would be a likely source of people who would visit your site.

Blogging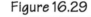

Blogging is a world unto itself. This form of Internet website, a portmanteau of web log, first emerged in the mid 1990s. Technorati (www.technorati.com), a recognized authority on what's happening on the World Wide Web, tracks over 100 million blogs. A blog is a regularly updated website that contains postings in chronological order. In essence, it's a running commentary on a topic that the blogger knows, likes, or is passionate about.

A blog can attract new clients and keep you connected with colleagues who share your interest in holistic wellness. The secret to blogging is building relationships. Think of it as a dynamic conversation that connects those who have information of value to share. Some key activities involved with linking on your blog include: listing blogs you like; commenting on others' blog posts; posting ideas, articles, resources and links from other bloggers and the Internet; and sending thank-you notes when someone gives you a link.

To make the best use of your blogging time and energy, talk to colleagues about their blogging experiences and opinion of what works and what doesn't work in the business realm. Also plan to spend some time visiting blogs of wellness practitioners. Blogging isn't a magic bullet. However, like any other marketing tool, if used skillfully it can help build your client base and strong, lasting relationships. The primary challenge for most wellness practitioners is finding the time to apply this tool to the marketing mix.

If you make customers unhappy in the physical world, they might each tell six friends. If you make customers unhappy on the Internet, they can each tell 6,000 friends.
— Jeff Bezos

Copywriting tips
www.copyblogger.com

Figure 16.29

Blogging Tips

- A blog is a great complement to your website, if you like to write and can find time to review and create postings frequently.
- A blog doesn't cost anything to create and requires minimal technical expertise.
- Consider hiring a graphic designer to fine-tune the look and feel of your blog. Emulate the best features of blogs you like, and align your blog with your website look. The typical cost ranges from $250 to $500.
- Post information about your healing philosophy on your blog. It is key to connecting with your target market.
- Make sure your blog writing reflects your professional image and offers good, useful information.
- Potential clients searching online will find you easier through a blog than a website. Search engines give blogs special treatment and higher rankings, provided you update your blog fairly often. For best results, plan to post to your blog at least twice a week.
- Aim to connect with other bloggers who share your values and vision of holistic wellness. Link to sites of other practitioners who may help your readers' with their health and wellness concerns.
- Drive traffic to your blog by writing articles and submitting them to free article websites. Be sure and include your blog address.
- List your blog in various blog directories based on your niche and area of expertise.

Online Discussion Groups •

Another way to gain visibility is to join newsgroups, listserves and forums that serve your target market. According to Web etiquette and group rules, it isn't appropriate to directly promote yourself in these venues. However, it's fine to list your website address or blog address as part of your signature line when you make posts that add value to the discussion topic. Posts that convey unique insights and useful information are appreciated and position you as a trusted and knowledgeable expert in your field.

A listserve is an automated email system that allows its members to send a message to a single address; that email is then sent to all the email addresses that are listed in the database file of the listserve. You must be a member on the listserver to send a message to members of the listserve. These systems usually have rules about what is and isn't appropriate to distribute to members.

Avoid business networking in personal online forums such as myspace.com, friendster.com and facebook.com. These sites are geared toward social networking and personal relationships, so it's best to keep business out of the mix.

e-Newsletters •

An e-newsletter, also known as an e-zine, is a great way to stay in touch with clients, announce special promotions and gain visibility without making a major dent in your budget. Other than nominal listserve management fees, it costs very little to send out an e-newsletter to hundreds of people. Unlike a print newsletter, no printing, mailing or design costs are involved.

Plan to send an e-newsletter either monthly or quarterly. The content doesn't have to be elaborate, just useful, interesting and geared toward helping your clients find solutions to their health and wellness concerns. Include a feature article, health tips, information about special promotions, newsworthy announcements and links to other websites of interest. Spotlight new services or products. You can also add a touch of humor or an inspiring quote.

Be sure to include your complete contact information, website address, and attach an email subject line that clearly identifies your newsletter so it won't be deleted as spam. Avoid creating a 10-page e-newsletter as it may not get read. Stick to a shorter format to ensure you don't lose time-pressed readers.

Make sure your e-newsletter is "opt-in," which means asking clients or associates first before adding them to your email list. Simply put, you need permission to market to clients on the Internet. Anything else is spam. You also need to include an unsubscribe option. Consider automating your e-newsletter distribution and list management with a communication company.

Discussion Groups
www.groups.yahoo.com

16

Use broadcast emails (other than e-newsletters) sparingly; otherwise they will be perceived as spam. Reserve these to highlight special promotions or articles of major interest, such as newsworthy research findings in preventive wellness and holistic health.

Online Distribution Companies
www.constantcontact.com
aweber.com

e-Newsletter Articles

www.ezinequeen.com/
articles.htm

> ### e-Newsletter Tips
>
> - Include a sign-up form for your e-newsletter on your website.
> - After a public speaking event, let the group know you have an e-newsletter. Ask them to give you their business cards if they would like to subscribe. It also works well to offer a giveaway, such as a discount coupon or special report for those who sign up.
> - If you're looking for a good way to get your articles published in other places on the Internet, put a blurb at the bottom of your newsletter that says people are free to use the material from your e-newsletter as long as they give you credit and include a link to your site.
> - Subscribe to other wellness practitioners' e-newsletters. Note what gets your attention and what bores you. Use what you learn to create content that engages your readers and keeps them looking forward to your next edition.

Figure 16.30

• Advertising •

Advertising is gaining public notice for your business through means that require direct payment. Some forms of advertising include: display ads in publications; radio and television commercials; classified ads; billboards; phone books; Internet ads; and bus-stop benches. Mass media advertising has typically been avoided by wellness providers, mainly due to the impersonal nature and the relatively high cost. Yet it's becoming more commonplace to hear ads on the radio, see billboards on the roads and even encounter television ads promoting wellness and complementary healthcare. Still, most of these advertising techniques are usually employed by larger clinics rather than individual practitioners, or are announcing a specific event. Classified ads tend to be the most productive form of advertising for practitioners. Your advertising venues contribute to your overall image, so choose them carefully.

Advertising is best used when your target market meets one or more of these criteria: your target is a mass market, your product or service is purchased frequently, the competition is high, or your goal is to quickly create awareness of a new service or product.

You can have brilliant ideas, but if you can't get them across, your ideas won't get you anywhere.
— Lee Iacocca

The two essential elements for successful advertising are consistency and quality. Quality relates to the ad's style, wording and visual impact. Statistics reveal that an ad needs to be seen at least three times before it's noticed and seven times before it inspires the reader to take action. It works better to place a smaller (or shorter) ad on a regular basis than to do a big splashy ad one time only.

The steps in designing effective advertising are: Identify your target market, grab the prospect's attention, highlight your differential advantage, list the benefits, state your offer, highlight the ad's features, request a response, and provide a means of contact.

Internet Advertising •

Whether you're a new wellness practitioner or experienced business owner, it's no small task to gain a working knowledge of Internet advertising. Many practitioners shy away from online advertising because of the perceived cost barriers and complex landscape. In many cases this is a wise move, but not always. Sometimes a closer look can reveal affordable and cost-effective ways to increase traffic to your website and bookings from new clients. For group practices with an ample advertising budget and an Internet savvy business owner, online advertising often amounts to a cost-effective way to boost profits.

A visit to Pay-per-Click Guru (payperclickguru.com) provides insights into the wide-ranging world of pay-per-click (PPC) advertising. PPC charges the advertiser only when a person clicks on a link to a text ad that leads to that advertiser's website. PPC allow advertisers to sign up and bid on specific keywords—relevant to the particular goods or services available on their website. This type of advertising is an art and requires both financial and marketing savvy.

You may want to visit Google (www.google.com) and click on "Advertising Programs" to get a picture of how Google AdSense and Google AdWords work. As Google is the top search engine, it's a worthwhile starting point. In short, Google AdSense automatically delivers text and image ads targeted to your site; Google AdWords lets you generate text ads that accompany specific search engine results.

To help you make smart decisions about Internet advertising, talk to friends and colleagues who have explored the territory, attend a seminar or read several resource books to help you make the most of your advertising budget. If your budget allows, work with an Internet marketing consultant even if only for a general orientation session.

The Online Advertising Playbook: Proven Strategies and Tested Tactics from the Advertising Research Foundation
by Joe Plummer, Steve Rappaport, Taddy Hall, Robert Barocci

Google Advertising Tools: Cashing in with AdSense, AdWords, and the Google APIs
by Harold Davis

Print Advertising •

Of all the advertising venues, print advertising, such as newspapers, magazines, trade journals and specialty publications, is the most preferred by wellness providers. Contact various print publications and request an advertiser's media kit. These kits contain rates for display and classified ads, demographic statistics and a sample of the publication. Compare rates and evaluate the best venues to reach your target audience.

Creating ad copy can be difficult. Most people think they should start with the headline. Unless you're struck by a bolt of advertising genius (hey, it could happen!), begin by making a list of your benefits, and determine the offer you want to make. Save the headline composition for last. Next write the body copy. Don't skimp on information. Studies show ads with more copy draw better than those with less. Then again, don't pack so much in that it requires a microscope to decipher the text.

In many ways the headline is the most critical element of an ad. People's choice of whether to read or ignore your ad is often based on the headline's impact. Five times as many people read the headlines as read the text. According to Cahners Advertising Research Report, ads with benefits in the headlines and copy are 2-3 times more likely to be remembered than ads that don't stress benefits.

Figure 16.31

Exciting Headline Styles

News: Use words such as "New," "Presenting" or "Announcing."

Instruction/Advice: Use words such as "How to," "Why," "Which," "You," "This" and "Discover."

Testimonial: Utilize strong quotes from satisfied clients.

Compelling Offer: Use words such as "Free" and "Limited Offer."

Curiosity: Ask questions to inspire readers to want to know more, such as "Do you feel (want, need, desire?)."

Claim: Relay a success story.

Figure 16.32

Display Ad Tips

- Include an attention-grabbing, benefits-oriented headline.
- If you use a photo, put the headline below it.
- Have the subhead elaborate the headline benefit.
- Incorporate a strong visual image.
- Photographs attract more readers than drawings. Before and after pictures are also quite persuasive.
- Identify your target markets.
- Personalize the ad to an individual reader.
- Keep the body text paragraphs short and visually attractive. Don't skimp on information—studies show ads with more copy draw better than those with less. Then again, don't pack so much in that it requires a microscope to decipher the text.
- Use language that's geared toward your target market.
- Include powerful words such as "new," "free," "save" and "now."
- Provide a guarantee.
- Offer incentives.
- Broadcast on station WIIFM (What's In It For Me).
- Back up benefits with key features.
- Demonstrate credibility and reliability.
- Include testimonials.
- State your offer in clear, simple terms.
- Compel readers to take action.
- If you're selling a product, make it easy to respond: include a toll-free number, fax number and other ways to contact you such as email or website; provide an order form; and offer to take credit cards.
- Include your logo, location and phone number.
- Border your ad—it makes small ads look bigger. Don't limit yourself to plain, straight-lined boxes, or use overly baroque designs.
- Make the layout attractive and inviting.
- Use color whenever possible. A second color (in addition to the black ink) can increase the ad's effectiveness by 25 percent. The most eye-catching and frequently used color is red. Full color ads provide four times the impact.

Figure 16.33 Sample Salon and Minispa Display Ad

Before

Godiva Salon and Minispa

• Bridal, Cosmetics and Hair Design • Body and Facial Waxing
• Customized European Facials • Hydrotherapy
• Manicures and Pedicures • Permanent Make-up

In Service Since 1979
196 E. Maine Terrace #129
Landtown, MO 94162

624-555-9721
www.godivaminispa.com

Problems
- No interesting, attention-grabbing header
- No benefits listed, only features
- Meaningless use of graphic
- No call to action
- Boring layout

16

strong
visual

After

Elegance & Rejuvenation
with Godiva Salon and Minispa

A full service salon and minispa for rejuvenating and toning the body. Licensed Estheticians on site

• Bridal, Cosmetics and Hair Design
• Body and Facial Waxing
• Customized European Facials

• Hydrotherapy
• Manicures and Pedicures
• Permanent Make-up

In Service Since 1979
196 E. Maine Terrace #129
Open Wednesday thru Sunday

Make An Appointment Today!
624-555-9721
www.godivaminispa.com

headline →
name →
benefits →
features →
added crediblity →
location and hours of operation →

call to action   easy to respond

Figure 16.34 Sample Massage Display Ad

Before

Total Health Through Massage

•Neuromuscular Therapy   •Swedish Massage
•Subtle Body Energy Work   •Deep Tissue

Leslie R. Vandruff
Licensed Massage Therapist

Call For Appointment
394-555-3692   **Introductory Offer!**
                            $30 an hour

Positives
- Call to action
- Incentive
- Clear name and title

Problems
- Too many fonts
- No significant graphic
- No list of benefits

attention grabbing
header

After

Total Health Through Massage

Leslie R. Vandruff, L.M.T.

Relieve stress, increase joint and muscle flexibility, release energy blockages, remove back and neck pain and increase your feeling of well-being.

• Neuromuscular Therapy   • Swedish Massage
• Subtle Body Energy Work   • Deep Tissue

Call For Appointment
394-555-3692   **Introductory Offer!**
                            $30 an hour

credentials stressed with "L.M.T." →
benefits →
graphic cleverly incorporated →
features →
call to action →

easy to respond   incentive

Figure 16.35 Sample Chiropractic Display Ad

Before

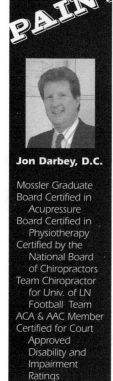

PAIN?

Jon Darbey, D.C.

Mossler Graduate
Board Certified in
Acupressure
Board Certified in
Physiotherapy
Certified by the
National Board
of Chiropractors
Team Chiropractor
for Univ. of LN
Football Team
ACA & AAC Member
Certified for Court
Approved
Disability and
Impairment
Ratings

If you're in pain and looking for fast, gentle results from a chiropractic physician you can depend on, call Dr. Jon Darbey. Gentleness in chiropractic may be a new concept to you as it was to me before I began my six years of training necessary for our doctorate degrees. During my studies, I learned how light pressure at precise locations can bring relief to pain. Don' t let your fear of pain stop you from receiving chiropractic treatment.

Gentle Chiropractic For:

Back Pain	Neck Pain
Painful Joints	Hip Pain
Headaches	Cold Hands/Feet
Arm/Leg Pain	Fibromyalgia

CALL DR. DARBEY
555-3216
Cortwell Medical Ctr, 139 Mordnar
(North of 5th)

Positives

- Interesting 3-D effect with "PAIN?"
- Photo as visual with clear name
- Call to action
- Purpose and features listed
- Location explained for convenience

Problems

- Too much unnecessary info in story text
- Started with "If"
- Font at call to action hard to read
- Too much text in credentials under his name
- Layout a bit funky due to no header at story text

attention
getting header

interesting 3-D effect with "PAIN?"

photo as visual

name and credibility

benefits listed

call to action

phone number bold and clear

features given

location explained
for convenience

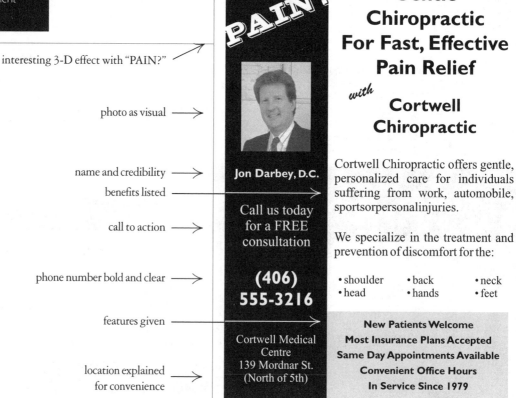

PAIN?

Jon Darbey, D.C.

Call us today
for a FREE
consultation

(406)
555-3216

Cortwell Medical
Centre
139 Mordnar St.
(North of 5th)

Gentle Chiropractic For Fast, Effective Pain Relief

with

Cortwell Chiropractic

Cortwell Chiropractic offers gentle, personalized care for individuals suffering from work, automobile, sportsorpersonalinjuries.

We specialize in the treatment and prevention of discomfort for the:

- shoulder
- head
- back
- hands
- neck
- feet

New Patients Welcome
Most Insurance Plans Accepted
Same Day Appointments Available
Convenient Office Hours
In Service Since 1979

Figure 16.36 Sample Counseling Display Ad

Before

Problems:

- No intriguing header
- No benefits listed
- Only lists number, no call to action
- Too much blank space, layout can be more effectively used
- Features OK, but is cold feeling
- Tag line—what qualifies better?

After

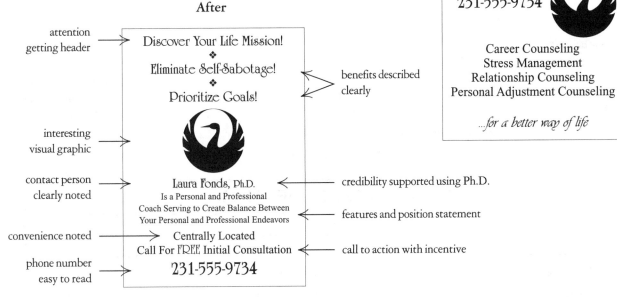

attention getting header

interesting visual graphic

contact person clearly noted

convenience noted

phone number easy to read

benefits described clearly

credibility supported using Ph.D.

features and position statement

call to action with incentive

Dr. Laura Fonds
Ph.D.
Certified Personal And
Professional Coach

231-555-9734

Career Counseling
Stress Management
Relationship Counseling
Personal Adjustment Counseling

...for a better way of life

Discover Your Life Mission!
❖
Eliminate Self-Sabotage!
❖
Prioritize Goals!

Laura Fonds, Ph.D.
Is a Personal and Professional
Coach Serving to Create Balance Between
Your Personal and Professional Endeavors
Centrally Located
Call For FREE Initial Consultation
231-555-9734

16

Figure 16.37 Sample Acupuncture Display Ad

Before

After

Liberate Your Life Energy With
Mia Lan Acupuncture

Acupuncture frees inhibited energy and aligns your chi for a beautiful life. It releases discomfort from:

- allergies
- arthritis
- stress
- body aches
- headaches
- sleeplessness

Call for appointment today
555-3271

Mia Lan, L.Ac.
Practicing Since 1971
Under Master Lee Wong

Liberate Your Life
Energy With
Mia Lan Acupuncture

Acupuncture frees inhibited energy and aligns your chi for a beautiful life. It releases discomfort from:

- allergies
- stress
- arthritis
- body aches
- headaches
- sleeplessness

Call for appointment today
205-555-3271

Mia Lan, L.Ac.
Practicing Since 1971
Under Master Lee Wong

Both have:

- Attention-getting header
- Interesting graphic
- Benefits described
- Credibility enhanced
- Features added
- Call to action
- Easy-to-read phone number

layout flows better

Classified Ads ● ●

Sample Classified Ads

www.businessmastery.us/
classifieds.php

Place listings in business directories, consumer telephone directories, trade journals, local publications, newsletters and special interest books.

Classified ads tend to be the most productive form of advertising for wellness providers. A classified ad is a concise, engaging description of your practice or announcement that is placed in a specific section of a publication. Classified ads are generally much less expensive than display ads—and you don't need to employ a commercial artist.

The major advantage of a classified ad is inherent in its definition. People look at those ads because they're interested in what's offered. Contrast this with display advertising in which you have to grab the reader's attention.

A catchy headline is required for your ad to stand out. Other ways to increase the visibility of your ad are to put the headline in bold capital letters, bold the whole ad, include some type of graphic design, add color or box the ad. Follow the same general design tips for display advertising.

Figure 16.38

CLASSIFIEDS

To Gain Leads

Sports Massage Therapy:

SPORTS CHAMPIONS! Keep your competitive edge with therapeutic sports massage! Visit www.CompetetiveEdge.com for a FREE *Health Tips for Athletes* pamphlet. Or call 394-555-5555.

Chiropractic:

BACK & NECK PAIN? FREE consultation. Call Cortwell Chiropractic Center for gentle, personalized chiropractic care. 555-5555, 139 Mordnar St. Ask for our FREE pamphlet on *Tips for a Supple Spine*. www.CortwellChiropractic.com

Counseling:

FEELING OUT OF SYNC? Create balance between your personal and professional endeavors. Call Dr. Laura Fonds for a FREE initial consultation. 231-555-5555 www.CreateBalance.com

Acupuncture:

FREE Acupuncture information pack. Release discomfort from allergies, headaches, stress, sleeplessness, arthritis, body aches and more. 555-3271 www.MiaLanAcupuncture.com

Nutrition:

FREE information! Learn how to achieve optimal health. Go online or call for your FREE copy of our *Healthy Living Guide*. 555-9643 www.NutritionNow.com

To Gain Clients

Sports Massage Therapy:

SPORTS CHAMPIONS! Keep your competitive edge! Therapeutic sports massage increases your performance, relaxes muscle spasm/strain, reduces injury and speeds up rehabilitation! Equipment travels to you! Call for a FREE *Health Tips for Athletes* pamphlet or for appointment. 394-555-5555 www.CompetetiveEdge.com

Chiropractic:

BACK & NECK PAIN? Do you suffer from work, auto, sports or personal injury? Call Cortwell Chiropractic Center for a FREE consultation. Gentle, personalized chiropractic care releases pain from your shoulder, back, neck, head, hands and feet. Most insurance accepted. Convenient office hours. 555-5555, 139 Mordnar St., Big Sky. www.CortwellChiropractic.com

Counseling:

FEELING OUT OF SYNC? Create balance between your personal and professional endeavors! Discover your life mission! Eliminate self-sabotage! Prioritize goals! Call Laura Fonds, Ph.D., for FREE initial consultation. 231-555-5555 www.CreateBalance.com

Acupuncture:

Acupuncture frees inhibited energy and aligns your chi for a beautiful life. Release discomfort from allergies, stress, headaches, sleeplessness, arthritis, body aches and more. Call Mia Lan Acupuncture for more info or for a FREE consultation. Downtown location. 555-3271 www.MiaLanAcupuncture.com

Nutrition:

Do you want to achieve OPTIMAL HEALTH? We can assist you in feeling strong, energetic and enlivened. Call Tracy Smith, N.D., for an appointment or to receive a FREE copy of our *Healthy Living Guide*. 555-9643. Also visit our informative website www.NutritionNow.com.

Telephone Directories • •

Telephone directories provide year-round visibility to every person in your community (actually they're worldwide with online directories). They are extensively utilized by the public for locating services. Look to see how other wellness providers list their practices. You needn't be overly concerned about an enhanced listing (additional lines of information) or a display ad if you live in a city where there are only a few people who provide your specific services. Then again, it could be a great opportunity for you to stand out.

If you decide not to place a display ad, consider purchasing an enhanced listing, using a second color or placing a border around it. Put your listing under the most logical category if you can only afford one listing; otherwise list under each applicable category.

Broadcast Advertising •

The broadcast media, such as radio and television, reaches a wider audience than print advertising and has immediate impact. Unfortunately, you need to repeat the ad frequently because of the likelihood listeners or viewers won't be paying attention when your ad plays.

Radio Advertising • •

Wellness providers are utilizing radio advertising more and more each day. Radio is still a personal medium and people respond well to it. This type of advertising is also relatively inexpensive. You can dramatically increase the effectiveness by using it in combination with another type of marketing activity. The most common reasons to advertise on the radio are to herald the opening of a new business, introduce new staff members, announce new services or products, and invite the public to attend special events such as workshops and open houses.

An option to traditional advertising is to sponsor a radio show or public service announcement. In return for sponsorship (which could be in dollars or services), your name gets mentioned during the show. For example: "The Monday Morning Alternative Music Hour is brought to you by Cortwell Chiropractic Center."

Many radio stations offer prize packages to their listeners. Donate your services as part of a prize package and you receive a lot of free airplay. For example, a massage therapist in Tucson offered one massage for the Mother's Day Package the station was giving away. Her name (which is unusual—so it's easy to remember) was mentioned several times an hour for two weeks! This is an example of a shrewd investment: minimal cost—extremely high return.

The greatest thing to be achieved in advertising, in my opinion, is believability, and nothing is more believable than the product itself.
— Leo Burnett

Figure 16.39

Tips for Radio Advertising

- Identify your service or product immediately.
- Highlight a benefit within the first few seconds.
- Mention your name at least five times within a 30-second spot.
- Keep to one topic or theme.
- Use appropriate background music or sound effects.
- Develop a radio persona.
- Capitalize on timely events, headline news items, weather, holidays and seasons.
- Be sincere.
- Develop a jingle.
- Make a compelling offer.
- Include a call to action.

Television Advertising ••

Television is a powerful advertising vehicle. It reaches more people than any other single medium. According to the Nielsen Report, the average household watches more than eight hours of television every day. While nationwide coverage is extremely expensive, local advertising is more affordable due to the abundance of cable networks and nonaffiliated stations.

The two keys to successful television advertising are placement and quality. In terms of placement, if one of your target markets is stockbrokers, running your ad on any station in the morning isn't going to net you high results (their attention is on Wall Street). Regarding quality, consumers rate the value of your services and products on the production quality of your commercial. You can damage your reputation if your commercial looks cheap or hokey.

Although most local television ads are designed to encourage the public to visit a location, such as a restaurant or a store, it's becoming more commonplace to see ads for wellness providers.

• Publicity •

Publicity is free media exposure for your practice. It is a powerful tool for any business, yet few people take advantage of this cost-effective way to gain visibility. Some examples of publicity are news releases, announcements, feature stories, interviews and press conferences. Publicity differs from advertising in that you don't pay for the exposure (although some media outlets do give news exposure preference to advertisers).

Publicity lends an air of credibility to a business that advertising cannot. People are more likely to utilize your services if they read an article about you, listen to an interview with you on the radio or watch you on television than if they see an advertisement about your business. When a respected journalist or reporter makes a positive statement about you, it has much greater impact than if you said the same thing about yourself.

Take a moment to reflect upon an interview you've read about a local businessperson. What were your impressions? Did you feel a connection with the person? Would you experience the same things by seeing that person's advertisement? Many people I know have increased their businesses significantly through their publicity efforts. Also, most wellness providers can't afford to place an advertisement that covers the same page space or airtime as an interview. Even if an interview doesn't generate a lot of direct business, you can still use it by framing a reprint on your wall, posting it on your website and including it your marketing packets.

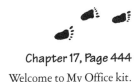

Chapter 17, Page 444
Welcome to My Office kit.

Developing Media Relationships ●

Publicity is a powerful marketing tool; to get it you must supply interesting, factual and newsworthy information to media outlets such as radio, television, newspapers, magazines, newsletters and specialty publications. While it's the media's job to inform the public about interesting people and events, they're flooded with press releases and media kits. You need to capture their attention. To get free publicity, you need to market yourself to the media. You must provide evidence that coverage of you or your business will benefit their readers, listeners or viewers. Media representatives tend to take interest in things that are new, have magnitude, contain an element of human interest or are beneficial to the community.

Press releases play an integral part in effective public relations. Generate ideas for press releases by thinking about what makes you unique—this is your "hook." In addition to your actual work, consider other aspects, such as how long you have been in practice, your location, your training, the equipment and products you use, the types of clients you work with, and any recent changes you've made to your practice. Familiarize the media with your business. Send out press releases on major business changes and events. The more often they see your name, the more recognizable you become. Your investment of a little time and postage can reap great rewards.

My philosophy is that not only are you responsible for your life, but doing the best at this moment puts you in the best place for the next moment.
— Oprah Winfrey

Become the Expert ● ●

Another idea for developing relationships with the media is to become the "expert in the field" who they reference as an information source. It is gratifying when someone from the media calls you for information or your opinion, even when the article isn't directly about you. To facilitate this, mail Rolodex-sized cards (with your name, business name, phone numbers and areas of expertise) to the editors and reporters of local publications, and to producers and hosts of radio and television shows. Put your major category of expertise on the protruding edge of the card. Also send this via email.

Be Newsworthy ● ●

You increase your odds of being interviewed if you offer something newsworthy. But what makes an event newsworthy? That all depends upon the specific media. This is why it's important to research the different media outlets in terms of their target markets and to list the types of articles they write or shows they produce that relate to you. For example, does the newspaper often run interviews of local businesspeople? If so, what types of business owners have been featured? Is there a segment on a television news program that highlights healthy things to do? Are there any specialty publications or shows aimed at people who would be interested in your services?

Some ideas for creating a newsworthy image include staging events, such as free demonstrations or "massage-a-thons;" disseminating information that is unique or useful to the general public, such as announcing a new wellness product or describing techniques to alleviate headache pain; forming a wellness group to study specific health-related topics; sponsoring a sports team by donating your services for pre- and post-events, and offering reduced rates for regular sessions; adopting a charitable cause; connecting with a celebrity; and giving an annual award or scholarship.

It is easier to get publicity if it's in an area that the media already covers. Ride the coattails of a national trend. Also note upcoming events that will most likely generate publicity, such as charity events, tournaments and expositions. Find a way to connect with these activities either by volunteering, becoming a sponsor or donating your services. Then send media kits. Check the newspaper for headlines that can be related to your services. Once you have developed an interesting angle, call the newspaper and offer your comments. Let them know you're available as a source for future related articles. Follow up this phone call with a letter, including your business card, the Rolodex-sized card and a brochure.

To get a mention in the media, such as a listing in the calendar of events, a press release suffices. If you want to announce a new location, additional staff, or an award, keep it simple and short. Some publications have a special section that highlights individuals and businesses in terms of being new, a change in status, relocation, staff additions, employee promotions and awards. These are usually 20 words or less. So, if you know what you want it to say, don't make it too wordy, lest you run the risk of the editor omitting crucial data. Send a photograph along with the press release, and offer to send a digital photo.

Media Hooks

- You are unique
- Launching new services or products
- Special events: grand opening, relocation, anniversary, milestones
- You can prove you do it better than your competition
- Receiving an award
- Your credentials
- Your cost is lower
- Process you use to get results
- Result is better, faster, cheaper, etc.
- Length of time in business
- Experience in this field
- First company in the field
- Testimonials from satisfied customers/clients
- Your mission
- Your market
- Your image
- Obstacles you've overcome
- Tie into something that has status
- Piggyback onto something that is already happening
- Consistent image
- You are the expert

Press Releases ●

Your chances of capturing a media representative's interest in what you're doing are greatly increased if the press release can be quickly assessed. Presentation is crucial with press releases. Type them (double-spaced) on high-quality paper, preferably letterhead. Make certain they conform to the preferred format standards of source information: the release date, a headline, the body and the conclusion. Keep your wording clear and conversational. Avoid using jargon.

One-page press releases work best. If it's more than one page, follow these guidelines: type "(more)" at the bottom of each page—except on the last page: type "End" or "30" or "###" after the final paragraph on the last page; and staple the pages together. After you have typed your press release, double-check to make sure that you have included important dates, times, locations and contact numbers. Then proofread, proofread, and proofread again.

Many news outlets prefer to receive electronic press releases. This way they don't have to retype the information. Find out the preferred format, and submit it in that manner.

Press Release Components • •

Source Information: Name, company, address and phone number. Put this in the top left-hand corner of the page.

Release Date: If the story or announcement can be printed as soon as it's received, type "For Immediate Release." If you want it posted on a specific date, type "For Release, Monday, October 7th." In general it's best to have press releases that state "For Immediate Release." Otherwise you take the chance of the media representative putting it aside and forgetting about it. Place the release date below the source information and to the right side of the page.

Headline: This is a succinct summary of the content of the release. Word it in such a way that you put the information that would capture your reader's attention first, without making it sound like hype. Always type the headline in bold capital letters. Two examples of headlines are: "FREE WORKSHOP ON INFANT MASSAGE" and "MELISSA BLUMENTHAL, NATIONALLY RENOWNED SPORTS PSYCHOLOGIST, HAS JOINED TOUCH, INC." Place the headline below the release date and center it between margins.

Body: This contains the details about the release. The first paragraph should be a concise statement, expressing the most important features first. Cover who, what, where, when, why and how. Use separate paragraphs for additional information or supplemental material. Write it in the "inverted pyramid style," as newspapers refer to it. That means placing the most important information at the top, as they cut from the bottom up. It's wise to use a multiple paragraph composition for the body because the space allotted for news stories and press releases constantly varies. This way, if they have extra space and you've provided them ample material, they will use it. Conversely, if their space is limited, it's easy for them to locate and use the vital information.

Conclusion: A separate paragraph indicating the action you want the reader, listener or viewer to take as a result of reading or hearing your story or announcement. You might type, "Call 555-5555 for more information" or "Stop by our Grand Opening on Saturday, October 12th from 10 a.m. to 2 p.m."

Press Release Distribution
www.netpost.com
ww.prnewswire.com

16

Sample Press Release
www.businessmastery.us/
press-release.php

Writing Effective News Releases....: How to Get Free Publicity for Yourself, Your Business or Your Organization
by Catherine V. McIntyre

Complete Publicity Plans: How to Create Publicity That Will Spark Media Exposure and Excitement
by Sandra L. Beckwith

Figure 16.40 Sample Massage Press Release

{Source Information}

Hands-On Massage

Francine Feelgood

359 Front Street
Anytown, WA
99243

732-HAND
(732-4263)

www.HandsOnMassage.com

Providing

Healthy Massage

for Your

Well-Being

{Release Date}
For Immediate Release

{Headline}

MASSAGE BAR OFFERS "DOUBLES"

{Body}

Doing business at Hands-On Massage just got better. The massage bar is now offering "doubles," in which two massage practitioners will do chair massage on a client.

Typically, the seated massage is done one-on-one with a single practitioner performing primarily upper-body massage on a client. With the new service available of "doubles," for an additional $10, clients may have two people working on them.

Hands-On Massage, owned by Francine Feelgood, opened her on-site massage "bar" in May. The business offers fully clothed seated massage to its clientele, ranging from athletes to executives.

"Instead of bellying up to the bar for a double shot of scotch, here you can double up on something healthy and rewarding for yourself," Feelgood said. Hands-On Massage also offers Happy Hour specials during the lunch hour and between 4:30 and 6 p.m. Sessions are offered in 10-, 20- and 30-minute intervals during weekdays from 10 a.m. to 7 p.m.

{Supplemental Information}

On-site massage, as this type of structured touch is commonly called, involves a fully-clothed person sitting on a specially designed chair, thereby allowing a practitioner full access to massaging a person's back, neck and arms.

{Conclusion}

For more information or to schedule an appointment, call 555-HAND (555-4263).

END

The Media Kit ●

If you want to be interviewed in print or on the air, send a media kit. Most wellness providers get interviewed as a feature segment, but if you're requesting an interview in connection with an event, it can become news coverage. Media kit components include: a cover letter; a press release (optional); a fact sheet; a photograph; a biography; a brochure; a business card; and supplemental information such as articles written about you or similar businesses, pamphlets stating the benefits of your services and a listing of previous media coverage.

If your "hook," or attention-grabbing value proposition, entails involvement with another event, include a summary sheet on the event. Papers can easily get misfiled, so it's wise to include identification such as company name, subject matter, contact person and telephone number on each piece of material. Ideally, put the information in a folder and enclose it in a 9"x12" envelope, labelled "Media Kit." Then mail it or hand-deliver it. You can also send an electronic media kit, but make sure to get permission from the intended recipient or it will most likely get trashed—particularly if it includes attachments. People are leery about opening attachments from unknown sources due to the plethora of computer viruses.

Cover Letters ● ●

The purpose of a cover letter (also referred to as a "pitch" letter) is to grab the media representative's attention so he reads the rest of the material in your media kit. State who you are, your hook, what you're sending, and ask for action. Ideally, this letter contains 100 words, but never more than 250 words.

Press Releases ● ●

(Please see previous section.)

Fact Sheets ● ●

Ensure accuracy by always including a one-page fact sheet that includes important, concise information. I use the following four categories: history, founder, awards and today.

History encompasses the technical information about the company, such as what the practitioner does, a mission statement and length of time in business.

Founder contains information on the wellness provider's professional background. Some practitioners may wish to combine the history and founder categories.

Under the **Awards** category, list honors received.

The **Today** category gives a bit more information on the practice and lists statistics such as the number of current clients, type of work the practitioner has done recently, hours and any new announcements.

The influence on others must proceed from one's own person. In order to be capable of producing such an influence, one's words must have power, and this they can only have if they are based on something real, just as the flame depends on its fuel.
— The I Ching

The unwritten rule is: always put photographs on the left side of the media kit.

Biographies ● ●

This is a short biography of you and your practice. Keep it more conversational in tone than the fact sheet and include the following: your philosophy; a description of the types of people you work with; the modalities you use; and special equipment and products you incorporate. Keep the length to two double-spaced pages. Some people omit the biography if their brochures contain this information.

Photographs ● ●

Affix a caption that describes the photograph and identifies all parties. This can be placed on the back or the front border.

Photographs convey a visual representation of who you are. Get professional publicity photos taken by a photographer. These should be kept current and updated every two to five years. In addition to digital images, keep a stock of color and black-and-white prints. Always put your name and phone number on the back of the photograph. If you're being profiled or listed under announcements, the publications often use the photo you send. When reporters conduct in-depth interviews, they usually bring along a photographer.

Stat Sheets ● ●

Whenever your hook involves another event or includes a connection with a newsworthy company, provide the media with a stat sheet. Stat sheets are one-page summaries. They outline the event or company background (e.g., mission statement, inception date), highlight activities, and list important dates, names and phone numbers.

Getting Interviewed ●

Print Coverage ● ●

Never underestimate the power of the written word. Many businesses have blossomed as a direct result of print publicity. Print media ranges from large daily newspapers to neighborhood weeklies, magazines, newsletters and specialty publications. Each publication has several departments, often with different editors. Some of the most common departments of interest for wellness providers are: business, education, events calendar, features, health, community outlook, news and sports.

Research all the local publications. Familiarize yourself with their styles, the types of articles they run, and the people profiled. Find out the names of editors and reporters for each department so you can send your publicity materials to the appropriate people. Plan your publicity campaign well in advance. Some publications, particularly magazines, have a long lead time between getting material and having it printed.

Call the person in charge of the section in which you would like coverage. Find out about their deadlines and preferred submission format. Be prepared to convey the essence of your story in 30 seconds. Then make certain that your media kit or press release is in the reporter's hands within 24 hours of your call. Call to confirm the material was received, and ask if the reporter needs any other information from you.

Guest editorials are spots for either individuals or representatives from a group to offer their opinions on major controversial issues. This is a good forum to educate the public about wellness concerns—particularly if something has occurred within your community that doesn't support alternative care.

Most reporters do their interviews on location (e.g., your office or home). Occasionally they will meet you in a public place. At the end of the interview, give the reporter a copy of your fact sheet to ensure that the vital information (e.g., names, numbers and statistics) gets correctly conveyed.

After you've been interviewed, send a short thank-you note to the reporter, stating how much you enjoyed the experience. Once the interview is published, send another follow-up. This time go into a bit more detail about one or two specific things (e.g., "I really appreciate the way you captured my philosophy by...."). Close the note by inviting the reporter to feel free to contact you in the future about this subject or similar topics.

Airtime ● ●

Radio and television interviews are great fun and can significantly enhance your public image. At the very least you'll be more recognizable to the general public after a television appearance. News programs, short features, talk shows, special programs and public service announcements are types of available air time.

Observe various programs to determine which ones would be the most suitable for your message. Cable television offers more opportunities than commercial stations. You can also produce or host your own show. Ascertain the following information for each show: program title, focus, day and time aired, producer's name and host's name. Call the station to find out who would be the appropriate recipient of your proposal. As with print coverage, when talking with the producer or host, ask about preferences for being approached, how much time you should allow to elapse before doing follow-up and deadlines. Give a 30-second highlight of your story and make certain that all follow-up materials are received within 24 hours.

Once you're slotted to appear on a TV or radio program, watch or listen to the show at least once beforehand. This is imperative for television shows so you can see what the set looks like from the audience's perspective. It also affords you the opportunity to notice the style of clothing the host wears, the positioning of the chairs and whether the cameras tend to do full-length body shots or mainly head and shoulder shots. Note the backdrop color so you don't wear similar-colored clothing—or else you will literally fade into the background. Watch the host's interviewing style: Is there active participation in the discussions? Do questions encourage lengthy responses or does the host tend to dominate the show?

If the publication is unable or unwilling to write an article about you, find out what the article submission guidelines are, and write the article yourself.

Many talk-show hosts ask the guest to submit a list of suggested questions. While this may seem intimidating, it's a great opportunity for you to shape the program. It gives you the power to ensure coverage of the most salient points about yourself, your business and your profession. It also solidifies the message you wish to convey. Have a friend or colleague coach you by asking the questions you submitted. This helps you clarify your responses so you won't fumble for words during the interview. Also have your coach toss in a few questions of her own, just to help prepare you for responding to unexpected or ill-informed inquiries (particularly if it's a call-in show).

Find out well in advance the directions to the studio, determine how long it takes to get there and verify the time you need to arrive (which is earlier than the actual taping time). If it's a television show, find out if the studio plans to provide you with a hair and makeup artist. Ask when the show will be aired, if they provide a copy of the program and when it will be available for you to pick up.

There is no such thing as "off the record."

When you go to the interview, bring a copy of the suggested questions, a fact sheet and any other supporting materials. Before taping, find out how the interviewer prefers to be addressed. If it's a television show, ask if you should look at the camera or the host.

When appearing on television wear rich, dark colors, other than blue. Avoid all white or "busy" patterns like checks, intricate, small designs or broad stripes. Jewelry should be simple and not flashy or dangling. Keep in mind that scarves tend to bring energy up to your face. Wear shoes that are darker than your hemline. Women: Apply makeup a bit heavier than normal and make sure your lipstick has a matte finish and matches the color of the inside of your lip. Men should also wear powder to reduce glare.

After you've been interviewed, send a short thank-you note to both the host and producer. Once the interview is aired, send another follow-up note. This time when you close the note, suggest additional topics and areas of your expertise that could be explored on future shows.

Watch the video and listen to the tape for evaluation purposes. Assess your strengths and challenges. Note how well and thoroughly you responded to the questions, your demeanor and any changes you want to make for future appearances.

Programs to Target • • •

News Programs: Getting coverage on your local news program may be the most difficult because reporters tend to cover hard news. The most likely angle to demonstrate newsworthiness is related to emergency situations, such as volunteering your services at an event that's already scheduled to be covered (e.g., providing free biofeedback sessions to firefighters during a record-breaking fire season).

Short Features: These segments last less than 10 minutes and are often included within a news program. Increase your odds of coverage by tying in your business with another soft news event, such as a health awareness week, the Great American Smokeout or a sporting event.

Talk Shows: Talk shows and live interview shows are excellent forums for introducing the public to your business and the benefits of your services. It is usually much easier to get coverage on a talk show than to arrange for a taped feature interview. Hosts are always looking for interesting guests. Some shows include audience interaction. As a wellness provider, you have an abundance of information to share with the public. Plus, if the show is on television, you can give a demonstration. I know of a massage therapist who managed to give a demonstration on the radio. He brought in a massage chair to the station and worked on the deejays while they were on the air. They relayed their experiences (along with their oohs and aahs of relaxation) to the audience while the therapist described what he was doing and the benefits of massage. The station's phone lines were ringing off the hook.

Special Programs: These programs are devoted to your specific business, your profession or your area of expertise. They last from 15 to 60 minutes. Usually you're the sole guest, but occasionally a producer chooses a program topic and slates several interviewees. Panels are another option for theme-centered shows.

Public Service Announcements (PSA): Although these announcements are usually reserved for nonprofit organizations, you can get PSA broadcast if it provides information that benefits the community.

Calendar Announcements: These announcements are often handled by the person in charge of public service announcements. The event must be free for a business owner to get it announced.

Planning Your Publicity Campaign • •

Research media outlets and design your public relations plan at least six months in advance to get the best results. Timing is critical. Sometimes publications have deadlines months before the distribution date. In some instances it may take you months or even years to get coverage.

Publicity coverage can dramatically increase your success. The disadvantage of utilizing publicity to build your practice is the lack of control. You can never be certain if or when you will get coverage or if the coverage will portray you the way you desire.

Be sure to coordinate activities to follow up your media coverage. Arrange workshops, introductory seminars and open houses to take place within three weeks and then two months after a scheduled publicity coverage.

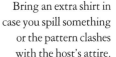

Bring an extra shirt in case you spill something or the pattern clashes with the host's attire.

Identify Media Outlets

Begin your media campaign by identifying at least 10 potential media outlets. Fill out the following information for each venue.

Print
- Publication Title
- Department
- Department Editor/Reporter
- Contact Information
- Notes

Radio
- Program Title
- Station
- Reporter/Host/Producer
- Contact Information
- Notes

Television
- Program Title
- Station
- Reporter/Host/Producer
- Contact Information
- Notes

How to Contact the Media ● ●

The mail, telephone, fax machines, email and personal delivery are all useful means to approach the media. The method chosen depends on the newsworthiness of your materials and the media representative's interest in them. Some prefer to talk with you first and others defer until they've seen your media kit. When you're confirming the media contact's name and address, you can ask the receptionist if he knows how the contact prefers to receive information.

Don't alienate the media by not playing according to their rules. Also don't hesitate to ask them what their rules are—although most of them follow certain guidelines, everyone has their own peculiarities and preferences. The most important thing to remember is to be patient, polite and courteous.

Mail ● ● ●

Mailing materials is the most common and generally preferred method to approaching the media. The major problem is the plethora of mail they receive. Call to confirm receipt of your press release or kit within two days after it should have arrived. Send the materials to a specific person. If you cannot get the name, address it to the relevant department, such as city desk editor, calendar editor or evening news producer. (See Figure 16.42 for a sample pitch letter.)

Time the mailing of your releases so they're appropriately received. Some publications have a deadline date of several months before printing. Daily newspapers prefer lead time of at least one week in advance of the date you want the announcement to appear.

Another suggestion for obtaining feedback is to include a stamped, self-addressed reply postcard. List the following questions: Are you planning to use this information? If so, when? Do you want more information? If so, what? Would you be interested in receiving materials of a similar nature in the future? Comments?

Telephone ● ● ●

At some point the media has to be contacted by telephone, either to make an initial contact or a follow-up call. Always find out first if the journalist/producer/host is free to talk. Then be brief and straight to the point. Find out which is preferred: talking about the story over the phone or sending (or resubmitting) written materials first. When making an initial contact, you're more likely to generate interest if you have several potential angles to your story. (See Figure 16.41 for sample scripts.)

Figure 16.41

Sample Telephone Scripts

Initial Phone Call

"Good morning, I'm Liza Montoya from Healing Touch Massage. Is this a good time to talk? I'm participating in a fundraiser for Health Awareness Week. I'm offering free demonstrations on self-massage techniques as well as donating five gift certificates for massages. Stress is the leading cause of illness, and massage is one of the best methods for reducing stress. I think your readers/listeners/viewers could greatly benefit by becoming more aware of the steps they can take to reduce stress and learning some simple self-massage techniques."

Follow-up to Pitch Letter

"Good afternoon, this is Liza Montoya from Healing Touch Massage. Is this a good time to talk? I'm calling about the media kit I sent, highlighting the Health Awareness Week fundraiser in which I'm participating. Health Awareness Week is approaching quickly and I was just wondering if there is any other information I can send you about myself or the fundraiser"

Subsequent Follow-up to Pitch Letter

"Good afternoon, this is Liza Montoya from Healing Touch Massage. Is this a good time to talk? We spoke several weeks ago about you interviewing me. You seemed very interested, particularly after you received my materials. We were going to discuss Oriental therapies, including techniques to relieve pain, such as headaches. Since we last talked, an article about ways to destress your life appeared in *Prevention* magazine. Taking personal responsibility for your well-being is a hot topic, and the information I can provide fits in well."

Additional Point if Contacting the Print Media

"If you're unable to do a feature, I would be willing to submit a written article."

Persistence Pays!

Faxes • • •

While faxed materials are acceptable, many people don't like to receive uninvited faxes. Plus, they never look as nice as materials printed on your letterhead. Use faxes for press releases but not media kits. When you call to confirm the name of a specific recipient, ask if that person likes to receive faxed press releases or prefers them mailed. Fax machines are more commonly used for sending follow-up materials and press releases that only request an announcement be made.

Email • • •

Like faxes, email is commonplace, but you can lose a lot of the emphasis of design layout (e.g., paper texture and color) and text italics and bolding if it isn't sent in html format or as an attachment. The positive aspect is that your release won't need to be retyped, so a harried reporter with space to fill might choose to publish your release out of convenience.

In Person • • •

Deliver your publicity materials in person to the media outlets that are the most important to you. The receptionist usually takes the materials and passes the materials to the reporter/editor/host. If you're lucky and can talk with the right person, be brief and to the point. Don't expect the person to conduct the interview right then.

Post Coverage Follow-up • • •

Whenever you get press coverage, send a thank-you note to the reporter who covered the story. Send thank-you notes to the host and producer whenever you appear on a show. It also never hurts to send a quick thank-you to the appropriate editors when your press releases get published. Acknowledgment is a vital element in building rapport. The greater your level of rapport, the more likely your next story will get the attention it deserves.

For events that you would like covered remind the newspapers, radio and TV stations the day before or the morning of the event.

Sample Television Pitch Letter

www.businessmastery.us/pitch-letter.php

Figure 16.42 Sample Print Media Pitch Letter

Healing Touch Massage

321 W. Prickly Pear Way
Needles, CA 92363
619-555-5555 • www.HealingTouchMassage.com

April 4, 2020

Alice Adams
The Desert Daily
111 Arid Lane
Needles, CA 92364

Dear Ms. Adams,

People of all ages are constantly looking for new ways to feel and look better. This search has contributed to a multibillion dollar health-food and vitamin industry. Instead of focusing on the newest, flashiest product to emerge in the marketplace, I'd like to propose an alternative viewpoint.

Massage is one of the best methods to reduce stress and increase circulation. It provides recipients with an easy, affordable manner in which to feel good. Touch has been around since the beginning of time; therapeutic touch has been around for thousands of years.

My name is Liza Montoya. I am a licensed massage therapist, in practice for six years. I specialize in Oriental therapies such as acupressure and shiatsu. I find that many people are fascinated by this approach to well-being. I believe your readers would benefit by increasing their awareness of wellness alternatives. I could also provide them with information on specific pressure points they can work themselves to relieve pain, such as headaches. If we do this as an interview, I could also arrange for you to watch a session or receive a treatment. This would provide you with a more direct experience of the work.

I've enclosed my brochure, some information on shiatsu, a fact sheet, a copy of an interview in which I was featured and a photograph.

I will call you next week to see if you're interested. I look forward to talking with you soon.

Sincerely,

Liza Montoya

Liza Montoya

Enclosures

• Community Relations •

Community relations increase your visibility and enhance your image, but only if it's clear you're doing the activities to serve the community and not just to build your business. You can cultivate these relations by: devoting your time and services to a charity or community organization; assembling a disaster relief team; giving presentations in public schools (career day, health education week); sponsoring an activity such as "adopt a highway" or a "massage-a-thon" for a special cause; developing a newsworthy persona outside of being a wellness provider; hosting your own radio show or public access cable show; giving free demonstrations; sponsoring a public interest program; and becoming a spokesperson for your profession (or even other activities you're involved in such as hobbies, sports or civic organizations).

Chapter 5, Pages 95-99
for tips on goodwill and
social responsibility.

Fundraisers •

One of the easiest ways to gain visibility and promote your practice while doing good is to donate your services for fundraising events. Target the appropriate groups according to your purpose (whether for professional advancement or personal gratification).

One idea is to choose a charity that has special meaning to you and donate a day's revenues. Send announcements to your colleagues, clients and the media informing them of the designated day and date. Depending on the type of service you provide, you could hold this "event" in a public place (check with your local zoning and licensing board first). You can make it a regular event such as once a quarter or even once a month.

*There are two ways of
spreading light: to be
the candle or the mirror
that reflects it.*
— Edith Wharton

Another option is to announce to your clients that for every specified dollar amount (say $50) they donate to your favorite charity, they get a free treatment (such as a half-hour session or an adjunct service). Caution: Communicate upfront the exact services you're offering. You may qualify recipients by requiring a copy of the check and a receipt for proof. Notify the charity and even the media.

If one of your major goals is to increase your visibility in the community, donate your services to events that are attended by people in your target market or those that are highly publicized. For major fundraising events, make certain your donation is substantial enough to be considered one of the top prizes: this increases the likelihood of you being included in all the various types of promotions, advertising and media coverage.

• Choosing a Graphic Artist •

The major promotional expense most wellness providers incur is the design and production of business cards, brochures and other visual promotional materials. Rarely is this process an easy one. Most of us "non-artists" don't know how to communicate well with people in the graphics or printing industry.

The first step is finding a good graphic artist who can take your ideas and transform them into exquisite printed materials. With the advent of desktop publishing, many people are calling themselves graphic artists when in reality they're adept word processors—they can make type look good on a page and even insert your artwork in an attractive manner; a true artist can turn your basic concept into a magnificent finished product.

To select an appropriate graphic artist, get recommendations from your colleagues. Interview prospective artists. Look at their portfolios. Find out the types of clients they have. Ask if they've ever worked with any wellness providers in general and your field specifically.

After choosing an artist, give the artist a sample session. One of the best brochures I had was designed by a graphic artist who was also a client. Since he had a direct experience of me and my work, he was better able to translate that into a brochure.

Some people are clear about what they want in their promotional pieces (particularly brochures), while others don't even know where to start. You can save yourself considerable time and money by giving your artist all (or most of) the written material. (Graphic artists aren't necessarily advertising copy geniuses.) Be certain that the design and content of your promotional pieces are appropriate for your target markets, establish your credibility, and focus on the benefits you provide.

Occasionally, things just don't work out and you need to cut your losses and find another artist. Personalities and communication styles don't always mesh.

Contents •

Most of the dissatisfaction involved in designing promotional materials stems from three areas: the final product not matching your expectations, the project taking longer than anticipated, and being charged more than you budgeted. The one step you can take to avoid misunderstandings is to create a written contract that clearly delineates the job and the responsibilities of both you and the artist.

Figure 16.43

Contract Tips

- A precise description of the project (e.g., design a two-color brochure with at least two photos and one graphic image; create gift certificates; design layout for office sign; and alter current letterhead, envelopes and business cards to match new brochure).
- A listing of the major steps involved and the person responsible.
- A timeline of target dates for all of the major phases and the final date of completion.
- A description of what exactly you're to furnish.
- A detailed estimate of the cost (including what constitutes possible additional charges—for instance, how many alterations are included in the base price).
- Clarification of who actually "owns" the artwork. If you don't put this into your agreement, you may discover (to your dismay) that you can only use items, such as a logo, on the specific materials designed by the artist.
- An explanation of how the final work will be done: Will you be given the final printed product, a computer disk or camera-ready art? If you're given art, will you be provided with color separations?
- A recourse policy if either party fails to meet stated responsibilities (e.g., the artist is three weeks late or you dislike the final product).

If you have concerns or ideas, don't wait to express them until you receive the final proof. Keep in mind that you can renegotiate along the way. If you or the artist decide to alter something, make sure you're advised of the possible repercussions in terms of time and cost. If a change is extensive, define what it involves in writing so both parties continue to have a clear idea of each other's expectations—especially the cost parameters. You may decide the proposed change isn't worth the cost.

Your printed marketing materials are your major promotional tools. They should be attractive and effectively communicate who you are and the benefits of your service. When you find an artist who is in sync with you and can translate your ideas into graphic images, invest the time in developing and nurturing that relationship—it can be invaluable to your career.

• Marketing Action Plan •

A marketing action plan defines goals for daily, weekly, monthly and annual marketing activities. Plan to invest at least 15 percent of your time in marketing activities to maintain your practice. To successfully grow your practice, you may need to spend two to three times this amount of time. The following sample marketing action plan is based on eight hours per week.

Figure 16.44

Marketing Actions

Daily
- Give clients samples, premiums, educational materials and discount coupons for friends.
- Confirm the next day's appointments.
- Place three phone calls to prospective clients, and follow-up calls to current clients.
- Demonstrate or incorporate at least one product per session.
- Review client files prior to each session.

Weekly
- Distribute 75 business cards, 50 brochures and 25 fliers.
- Call one allied wellness provider to initiate an affiliation or to follow up.
- Attend one networking function.
- Spend at least one hour working on a long-term project.
- Contact one group regarding a future speaking engagement.
- Send birthday cards and notes to clients.

Monthly
- Spend at least two hours reviewing your marketing plan and doing research.
- Meet with a business support group twice.
- Send two letters of introduction to allied wellness providers.
- Meet with two allied wellness providers.
- Give two presentations.
- Send out press releases about your public speaking engagements.
- Donate services to your favorite charity.
- Tabulate information from Client Comment Cards and make necessary changes.
- Work with the media: send press releases and kits, do appropriate follow-up.

Quarterly
- Hold one open house, do a "party," and sponsor an event.
- Update client educational materials and rearrange the product display area.
- Send a newsletter to clients, colleagues and prospects.
- Offer some type of special promotion, and do a cooperative marketing project.
- Read at least one practice-building book.
- Get interviewed by the paper, radio, television or a specialty publication.

Annually
- Participate in at least two trade shows, fairs or expos.
- Send out a client survey.
- Attend at least one practice-building workshop.

• Marketing Ideas from A to Z •

A

- **Acknowledgments:** Always thank the person, company or organization that refers a client to you. Make sure to acknowledge others when they've been helpful—either in writing or with a small token of appreciation.

- **Advice Column:** Write an advice column regarding your field for a local publication. Not only is this educational, it builds your credibility by demonstrating your degree of expertise.

- **Announcements:** Inexpensive promotional tools to enhance your visibility and keep you connected. Send to your current clients and select prospective clients to announce special offers, speaking engagements and changes that occur in your practice.

- **Articles:** Write articles for magazines, newspapers, trade journals, in-house publications and newsletters published by other organizations.

- **Auctions:** Donating services/products for silent and not-so-silent auctions provides you with free exposure and support for your community.

B

- **Bags:** Imprint bags with your company name, logo and position statement. Many people reuse bags, so your information gets seen repeatedly.

- **Banners:** Used at a booth or special event, they can include your name, slogan or logo.

- **Benefits:** Donating services or products as door prizes gives you publicity and shows your interest in helping in your community.

- **Billboard Advertising:** Seen by many people and is a good way of informing the public about you and your services. Look for high-traffic locations such as well-traveled main streets and intersections. Keep your copy short and to the point.

- **Breakfasts:** Speak at local business "breakfast" clubs. Having breakfast with potential networking associates is a great way to start your day.

C

- **Canvassing:** Take brochures, cards or fliers to area businesses letting them know you're there, who you are and what you can do for them. Distribute information to your target markets.

- **Celebrations:** Celebrate milestones (e.g., opening, moving, anniversary, 100th client), and invite your clients, colleagues and prospective clients to celebrate with you. Provide refreshments, music and fun.

- **Classified Ads:** There are many possible places to place ads such as newspapers, trade journals, magazines, local business and health papers and event programs (e.g., tournaments, concerts, fundraisers).

- **Columnists:** Some write stories or series of articles on health-related issues; find out about the columnists in your area and propose an interview or provide information to them.

- **Comment Cards:** Give your clients the opportunity to voice their opinions about you and your company. Include one in your Welcome Kit, stack them in the waiting area, and mail them to all your clients at least once a year.

- **Conferences:** Attending or participating in service- or product-related conferences is another form of marketing and public exposure. Again, use that booth you designed to your best advantage.

- **Connections with Others:** Let other related businesses know you will display signs and have information available in your office if they do the same for you.

- **Consultations:** A free consultation gives you the opportunity to demonstrate your expertise, answer questions and hand out information. Also, offer free services for local special events.

- **Contests:** People love to play games! Contests bring attention to your business and add names to your mailing list. It's best to get people to come to your business to enter.

- **Coupons:** Terrific for marketing to prospective clients (e.g., 50 percent off the first visit) and rewarding loyal ones (one free session after each 10 visits). Coupons don't cheapen your practice if they're tastefully done. Many wellness providers offer introductory specials.

D

- **Demonstrations:** Allow prospective clients to experience firsthand your services and products.

- **Direct Calling:** Speaking directly with potential clients, other professionals, networking associates and your clients adds the personal touch to your marketing strategy.

- **Direct Mail:** Postcards, fliers, catalogs, notices and announcements are inexpensive methods of staying in communication with your clients.

- **Direct Mail Coupons or Card Packs:** Coupons are given to and compiled by companies and mailed to target markets; participants share in the mailing costs.

- **Direct Referrals:** Referring clients directly to other professionals is one of the strongest threads in networking and is usually reciprocal. Setting up a network of related services and products is one of the best tools for effective business growth.

- **Directories:** Take out listings in appropriate directories. Publish a directory of local allied wellness providers to be given away at major events, mailed out in promotional campaigns and distributed to other wellness providers.

- **Discount Sales:** Giving a discount can help a prospective client decide to try your services and products. Used for rewards, introductions and referrals.

- **Display Kudos:** Frame and display any press, complimentary letters and awards where they can be seen. This allows others to see your dedication and service to your profession. If you have too many to display at once, rotate them regularly.

- **Donate Services to Charities:** Even donating an hour a week to a community cause or charity creates goodwill and word-of-mouth marketing.

E

- **Emergencies:** Coordinate an emergency response team of wellness providers to be ready during tough times like floods, hurricanes, fires or blizzards.

- **Expos and Health Fairs:** Participating in these events is an excellent venue for networking: gives you exposure to other professionals in your field as well as their products and services; provides an opportunity to meet potential clients; and makes use of that booth you created.

F

- **Flea Markets:** This is a place where you can reach large numbers of people while demonstrating your products and services.

- **Fliers:** Announce upcoming events, sales and changes in service; whatever is happening with your business that the public needs to know about. In addition to posting them around town, mail at least 25 per week to prospective clients.

- **Free of Charge:** Once in awhile, do something free of charge for your clients; perhaps a modality such as a hot pack, or upon seeing they're enjoying having their feet rubbed, let them know and give them an extra five minutes.

- **Frequent Buyer Cards:** Offer an exclusive discount on products or services to frequent clients. Give a free session or product after a set number of sessions (e.g., "Your 11th session is free!") or dollar amount of purchases.

G

- **Gifts:** Instead of always giving candy or food as gifts, help enrich someone's mind with a book, an inspirational bookmark or a mug with a meaningful message. Establish goodwill and loyalty by giving small gifts to employees for work well done or for when the go that extra mile they go for you.

- **Gift Certificates:** Wonderful way for clients to share their experience with others and a great marketing tool for you. Keep in mind that the profit isn't generated from the sale of the certificate but from the subsequent sessions.

- **Golf Resorts:** Post a sign offering a free session to members who have made a verifiable hole-in-one.

- **Grand Openings:** This is a "grand" way of letting people know who you are, where you are and what you're all about.

- **Greeting Cards:** These are a good method of connecting with clients, networking associates and referring professionals just to wish them good tidings.

H

- **Health Clubs:** Submit a proposal for the health club to purchase gift certificates to give as an incentive to new members who pay in full upon initiation or when members reach a milestone goal.

- **Holidays:** Decorate your office to match the holiday, offer special discounts for holidays, and give specialty gifts (e.g., cinnamon-scented oil for Thanksgiving, sports bottles for the Summer Solstice).

I

- **Introductory Letters:** Send letters to allied wellness providers to develop mutual referrals. Send at least two letters each week until you have amassed your desired network.

- **Introductory Seminars:** The focus is introducing your services or products to prospective clients. Having introductory prices available helps fence sitters make a move in your direction.

- **Invitations:** Can be hand-delivered, verbal or mailed. Invite people to see your facilities, come to a free demonstration or call for information.

J

- **Jargon:** Avoid using jargon unless you're certain your listener knows the terminology.

- **Jingle:** Create a catchy tune and phrase that easily identifies your company (particularly for radio and television advertising).

K

- **Keynote Speeches:** Advise your professional associations and community organizations that you're available as a keynote speaker.

- **Kiosks:** Post promotional materials on kiosks at malls, colleges and pavilions. Check for regulations first.

L

- **Lectures:** Giving lectures on your service or products provides credibility to you as a professional, educates the public and becomes a vehicle for sales.

- **Little Things:** Make doing little things for clients a matter of business policy. These little things help establish client loyalty.

- **Location:** This is an important component to the success of a business. A poor location can break a business even if your service and products are good. If you're in an area that is inconvenient or unsafe, people will seek out other providers.

- **Logo:** A graphic representation of your business that helps people quickly recognize your company.

M

- **Mailing Lists:** Keep accurate lists of clients, prospects, practitioners, networking associates and companies or individuals in related fields. Trade lists with others who provide services or products to your target markets.

- **Memberships:** Join professional associations, business groups and service organizations.

- **Mistakes:** We all make them, and the best way to handle them is with no excuses—just plain honesty. Create a "goof gift" to give to clients when you or a staff member makes a mistake.

N

- **Networking:** Join networking organizations, community organizations, clubs; and participate in community special events. Networking is a great way to establish trust and build professional relationships.

- **Newcomers Welcome Kit:** Send a kit to new clients as soon as they book their first appointment. Include several business cards, brochure, pertinent information, product samples and educational or promotional materials on the benefits of your services or products.

- **Newsletters:** Used as a consistent marketing tool, they establish your expertise and educate the public. Newsletters can also be sent to other health professionals and potential clients for marketing purposes. Another idea is to write articles or place ads in others' newsletters.

- **Newspaper:** Submit opinion pieces, articles, letters to the editor, press releases and calendar listings. Get a newspaper reporter to interview you. Also place display and classified ads.

O

- **Open Houses:** Hold quarterly and special holiday open houses for colleagues, businesses in your community, prospects and clients.

- **Order Forms for Product Sales:** Have these available for quick, impulse sales as well as for those who like to ponder. The elements to successful product sales are quality, availability and convenience.

P

- **Painted Cars and Car Signs:** Provides great coverage as you go through your day; draws attention as it's unusual to see unique, eye-catching things on cars.

- **Package Deals:** Putting together packages for services and products that save clients money can improve sales without increasing marketing costs.

- **Pamphlets:** Detailed information about you, your services, philosophy, mission statement, benefits, specific techniques and health tips.

- **Park or Street Bench Advertising:** Place ads on benches that are seen by your target markets (e.g., in front of stores they patronize).

- **Personalized gift items:** Also known as premiums and specialty advertising. Keep an assortment of inexpensive, fun, useful items to give away.

- **Postcards:** Fast, easy and inexpensive method of reminding clients of follow-ups, appointments, announcements or just saying hello. Also a good technique for generating new clients.

- **Professional Journals:** Not only a good place to advertise, but also to write articles and make yourself known. Writing adds to your credibility as a professional.

- **Public Service Tie-In:** Sponsor events such as the blood donor mobile unit, police fingerprint unit for children or fire department home safety seminars.

- **Public Speaking:** Give talks at business associations, clubs and public service organizations. Join an organization like Toastmasters to learn platform-speaking.

Q

- **Qualify:** Design your marketing materials so that they actually pre-screen clients.

- **Quotes:** Use quotes from people who are prominent within your target market.

R

- **Radio:** Take an ad, sponsor a program, become a guest speaker on local talk shows or host a wellness talk show.

- **Raffles and Prizes:** Providing services or products for special events for raffles and prizes helps in getting your name out to the public.

- **Referral Cards:** These cards encourage clients to promote your practice.

- **Referral Networks:** Essential as a marketing tool; not only benefits you but provides the opportunity for you to assist others with their growth and prosperity.

- **Rewards, Incentives and Gifts:** Submit proposals for companies to offer your services for customer or employee rewards. They could offer certificates for sales incentives, to honor employees of the month, to use as premiums with their customers and to give as holiday gifts for employees (it's certainly classier than a gift certificate for a frozen turkey).

S

- **Scholarships:** Sponsor an academic or sports scholarship for children, young adults or members of your target markets.

- **Scripts:** Providing your employees with scripts for various circumstances helps guide them in representing your business to its optimum and aids in deterring the disasters "winging it" can create.

- **Seminars:** Establishes you as an authority in your field, lends credibility, provides a catalyst for your services and products, and educates the public.

- **Sign Language:** Learn to communicate in sign language so you can offer services to the hearing impaired.

- **Signs (Indoors):** Hang signs and posters announcing specials. Emphasize services such as "Gift Certificates Available."

- **Signs (Outdoors):** Your sign should be clear and large enough to be easily seen. Include your logo if economically feasible. Your location sign needs to be easily and quickly identifiable.

- **Special Events:** Encourage publicity by being a sponsor of (or participating in) local events or holding unusual events at your place of business.

- **Special Promos and Displays:** Boost marketing efforts with "in-store" displays featuring your products, cards, brochures and fliers that explain your services and benefits. Attract business by providing discount fliers that can be redeemed at the time of the appointment.

- **Sponsor an Athletic Team:** Print T-shirts with your name and logo for the team to wear; show up at the games to support your team; and display a sign in your office that says, "Proud sponsor of the ABC Cycling Team!"

- **Sponsor an Event or Community Activity:** Involves your business in the community and helps you meet potential clients.

- **Sporting Events:** Volunteer your services at local sporting events, Senior and Special Olympics.

- **Statement Stuffers:** Include information about specific products or services whenever you send out statements to clients. You can also place your brochure in other people's billing statements (just make sure they go to your target markets).

- **Surveys and Questionnaires:** Great way to get the "pulse" of your clients and discover what you're doing right and what needs to be changed: find out what clients want, like, dislike and their opinion of your services.

T

- **Television:** Become a guest on local television shows. Place commercials which demonstrate your services or products and their benefits—fully utilize the dynamics of music, words and pictures.

- **Testimonials:** Nothing hits home like personal accounts of the success of your products and services; use in marketing tools, advertising and seminars. Always use full names and if possible the title, company and city.

- **Theme Festival:** Band together with nearby businesses and hold a gala event such as "Spring Festival" or "Winter Warm-Ups."

- **Theme Week:** Devote a week to a particular activity (e.g., Mobility Week), and set up activities centering on mobility issues. Coordinate with your local government to sponsor city-wide events.

- **Trade Directory:** Advertise in local trade directories. They are usually the first place people look when they want your specific service and/or products.

- **Trainings:** Training other professionals establishes your credibility and expertise. They range from an evening class to a weeklong intensive training.

U

- **Umbrellas:** If you live in a rainy city, purchase a stock of umbrellas with your logo imprinted on them to loan or give to clients who forget their own.

- **Uniforms:** Create a unique, professional image by putting your logo, position statement or favorite design on clothing.

V

- **Vacation Nights:** Sponsor a "health" vacation with guest speakers, activities, drawings and show slides (e.g., spa destinations, great places to hike and boat).

- **Videotapes/DVDs:** A unique method of presenting and demonstrating your services and products which can be left with other professionals for marketing; have clients view them while waiting to see you; use as part of a proposal for a corporate contract; and show as an educational tool for the public.

- **VIPs:** Turn your customers into VIPs. Give them the opportunity to avail themselves of special sales and promotions.

W

- **Welcome Wagon:** This organization greets new residents in specific neighborhoods and delivers gifts and coupons from local businesses.

- **Window and Store Front Displays:** Create an inviting display showing your services or products; make it colorful and catchy to grab the public's attention, and change it frequently. These can also be created at related businesses, not just your own. Some malls even rent "Window Display" areas in front of vacant stores or have special display alcoves.

- **Word-of-Mouth:** One of the most powerful resources for business; satisfied and dissatisfied clients talk and talk and talk....

- **Workshops:** Conduct workshops or classes in your area. Advertise in newspapers and local magazines, mail fliers and hang posters. Do free lectures which you can advertise at no cost by sending out PSAs to print media and radio stations.

- **Writing Articles:** Good method of demonstrating knowledge in your field, educating the public and making yourself known.

X

- **X-Rays:** If you're a chiropractor or dentist, offer free x-rays as part of the initial visit.

Y

- **Yellow Pages:** Used extensively by the public for locating services. Place your listing under the most logical category if you can only afford one listing; otherwise list under each applicable category.

Z

- **Zoological society:** Sponsor an animal or event at your local zoo. Sponsorships are often published in the society's newsletters, and if the contribution is significant, the zoo might even place a plaque (with your name) on its premises.

Client Retention

17

• Beyond Customer Service •

A thriving practice consists of a strong base of clients who receive your services regularly, as well as a steady stream of new clients. Unfortunately, many practitioners become so focused on efforts to attract new clients that they overlook simple ways to enhance client retention. It is easy to understand how this can happen—new clients are vital to growing a business. However, this is only half of the success formula; retaining existing clients is the other half.

The good news is that you can easily master the art of retaining valued clients with a minimal investment of time and effort. The trick is that the effort must be consistent to succeed. This chapter highlights time-tested ways to enhance your customer service so you can avoid the mistake of underemphasizing client retention.

The core of client retention is a solid customer service plan. At the heart of all top-notch customer service plans is one thing—a consistent, careful and creative effort to build strong relationships with clients. In marketing lingo this is referred to as relationship-based marketing, and it involves truly caring about how you can best serve your client's needs. In essence you become your client's partner in wellness. It isn't about convincing or selling; it's about listening, planning, educating and being proactive. It means going the extra mile to attune to your clients' needs and taking the time to express your appreciation for their business.

People will forget what you said. People will forget what you did. But people will never forget how you make them feel.
— Bonnie Wasmund

Figure 17.1

What Clients Want

- Convenience
- Safety
- Efficiency
- Understanding
- Value
- Accessibility
- Courtesy

- Reliability
- Compassion
- Integrity
- Attention
- Acceptance
- Professionalism
- Expertise

Customer Service Levels •

As in any business, levels of customer service in the wellness field can vary. To give you a picture of these levels, following is a brief description of minimal customer service, good customer service and exceptional customer service.

Minimal Customer Service • •

According to Tom Mills of Howard Services (the company's specialty is "mystery shoppers"), nine out of 10 people who have a bad experience won't tell a manager. Seven of those people won't return.

For wellness providers, minimal customer service means that you care about your clients, they feel comfortable and safe, your actions are professional and you meet reasonable requests.

Facilitate Clients' Achieving Their Treatment Goal • • •

Concentrate on addressing clients' major goals; if you're a somatic practitioner, focus on the specific requested areas or incorporate other modalities. Keep accurate client files, customize each treatment, stay focused during sessions and be prompt and prepared. Do good work, be a good listener and respect clients.

Use High-Quality Products • • •

Purchase a reliable, sturdy table (with side or length extensions if the table is too small for some of your clients). Provide a variety of lubricants and skin care products and keep an ample supply of clean linens and accessories such as sheets, gowns, bolsters, blankets, pillows, towels and tissues. Maintain a wide selection of music.

Run Your Practice in a Manner That Demonstrates Your Concern • • •

Greet clients cheerfully with a smile and a handshake. Have water for clients to drink before, during and after their session. Share information and resources. Send thank-you notes for referrals. Adhere to a code of ethics. Have an appointment schedule available. Return calls within 24 hours and make confirmation calls. Send appointment reminders when sessions are more than one month apart and call new clients within two days after their initial session. Inspire trust and keep confidences. Be enthusiastic about every meeting—whether it's the first or fiftieth.

Good Customer Service • •

Good customer service includes all of the activities under "Minimal Customer Service" plus going the extra step to meet requests. For example, a client shows up for an appointment experiencing a headache. A baseline customer service response would be to focus attention on that condition. Good customer service would include utilizing modalities, equipment or products that aren't necessarily part of your usual routine, and lengthening the duration of the session if necessary (and appropriate) until the headache is alleviated.

Quality is meeting customer expectations at a competitive price.
— Thad Barrington

Take a Client-Centered Approach • • •

Develop a long-term wellness/treatment plan with each client. Respond to requests, such as those regarding pressure or modalities. Provide referrals to other practitioners who could do even more with your client. Refrain from talking too much about yourself and keep conversations client-oriented. Conduct thorough intake interviews with regular follow-up assessments. Utilize appropriate equipment. Demonstrate self-care techniques (e.g., stretches) and provide handouts. Review client files prior to appointments.

Make Your Office Environment Comfortable and Inviting • • •

Install a dimmer control for the lighting and use flannel sheets in the winter. Place an oversized stepstool near the table and hang a hook or shelf on the wall for clients' personal belongings. Use clients' favorite types of products. Allow clients a few minutes to just lie there before having to get up. If you are a touch therapist, provide access to a shower on premises and towel off oil if necessary.

Exceptional Customer Service • •

Exceptional customer service requires that you be proactive—anticipating what your clients want—and making those services available. You must know your clients well. This involves taking the time to ask clients about their preferences and thinking ahead about what they might want. When you provide what they need before they know it, your clients appreciate your extra attention and think the world of you. Exceptional customer service incorporates all the activities listed above plus the following communication, session-oriented activities, practice management and support activities.

Mastery is not something that strikes in an instant, like a thunderbolt, but a gathering power that moves steadily through time, like weather.
— John Gardner

Elevate the Therapeutic Relationship to a Wellness Partnership with Clients • • •

Always review a clients' charts before their sessions. Before you do any hands-on work, update the clients' long-term treatment plans and set specific goals for the current sessions. Depending on the type of work you do, consider taking before and after photographs to visually document progress. Take the time to research potentially effective techniques or other recommended services for specific client conditions, and prepare handouts of resources and referrals of other wellness providers. Place a check-in call the day after the first session and whenever a client experiences dramatic changes from your work.

Take a Proactive Approach to Communications • • •

Practice active listening and encourage feedback. Recognize that some clients may have difficulties at times in clearly expressing their needs. Be prepared to act as a communication coach.

Pamper Your Clients • • •

Pamper your clients with state-of-the-art equipment such as a hydraulic table, ergonomic positioning cushions and a luxuriously padded face cradle. Use fine linens, heated booties and mittens, and specialty products (e.g., aromatherapy, sports creams, custom-blended oils, personalized skin care formulations and customized herbal formulations). Provide an assortment of beverages such as juices, herbal teas and personal bottles of filtered water (with your sticker attached to the bottles). If it's cold outside, warm the table or chair with a full-length heated mattress pad and take the chill off any equipment. If you are a touch therapist, have hot packs ready and prepare a warm foot bath. If the weather is warm, be sure that the room temperature is mild and the lights are dimmed. Touch therapists can also offer clients a cool foot bath and a chilled eye pillow in the summer.

Design a Luxurious Office Environment • • •

Furnish your office comfortably, including a private area where clients can put their belongings. Appeal to your clients' senses by hanging beautiful artwork, and calm them with soothing sounds from an in-room water fountain and an excellent sound system.

Raise the Bar in Your Practice Management Activities • • •

Incorporate excellent customer service into the day-to-day running of your practice. Return phone calls within two hours. Provide insurance billing. Refer people to your clients' businesses. If you know a client prefers a specific time slot, do your best to keep it available. Send personalized letters to your potential clients, announcing who you are and what you do. Undergo semi-annual peer review, and have your clients evaluate your services annually. Review all client files monthly; look for trends, note if several people are making similar requests, and initiate appropriate changes.

Make Your Clients Feel Special • • •

Offer a free treatment, product or adjunct service on special occasions such as birthdays. Send an anniversary card from their first appointment with you. Give clients something for every referral—either a sample product, a 15-minute session or a free adjunct service such as a paraffin treatment. Ask clients to give you feedback either verbally or on a comment card. Invite clients to test a new product or service before you offer it to the general public. Offer incentives (see Figure 17.6) and freebies. Post published newspaper or magazine articles about your clients' achievements in your office and on your website (with their permission, of course, so as not to violate confidentiality).

The ultimate lesson all of us have to learn is unconditional love, which includes not only others but ourselves as well.
—Elisabeth Kübler-Ross

Support Client's Well-Being Outside of Sessions • • •

Stock books and products that can be beneficial to clients—particularly items that aren't readily available at local emporiums: books on stretching, wellness, carpal tunnel syndrome, workplace ergonomics and self-massage; stretching equipment such as exercise balls and bands; herbs and poultices; massage tools such as rollers and eye pillows; and specialty lotions, sports creams, skin care products and aromatherapy supplies. Keep in touch by sending clients announcements, newsletters, and newspaper or magazine clippings on topics in which they've expressed interest. Hold events such as monthly open houses, demonstrations and free workshops for clients and their guests.

Customer Service Action Plans •

Customer service action plans grow and evolve throughout your career. The first step in developing a plan is to create a customer service mission statement. It might help to ask yourself what you want clients to say about your level of customer service. If you have been in practice for a while, also survey your current clients for feedback on the items they deem important.

Client Comment Cards • •

Client comment cards are a great tool for obtaining feedback on how your clients feel about you and your practice. These cards make it safe and convenient for clients to share suggestions, compliments or complaints.

They are easy to produce and usually cost-effective. Most people complete comment cards—whether it's for the offered premium, the opportunity to vent, or simply because they want to assist you in improving your practice. It works best to mail these cards to clients' homes. Print them as postage-paid response cards to make it convenient for clients to send their comments to you. The next best option is to put a "Client Comment" drop box near the exit.

Remember, on the average it costs six times as much money and takes three times the effort getting a new client as retaining one.

Figure 17.2

Comment Card Design Tips

- Use high-quality card stock and make sure the type is large enough to read.
- Create an attention-grabbing headline.
- Mainly ask questions for which the responses can be checked off or filled in with a rating.
- Ask several open-ended questions.
- Request a name, address and phone number.
- Include your name (or someone else in your office) on the return address.

Customer Service Action Plan

- Draft your customer service mission statement.
- Outline your goals and list the actions you commit to take.
- Answer the following questions for each activity:
  1. Is this important to my clients?
  2. How will this add value for my clients?
  3. Is this the best use of my time and resources?
  4. How will my clients know about these actions?

Customer service techniques are only powerful if your clients are aware of them. You could implement major changes, but if your clients aren't directly informed, they might never notice.

There is one caveat to customer service actions: Never implement a customer service activity that you aren't willing to consistently continue. Once your clients become accustomed to a certain level of treatment, they expect it and are offended if you are remiss. Ultimately the key to going beyond customer service is to inspire your clients to move from a space of client satisfaction to one of client enthusiasm. Ideally this results in "glowing reviews" that naturally translate into word-of-mouth referrals.

Figure 17.3

10 Phrases for Poor Customer Service

"I don't do that."
"Can you call back later?"
"That's not my problem."
"It's against policy."
"You don't understand."
"What do you expect me to do about it?"
"Let me put you on hold."
"I'll get around to it."
"No one's ever complained before."
"Make it quick."

• Prevent No-Shows •

The client retention process begins before you actually see a client for the first time. This is where the pre-interview comes into play. Whenever new clients book an appointment, take the time to make them comfortable. Ascertain if they have any concerns or questions and address them. Get them involved from the beginning. Find out what they need and explain how your specific abilities can support them (or refer them to an appropriate allied professional).

Just because a new or returning client schedules a session, it doesn't mean he will show up. You can reduce the number of no-shows by incorporating the following tips into your office procedures.

Figure 17.4

Tips to Reduce No-Shows

- Send a welcome letter, your brochure and information about your practice prior to the first appointment (preferably immediately after the telephone call when the session is booked).
- Ideally, send a "Welcome to My Office" kit (see Figure 17.5). Items to include in this kit are: a personalized welcome letter; your specific practice brochure; a pamphlet describing (in friendly language) what a client can expect from your services, what they need to do to prepare for the session, your policies and your procedures; several business cards; client intake and health history forms; a sample gift certificate, your recent newsletter; a map to your office (if it's not already on the back of your brochure); and other promotional materials (e.g., a copy of a published interview). This may sound like a lot of material, but the few dollars it costs to assemble and mail this kit demonstrates your professionalism and concern about your clients.
- Confirm appointments by telephoning your clients the day before their sessions, sending reminder notes or both.
- Give clients an appointment reminder card to take home. Include your cancellation policy on this card.
- Give clients a copy of their treatment plan.
- If applicable, offer home assignments or a list of wellness tips that are designed to assist clients in attaining their wellness goals.

Sometimes we stare so long at a door that is closing that we see too late the one that is open.
— Alexander Graham Bell

If you follow these steps, you will minimize the no-show factor and won't be so disconcerted if the occasional last-minute cancellation or no-show occurs. I've found that when this has happened to me—it was perfect. Either I wanted to do something else anyway or another client would call wanting to come in right away (and fill the vacant appointment slot).

Figure 17.5 Welcome to My Office Kit

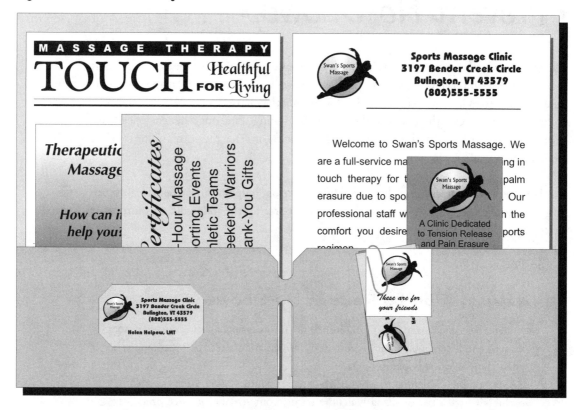

The Client

... is the most important person in our business.

... is the reason for our work, not an interruption.

... is doing us a favor by purchasing our services and goods.

... is a feeling human being.

... is someone who wants a break—to be taken care of.

... is the person who enables us to earn an income.

... is deserving of the best service we can offer.

• Incentive Programs •

Incentive plans serve to reward loyal clients and to create a way to increase the session frequency for others who simply can't afford to receive treatments as often as desired. The following ideas are geared to spark your creativity. Adapt them for your specific needs and desired results.

Figure 17.6

Top 10 Incentive Ideas

- Offer prepaid package discounts such as: purchase three sessions and receive a 10 percent discount; seven sessions qualifies for a 20 percent discount; purchase eight sessions and receive two for free.
- Present clients with a Frequent Buyer Card. This can be done in two ways: clients receive a free session after seeing you for a set number of sessions, (e.g., "Buy 10, Get Your 11th Session Free!"); or give a free session for a specific number of sessions a client receives within a certain period of time (e.g., "Receive 5 Treatments in 2 Months and your 6th treatment is Free!").
- Provide a certificate for 50 percent off the client's next session whenever a client refers a new client.
- Send clients an "I Enjoyed Working with You" packet. After a client's first visit, send a greeting card that states it was a pleasure working with her and that you look forward to helping her achieve her wellness goals. Include a coupon for a complimentary adjunct service or product to be used with her next appointment.
- Give clients a half-hour session certificate for every referral.
- Give clients an adjunct service for every referral.
- Have clients sponsor a demonstration party—and thus receive at least one free session, with the potential for many more.
- Offer holiday specials: For example a touch therapist could allow clients to purchase half-hour certificates at half price with every full-hour session they purchase. These half-hour certificates can be combined for full sessions or given as gifts.
- Give a free mini-session for birthdays.
- Offer a two-for-one Valentine's Day special.

Your incentive program need not be limited to your hands-on work. For all the previous examples you can substitute products, adjunct services and seminar registrations.

These incentive suggestions serve a dual purpose—they acknowledge your current clients, and many of the ideas provide a means to inspire referrals from your clients. It's wonderful to combine client retention techniques with your promotional endeavors. However, don't rely on your clients to build your practice. It isn't their responsibility. They may be uncomfortable telling others about your services—many consider their wellness an extremely private matter.

• Rebook Clients •

The rebooking process is a natural extension of your session. People rebook when they feel comfortable with you, value your services and are confident that they will get their desired results. I can count on one hand the clients that weren't regulars throughout my career as a massage practitioner and a rebirther. I took the position that I would work with clients until their goals were accomplished, which, in massage, can be a lifetime commitment! I attracted the clients who felt the same way. The exceptions were if I knew in advance that I would only work with them once or twice (e.g., they were visiting from out of town).

The situation is similar in my coaching practice. Occasionally, someone sets up a one-time appointment to discuss specific concerns or questions, but most of my clients work with me until they've reached the next level in their business. The rest consult with me when they need it (e.g., once a quarter or even once a year). Some of these client relationships have continued for decades!

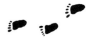

Chapter 6, Pages 116-117

for tips on creating treatment plans.

If you do thorough intake interviews in which your clients identify their long-term and short-term wellness goals, and you develop a treatment plan together, then you already know if they want to book and approximately how often. Sometimes practitioners feel awkward asking when a client wants to return. Avoid saying, "Would you like to book another session?" A better way to phrase the question is, "When would you like your next session?"

Session Completion Protocol •

Your session doesn't really end until your client walks out the door. After the technical one-on-one work is done (e.g., the massage is over, the nutritional consultation is conducted, the movement instruction is finished), it's time to do the session completion protocol. Briefly review what occurred in the session, highlight some of the client's major goals, assign homework, give the client an opportunity to ask questions, make any necessary referrals and schedule the next appointment. Give the client several of your cards and brochures, a copy of his treatment plan (or offer to email it later) and any appropriate educational handouts.

If you don't follow a session completion protocol, I still recommend asking the client, "When would you like to schedule another session?" If the client appears hesitant, suggest he calls you back when he has his appointment book handy. Don't be pushy. Tell him that you hope to hear from him soon and send him off with the appropriate educational and marketing materials.

Post Session Follow-Up •

Follow the action items defined in the Exceptional Customer Service section, such as placing a check-in call the day after the first session and whenever a client experiences dramatic changes from your work. A couple of days later, send an "I Enjoyed Working with You" packet. If the client still doesn't rebook, follow the steps below on how to reconnect with past clients.

Figure 17.7

Rebooking Materials

- Welcome to My Office kit
- Appointment Book
- Appointment Reminder Card
- Client Treatment Plan Copy
- Brochures
- Business Cards
- "I Enjoyed Working with You" packet
- Frequent Buyer Cards
- Greeting Cards
- Newsletters
- Coupons
- Client Comment Cards
- Client Survey Letters
- Educational Handouts

• Transition Practicum Clients •

You can jump-start your practice by building business with clients you worked with while in school. Keep in mind that it can be a shock for clients to make the transition from paying nothing or a nominal fee to your standard rate. Upon graduation you may lose many clients if they're abruptly required to double or triple that amount. Ease this transition by offering them a lower rate that gradually increases over time until they are at the standard rate. You never know, they may offer to pay your standard rate anyway.

Shortly before you are ready to open your practice, send a thank-you letter to your practicum clients to formalize your new status as a credentialed wellness practitioner, and offer a special transition program. See Figure 17.8 for a sample letter to help you transition practicum clients to your standard rate in a gracious and businesslike manner. It is highly likely your clients will appreciate your professionalism and special consideration, and choose to schedule ongoing sessions.

There are no traffic jams along the extra mile.
— Roger Staubach

Figure 17.8 Sample Transition Letter

Essential Wellness
123 Breezeway • Tucson, AZ • 520-555-8787
essentialwellness@example.com • www.essentialwellness.com

December 14, 2020

Susan Mountain
1212 Winding Way
Tucson, AZ 85750

Dear Susan,

I greatly appreciate your confidence in me and the support you've given me throughout my schooling. Now that my educational program and cerification are complete, my rate for new clients is $60 for a one-hour session. Because I value your longstanding support, I am pleased to extend you the following special rates: For the next three months, your rate will be only $35 per session: the following three months, your rate will be $50 per session. After that, the rate will be $60 per session. This special rate takes effect as of January 1st.

Wishing you health and happiness,

Marie Everybody

Marie Everybody

• Recapture Lost Clientele •

At this point you may be thinking, "It's time to increase my effectiveness and work smarter by incorporating a customer service plan and a client retention program for active and new clients." Excellent plan, but what about those inactive clients—the ones you haven't seen in months or perhaps even years? You may still retrieve your "lost" clients and renew your therapeutic relationships.

Every practice experiences an ebb and flow of clients, yet many wellness providers work under the false assumption that if a client doesn't return within three months, then that client is lost forever. Another potentially hazardous belief for practitioners is that as long as they are attracting new clients, it's okay to become complacent with customer service and accept a higher attrition rate.

To keep a lamp burning we have to keep putting oil in it.
— Mother Teresa

Why Practitioners Lose Clients •

The reasons we lose clients are numerous and may have nothing to do with us. Clients relocate, their financial situation shifts, their lifestyles change, their schedules become so filled that it's difficult to book sessions, or the treatment series reaches its natural conclusion.

Then again, it may have to do with your particular kind of work, something you said or did (or didn't), your office environment or your business management.

Ninety percent of unhappy clients never return. Most won't even tell you why, but they will tell 10 other potential clients. Every time the story is relayed it gets worse.

The Results from Your Work ● ●

In some cases, clients may not return because they received what they intended from your work. For example, if the focus of your work is pain relief, once a client no longer experiences pain, he probably won't return.

Another reason for losing clients is that they may not have received what was wanted or needed. For instance, a client says he wants a lot of work done on his feet, yet you spend very little time there. Perhaps clients weren't asked for regular feedback, so they went elsewhere without stating complaints or preferences. Maybe the work was too challenging. Or maybe these clients are simply experimenting with other types of wellness services.

Professionalism ● ●

Lack of professionalism can lead to a loss of clients. Practitioners sometimes cross boundaries or inadvertently offend. Do you greet your clients appropriately, with direct eye contact and a handshake? Do you wear appropriate attire, maintain good hygiene, and avoid wearing strong perfumes or scents that may cause discomfort to those sensitive to or allergic to scents? Do you follow up on commitments, such as researching topics and sending materials? Do you schedule ample time to see clients and regroup between sessions? Do you talk too much during sessions? Do you return phone calls within 24 hours? Do you break confidentiality by talking about other clients?

You also may lose a client because the receptionist or another wellness provider in the office was curt, mishandled the client's records or made an error when scheduling appointments.

Convenience and Comfort ● ●

Lack of convenience or comfort are reasons for clients not to return. Your office may not be conveniently located for your target market. There may be scheduling difficulties due to either your hours of operation being inconducive to a client's schedule or because a client opted to be more spontaneous rather than planning in advance for a session and was never able to book on short notice. There may be accessibility concerns for people with disabilities, such as those who may have difficulty climbing stairs. Even though you may do great work, you could lose clients to another wellness provider who has better equipment, supplies, accessories or products than you do (e.g., a hydraulic table, an aromatherapy diffuser, hydrotherapy equipment, warm linens, organic skin care products, a full herbal pharmacy). Or there may be visual, auditory or olfactory disturbances associated with your office setting that prevent clients from returning, such as being located next to a perfumery, a music studio, a day care center, or a psychotherapist who specializes in anger release.

The trouble with most of us is that we would rather be ruined by praise than saved by criticism.
— Norman Vincent Peale

Finances ● ●

Financial interactions can be a source of miscommunication. There could be billing problems (particularly when it comes to insurance reimbursement). Be sure to keep track of package deals and gift certificate redemption. Be extremely careful of your wording and tone when questioning clients about their accounts; otherwise you could easily offend. Another reason clients don't return is their financial situation may have changed and they cannot afford your services.

Psychological Needs ● ●

A psychological component exists regardless of the main reason people schedule treatments (e.g., general wellness care, pain relief, stress reduction, relaxation, sports performance or a specific health condition). For most people, wellness services are also a way for them to honor themselves, give themselves a reward or provide a time of nurturing that's just for them. It is their opportunity to be the center of the universe. If you aren't giving your full attention to your clients, you may lose them. For instance, if you allow your mind to drift during a session for too long or too often, your client will notice the lack of connection. Do you leave your own troubles at the door? Also, if you answer the phone while working, you're essentially communicating to the client that she isn't very important.

Page 441

for information on Client Comment Cards.

Tools to Determine Why Clients Leave ●

The first step in analyzing the possibilities behind your clients not returning begins is to perform a self-inventory to evaluate your communication skills, your professional demeanor and your office operations. Identify the specific actions you take to provide excellent customer service and pinpoint the areas most likely for miscommunication or problems. (You can also hire a colleague or business coach to analyze your practice.) This is a good time to consider what proactive efforts you can take in your practice for continued improvement. Don't be misled by the "If it ain't broke, don't fix it" philosophy. There is always room for improvement.

Survey Clients ● ●

The best source for information about your practice is your current clients. Send them a short client survey, including a self-addressed, postage page return envelope, and inform them you're evaluating your practice and ways to enhance your service, and would appreciate their feedback on the following questions:

- Why do they continue receiving treatments from you?
- What do they like about you and your practice?
- What are their suggestions for improvement or added convenience?

You could also assemble a focus group of current and previous clients. The purpose of a focus group is to elicit honest feedback. Ideally, the group size is between eight and 10 people and is led by an outside facilitator. You can be present to welcome the group and return at the close of the meeting. The facilitator is crucial to keeping the dialogue on track and providing an atmosphere of trust and confidentiality. When you invite people to attend, tell them that you are looking for ways to improve your practice and would appreciate their input. You will fill the group faster if you provide some type of compensation and a meal or snack. Make a list of questions for the facilitator to ask (refer to your self-analysis).

The feedback you receive may offer insight into why some of your clients left and thus assist you in making necessary changes. Even if you are unable to renew many of your previous clients, these changes will help you avoid losing any more.

Another idea that helps you discover why clients don't return is to send a personal letter to your inactive clients (see Figure 17.9). The letter also serves as a way of renewing relationships.

Greeting Cards
www.koglecards.com
www.watercolorscards.com
www.info4people.com

17

Reconnect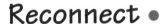

To inspire clients to return, you need to grab their attention. Send a postcard or letter with an incentive. For instance, you could send a $10 discount coupon or offer a free adjunct service with their next appointment. Sometimes a simple reminder is all that's needed. A massage therapist sent me a custom-printed card that had a funny cartoon emblazoned on the front and the caption said, "Remember to take care of yourself—schedule a massage today!" Right below it had her name, address and phone number. A note of caution: you can only use copyrighted or syndicated cartoons with written permission (and there's usually a fee assessed). Several companies make cards that can be used as client reminders.

If your client surveys pointed out problem areas that you were unaware of, you could send a note to your inactive clients saying you just want to touch base to let them know about some changes you are making in your practice (e.g., a new location, extended hours, additional services or treatment program assessment). You could also invite previous clients to come in for a free in-depth assessment and treatment plan (this is particularly effective if you weren't doing thorough treatment plans previously). Another idea is to create a special maintenance program and encourage previous clients to participate.

It may take several interactions to inspire a client to return. You can maintain connections by sending newsletters every quarter, mailing postcards that announce specials several times per year, holding open houses, and giving presentations. These are also great techniques for keeping current clients and enlisting new ones.

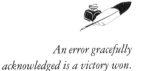

An error gracefully acknowledged is a victory won.
— Caroline L. Gascoigne

Remember that part of realizing how you may have lost clients is a valuable key to keep those you have from leaving. It is never too late to reconnect with a lapsed client. A phone call may be all that's needed. Sometimes people get overwhelmed with life and forget to take time for themselves. Others haven't made a commitment to receive regular wellness care. In either case, they may appreciate your follow-up call. It can be the ticket to their return.

Figure 17.9 Inactive Client Survey

The Relax Depot

954 Miramond Way • Grand Junction, CO 81501
970-555-9712 • Fax: 970-555-9713
www.relaxdepot.com • ccross@relaxdepot.com

February 2, 2020

Phyllis Forgotten
123 Prodigal Way
Anytown, CO 81506

Dear Phyllis,

Hello! It has been a while since I've seen you. You are a valued client and your satisfaction is important to me.

I aspire to establish and maintain good client relationships. Your feedback and suggestions will help me to better serve you and my other clients. Would you please take a moment to answer a few questions? Please be honest, as I desire accurate information.

What did you like about your sessions?
Did you feel that your needs and goals were met?
What are the main reasons you haven't had a session lately?
If you could change anything about our work together, what would it be?
What would encourage you to return?

Please rate my services on the following, using a scale of 1-10 where 1 is the lowest score and 10 the highest:

_____ Professional competence (e.g., the scope of services offered and your confidence in my abilities).

_____ Session quality (e.g., the manner in which services are provided, communication and compassion).

_____ Ambiance (e.g., room temperature, comfort of equipment, lighting and music).

_____ Overall customer service (e.g., scheduling, attention, providing educational materials and follow-up).

_____ Competitive pricing (e.g., are the results you receive from my services comparable to what you pay for other services, products, medications or supplements that address those same concerns?).

Please return this to me by using the enclosed self-addressed, stamped envelope. Your answers are confidential. Thank you for your time. Enclosed is a $10 coupon toward a session to be redeemed by you or a friend.

Sincerely,

Chris Cross

Enclosure

P.S. I am holding an open house on Friday, March 13 from 4-7 p.m. I will be demonstrating several self-relaxation techniques as well as displaying some nifty new equipment and products. I hope to see you there!

Relax Your Body Into Good Health

Epilogue

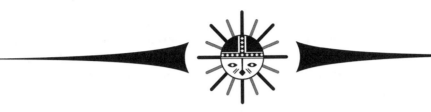

10 Best Ways to Guarantee Failure

Ever wonder how the most successful practitioners seem to magically attract new clients and build a thriving practice? What is their secret? Although each success story is unique in its own way, strategic plans, business savvy, a knack for marketing and dedication are common themes.

One thing is for sure, if you follow the 10 activities listed below, you are guaranteed to fail. Maybe a little tongue-in-cheek tour of these fatal errors will illustrate why the most successful practitioners, as highlighted throughout *Business Mastery*, follow a very different path to success.

1. Open an office next to a martial arts studio or a violin instructor

So what if your clients have to park four blocks away, fend off the stray animals that congregate by your front door and then walk up a flight of rickety stairs to get to your office, not to mention the peculiar noises that crescendo at the oddest times. Who cares about a little inconvenience and a few unpleasantries?

In the wellness field, location is everything. A tranquil and comfortable setting works wonders to help your clients relax and best enjoy the benefits of your sessions. Carefully evaluate the surrounding area and business setting. Look for locations where the adjacent businesses complement what you do (or at least don't detract from your work). You don't wield much control over what new businesses open after you are set up, although you could request a provision in your lease agreement that certain types of businesses not be allowed.

Image also plays a crucial role in your success. Create a comfortable and safe indoor and outdoor space so clients will want to return. Aim for a clean, organized, quiet and private office space. Create an office environment as comfortable as possible for yourself and your clients. Also, look for ways to differentiate yourself from other practitioners (e.g., a decorative fountain for soothing sounds of water, flannel sheets in winter, and an assortment of juices and filtered water).

2. Be a Chatty Cathy

Talk non-stop about yourself. Don't listen to your clients' concerns. In fact, purposely eliminate addressing a health concern that they point out needs extra attention. Ignore information offered about clients' personal lives, and when brought up, interrupt with a story about how good or bad YOUR day was. When meeting someone new, babble on before you're even asked about how you got into the field and drone on about every technique you utilize in your sessions.

All successful practitioners have highly developed listening skills. This means treating clients as though they are the center of the universe. It also means paying attention to nonverbal as well as verbal communication. Ask open-ended questions, not just ones that require Yes or No responses. Also, though it may seem natural to talk about yourself, limit self-disclosure and continue to bring any conversation back to the client in the room. Encourage your clients to share their wellness goals with you. Develop treatment plans jointly with them. This helps to clarify the type of work required, set boundaries, and ensure your clients' unique needs are met. It also greatly boosts client retention.

Many people become either tongue-tied or drone on forever when asked what it is they do. Script a carefully prepared 30-second introduction about who you are and what you do. This isn't meant to be a sales pitch. Keep it simple, honest and dynamic. Include a few benefits of the work you do and something that expresses who you are. By having this memorized introduction, you are free to focus on listening to the other person.

3. Stay at home and wait for the universe to support you

After all, many wise leaders have claimed that if you do what you love, money will flow to you. And if it's meant to be, then it will happen.

Karmic laws may rule, but belief without action will bring only a fraction of the potential results. The key word in the phrase, "Do what you love and money will flow to you," is the word *do*. Creatively planned effort with sincere intention will reap many future returns. Most businesses fail because of a lack of planning and/or undercapitalization. If you are doing what you love, tell others and this becomes marketing in the truest form. If you are in the building phase of your practice, get your hands on as many bodies as possible. Do demonstrations, donate your services for worthy events, and offer your services to people in need. Loving what you do will become obvious to those who receive your work and may inspire clients' word-of-mouth referrals to you. But these are just the beginning. It doesn't take a lot of effort, but consistent, disciplined and conscious attempts to reach out to existing and new clients are required.

4. Don't return phone calls

Assume that if a current or potential client really wants to talk with you or book a session, he'll call back. It's also okay to answer the phone while in session with a client. Your client won't mind you taking a few minutes of the time she's paid for so you can talk to someone else.

Since the phone is one of your primary communication links to customers, it is imperative that you establish times during the day to return phone calls. Usually when people call to schedule a session, they want it as soon as possible. So if you wait too long to call back, the opportunity may be lost. Return all phone calls within 24 hours or sooner. Keep necessary supplies, appointment book and information close to the telephone so that you won't keep anyone hanging while you're fumbling for them. Greet callers courteously and enthusiastically.

It is inappropriate to answer the telephone while working with a client. That client has paid for your undivided attention during a specified amount of hands-on time. If need be, utilize an appointment service to book sessions or employ a receptionist. You could also subscribe to a voice-messaging service, buy an answering machine or use online appointment booking software. Whichever method you choose, make certain that the phone can't be heard in the treatment room.

5. Toss Receipts

It's such a hassle, so why bother, right?

Consider being a "receipt cop" a part of doing business. It's a way to increase your net income by offsetting gross income from paying clients. Most therapists keep track of the bigger items (usually paid with a check or credit card) such as equipment, telephone, stationery, advertising, office supplies, dues and rent. But those little cash expenses add up (e.g., meals, taxi fares and tips while at a convention, bottled water or juice bought while doing work at a corporate account, and gasoline or mileage expenses for business use of your car).

Keep a copy of checks, money orders or credit card payments for tax records. Sometimes you can't get a receipt for cash purchases (particularly from vending machines), so keep a cash journal that documents the type of business activity you were doing while making the purchase and the details about the actual purchase (i.e., item description, place purchased, date and amount). Financial management is crucial for long-term success.

6. Be late for appointments

Time is relative (ask Einstein). The session can't begin without you anyway. Also, people are always glad to have some unexpected free time to contemplate their navel. Besides, it's not as if clients never keep you waiting. What's a few minutes?

Without a doubt, lateness conveys the attitude that your time is more important than your clients' time. It clearly registers as disrespect. If you arrive at the same time as your client, you're late. Being timely means allowing ample time to review client charts, set up your room and get centered. Schedule yourself wisely so that you work at a comfortable pace and allot time for breaks. Timeliness is an admirable quality, especially given the personal nature of this field.

7. Assume that the whole world is your market

Attempt to make everyone your client. After all, everybody benefits from your work. If you narrow your market, you might starve to death. Place display ads, business cards and brochures everywhere, and hope that your phone rings off the hook.

It's true that almost anyone can benefit from wellness care, but to work smarter—not harder, it's vital to focus your promotional efforts on several target markets. Decide whom you would like to work with and pursue those markets. Many opportunities exist in this world, and it's impossible to follow them all or be everything to everyone. Given that, like most practitioners, you have limited marketing resources, so it's important to know where to focus your time and money. This doesn't mean that you must refuse to work with people who don't fit your target market profile, just that you don't randomly expend your resources.

8. Never think twice about exiting clients

Once they walk out the door, forget they exist. Keep looking for more clients. You don't want to get bored by working on the same people all of the time.

Client retention is the foundation of a stable, thriving practice. It costs six times more to go after a new client than to retain an existing one. Pay attention to nurturing current clients. Build rapport by showing interest in your clients' ongoing well-being. Work with clients to create effective treatment plans and customize your sessions. Continue your customer service through appropriate follow-up. Some ways to show concern are: check in with clients the day after their session; send special occasion cards for events such as birthdays and anniversaries; make confirmation calls; and gather information, referrals or resources for topics of concern to your clients.

9. Be a lone ranger

Become as isolated as you can. Don't share any of your ideas because someone might steal them and become successful. Don't bother with continuing education, because your original training meets the local requirements (and you're such a wonderful healer that you don't need to learn anything else).

Even though we see clients, the work of most wellness practitioners is rather solitary. Rarely do practitioners work in an environment that involves case management or discussions with peers. It's vital for your personal well-being as well as your business success to establish a support system. Meet with colleagues on a regular basis, choose advisors, attend networking functions, and get involved with local health-oriented activities. Seek opportunities to engage in cooperative marketing ventures.

Continuing your education is another aspect of involvement in your profession. Stay on the cutting edge of technical knowledge as well as professional development skills. Two side benefits of attending workshops are meeting other like-minded people and renewing your enthusiasm for your work.

10. Never receive any somatic wellness treatments

You don't have time to get worked on. Besides, nobody does your style of work, which is your favorite, or if they do, they certainly aren't as good as you. What you want is for clients to knock down your door, asking for your work. If you keep this up, you'll be making all sorts of money.

Think about how much you use your body. Walk your talk. Receive regular wellness treatments so you can stay healthy and strong. It's the only way to realistically sustain a long-term practice and your well-being. This can be difficult, particularly for those of you who live in isolated areas. But if you don't receive regular treatments, how can you ethically encourage others to do the same?

I wish you great success in all you do!

Cherie

Endnotes

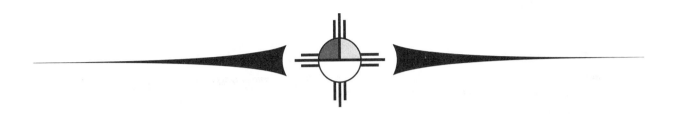

Chapter 1: Getting Started

1. www.score.org/small_biz_stats.html.

Chapter 3: Success Strategies

1. Jim Lundy, *Lead, Follow, or Get Out of the Way* (The Berkley Publishing Group, 1986).

2. Ron Dalrymple, *The Inner Manager: Mastering Business, Home and Self* (Celestial Gifts Publishing, 1987).

3. Dr. C Diane Ealy, *The Woman's Book of Creativity* (Beyond Words Publishing, Inc. 1995) 229-234.

4. Ealy 89.

5. Michael J. Losier, *The Law of Attraction*: *The Science of Attracting More of What You Want and Less of What You Don't* (Michael J. Losier Enterprises, 2006).

6. *What the Bleep Do We Know!?* Captured Light & Lord of the Wind Films, LLC, 2004.

7. Masaru Emoto, *The Hidden Messages in Water* (Hillsboro, Oregon: Beyond Words Publishing, 2004).

8. Ealy 241-245.

Chapter 4: Boost Career Longevity

1. Randall S. Hansen, Ph.D., career counselor www.careerdoctor.org.

2. A.T. Ferrell-Torry and O.J. Glick, "The use of therapeutic massage as a nursing intervention to modify anxiety and the perception of cancer pain." *Cancer Nurs.* 1993 Apr;16(2):93-101.

3. C.M. Olney, "The effect of therapeutic back massage in hypertensive persons: a preliminary study." *Biol Res Nurs.* 2005 Oct;7(2): 98-105.

4. Les Kertay, "Ethical considerations for bodyworkers who counsel," *Massage Magazine* July/August 1998.

5. Napoleon Hill, *Think & Grow Rich* (Fawcett Crest Books, 1960) 168-169.

Chapter 5: Conscious Practice

1. Thomas J. Peters, "Ethics is everyday, lifetime endeavor," *The Arizona Daily Star*, 26 September 1989.

Chapter 6: Therapeutic Communications

1. Marshall B. Rosenberg, *Nonviolent Communication: A Language of Life: Create Your Life, Your Relationships, and Your World in Harmony with Your Values* (PuddleDancer Press 2003) 96.

Chapter 7: An Insider's Look at Work Settings

H. Barry Waldman, D.D.S., M.P.H., Ph.D. and Steven P. Perlman, D.D.S., Msc.D., "Patient-centric practices-no matter the size!" *AGD Impact*, November 2006:32.

Chapter 8: Employment Fundamentals

1. Dan Baker and Cathy Greenberg, *What Happy Companies Know: How the Science of Happiness Can Change Your Company for the Better* (Collins Hemingway; Pearson Education, Inc., 2006) 202.
2. Baker and Greenberg 197.

Chapter 9: An Insider's Look at Practice Settings

1. *Employer's Guide to a Healthy Organization*, special report published by The Health Fitness Corporation, Minneapolis, MN. www.hfit.com.
2. Jean Ives, "Massage Is In Business" Massage Therapy Journal, Spring 2004.

Chapter 11: Create a Dynamic Business Plan

David M. Anderson, "Deadly Sins," *Entrepreneur*, August 2001.

Chapter 12: Practice Managment

1. *Case Study: Delane's Natural Nail Care.* Small Business Technology Institute, San Jose, CA. www.sbtechnologyinstitute.org/consulting/caseStudiesTAP.htm.

Chapter 14: Financial Management

1. Suze Orman, *The 9 Steps to Financial Freedom* (Crown Publishers, Inc. 1998).

Chapter 15: Marketing Fundamentals

1. Marsha Sinetar, *Do What You Love and the Money will Follow*, (Dell Publishing, 1987).
2. Faith Popcorn and Lys Marigold, *Clicking: 17 Trends That Drive Your Business—And Your Life* (HarperCollins Publishing, Inc.1997).
3. David A. Aaker, *Managing Brand Equity* (The Free Press, 1991) 14.

Chapter 16: Marketing in Action

1. Michael Port, *Book Yourself Solid: The Fastest, Easiest, and Most Reliable System of Getting More Clients Than You Can Handle Even if You Hate Marketing and Selling* (John Wiley & Sons, Inc. 2006) 159.

Index

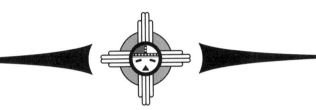

Other Offerings

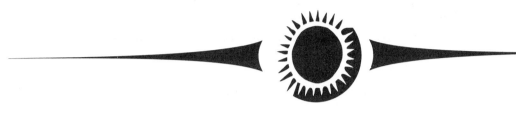

About Sohnen-Moe Associates, Inc.

Sohnen-Moe Associates, Inc. provides convenient, affordable, state-of-the-art information and tools to help you grow your business and make your dreams come true. Having the technical skills to be an excellent wellness practitioner is necessary but insufficient for business success. It takes very different skills to cultivate a profitable practice. You can gain these skills through studying and working with an experienced coach who knows how to support people in achieving their goals. We offer the following innovative, practical, time-tested resources to increase your success: home-study courses; books; workshops; coaching services; Teacher's Aide Newsletters; and two information-rich websites (www.sohnen-moe.com and www.businessmastery.us).

We are committed to supporting small business owners (particularly those in the wellness fields) to develop profitable, enjoyable businesses. We assist people to do what they love and prosper. We look forward to supporting you in working smarter, increasing your client base and bringing home the income you deserve!

Workshops

Our skill-building courses are interactive and experiential. Each seminar is custom designed to achieve the results you desire. The most popular workshops that Cherie Sohnen-Moe presents include Marketing From Your Heart, The Ethics of Touch, Business Mastery, Present Yourself Powerfully, Therapeutic Communications, Taking Your Practice to the Next Level, The Four Keys to Publicity, and Creative Teaching Techniques.

Cherie is a dynamic presenter, and her workshops are highly rated by participants. Sponsors may mix and match topics from any workshop description to design a seminar that meets their specific goals. Sohnen-Moe Associates is approved by the NCBTMB as continuing education (Provider No. 031932-00). Our courses are accepted by the AMTA, ABMP, Florida State Department of Health (Provider No. MCE477-05) and many other practitioners' national and state boards.

Coaching

Feeling puzzled about how to create and maintain a successful business? Get yourself a coach! Acquire skills and knowledge, and benefit from ongoing support, inspiration and encouragement. Working with Cherie Sohnen-Moe or one of our business coaching associates is a great way to increase your success by leaps and bounds.

Coaching provides support in resolving problems and provides suggestions to implement change for a more efficient, vital and flourishing business. No successful athlete would be without a personal coach to ensure victory. There is no wonder why most prosperous business owners have worked with a consultant or a mentor to advise and support them along the way.

If you experience any of the following scenarios, you can benefit from coaching.

- You are so intent on "doing it yourself" that you never get it done.
- You puzzle over the best way to grow your business.
- You lack satisfaction in aspects of your work.
- You want more clients or customers.
- You have difficulty promoting yourself.
- You feel stuck and don't know how to move to the next level of your business.
- You work very hard, yet don't earn what you want.
- You have difficulty retaining clients or customers.
- You want to buy or sell a practice but aren't sure how to proceed.
- You want an objective opinion on a specific issue.

Cherie brings more than 30 years of experience working with people to establish businesses that successfully reflect their individual goals and values, create more personal time, and increase their income. Her clients include members of the massage and bodywork professions, estheticians, restaurateurs and artists, as well as businesses in the industries of education, retailing, automotive, spas and salons.

What Others Say

"Thanks to Sohnen-Moe Associates, Inc. for the accurate evaluation of my massage therapy practice. Because of Cherie's availability and willingness to advise and answer questions, I was able to market, negotiate and sell my practice for much more than I realized it was worth."
—Sue Baker, Massage Practitioner

"I didn't want to admit that I didn't know what I was doing. I am more creative than business-oriented, and Cherie has a way of taking ideas and putting them to work. She makes sure that I know and can justify what I am doing. There's something zen to it . . . she's not a traditional business consultant. I wish I had gone to her before I had started out."
—Jennifer Utken, The Well Rounded Woman

How to Schedule a Coaching Session

You can schedule coaching sessions on a one-time basis, weekly or quarterly, with sessions taking place either by telephone or on-site. Fees range from $100 to $175 per hour. As a purchaser of *Business Mastery*, you're eligible for a special introductory coaching rate of $75 for the first hour or $35 for the first half-hour. Call us at 800-786-4774 or email sma.coaching@sohnen-moe.com.

Website: www.sohnen-moe.com

Our website offers you fast and easy access to our products, services and resources. Take a tour through this excellent resource for business success! Be sure to visit these exciting sections:

Professional Development Catalog
We carry 40+ books, software and other items to assist your business development, marketing and practice management.

81 Home Study Courses (2-6 contact hours each)
Our courses use *Business Mastery* and *The Ethics of Touch* as the reading material. The *Business Mastery Continuing Education Series* (36 courses) helps new practitioners establish thriving practices and seasoned practitioners take their businesses to the next level. *The Ethics of Touch Continuing Education Series* (45 courses) takes an in-depth look at ethical issues through reading materials and reflective exercises. They are designed per the NCBTMB Standards of Practice requirements.

Business Tips
Each week we give you new ideas: marketing tips that are inexpensive and simple to do; suggestions on how to manage your practice more efficiently; and insurance tips.

Free Forms
Download a wide array of forms to make your practice more functional. Available as PDFs or as WordPerfect, MSWord, or RTF documents so you can customize them!

Workshops
Descriptions of our workshops, how to be a sponsor and updated travel schedule.

Marketing Mastery
Effective and consistent marketing is a major key to a successful career. Register for our free Marketing Mastery subscription service. We start off with an overall marketing plan and then email you monthly goals and weekly reminders for marketing activities. Use all or part of this plan to expand your marketing and networking efforts, elevate your visibility in the community, and, of course, increase your client base.

Resource Directory
A comprehensive collection of 1,000+ products, services, associations and organizations related to your profession.

Teacher's Corner
We post the following resources to assist teachers in making their jobs easier, more effective and fun: back issues of our Teacher's Aide Newsletters; upcoming teachers' workshops; teaching tips; the *Business Mastery Teacher's Manual;* and *The Ethics of Touch Teacher's Manual.*

Website: www.businessmastery.us

This website is the online companion to *Business Mastery.* It offers you fast and easy access to additional information on topics covered in the book, a downloadable *Business Mastery Workbook,* reference materials, resources and website links. Be sure to visit regularly as we plan to continually update these sections:

Business Mastery Workbook
This workbook includes all of the written exercises and checklists from *Business Mastery.* To download your free copy of the *Business Mastery Workbook,* go to www.businessmastery.us/workbook.php.

Chapter Supplements
We have so much information to share that it could not all fit into the *Business Mastery* book without making it unwieldy. This section includes supplementary information on some of the topics covered in the book; marked with the ✋ symbol.

Chapter Resources
Each chapter has a separate webpage with margin resources from the book, additional website links, articles and books.

Teacher's Resources
We offer extensive ancillary support materials for schools that require *Business Mastery* as a text: The Art of Teaching, a 60-page teaching guide; a test bank; handout and overhead masters; 16-, 36- and 70-hour syllabi, complete with lesson plan builders (goals, objectives, activities).

Forms
All of the forms mentioned in the book plus more!

Other Items Published by Sohnen-Moe Associates

Business Mastery Supplement
Work smarter—not harder! This text-based computer CDROM helps you easily update your business plan, save time in creating professional letters, and spark creative marketing ideas. It includes a 50^+ page massage practice business plan and more than 150 letters (including primary care correspondence, cooperative marketing suggestions and client communications) and checklists commonly needed by practitioners in professionally managing their business.

Present Yourself Powerfully, by Cherie Sohnen-Moe   7-page manual and 14 handout masters
Public speaking is one of the best ways to build your business. This presentation kit makes it easy to give talks, workshops and demonstrations. The manual explores topics such as: the keys to giving successful presentations; analyzing the audience's needs and preferences; designing exciting presentations; utilizing audio-visual materials; developing an engaging self-introduction; managing the physical environment; enhancing verbal communication skills; doing fun, effective demonstrations; getting your audience involved; increasing the impact of your nonverbal communications; tips for continuing connections made through your presentations; and how to make money through public speaking. It also includes a variety of checklists to encourage further exploration, and two, 20-minute, scripted massage/bodywork-oriented presentations, complete with handout masters.

The Ethics of Touch: The Hands-on Practitioner's Guide To Creating a Professional, Safe and Enduring Practice, by Ben E. Benjamin, Ph.D., and Cherie Sohnen-Moe   320 pages
Ethics is an exciting, vital field of study for all professionals. Our lives are more fulfilling and our practices are more successful if we live with honor and integrity in all our relationships and business dealings. This book defines core psychological principles; teaches methods for resolving ethical dilemmas; supplies specific techniques for maintaining healthy boundaries, enhancing communication and fostering a sense of safety; examines dual relationships; provides a protocol for working with survivors of trauma and abuse; clarifies the role of supervision; and furnishes strategies for managing an ethical practice. Each chapter concludes with numerous thought-provoking questions and activities.

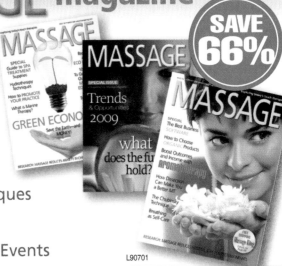
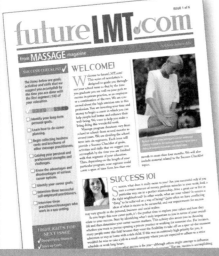
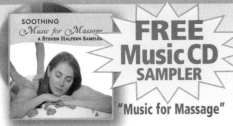

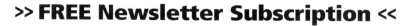

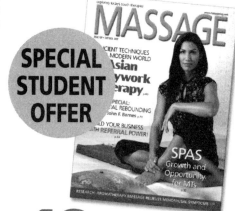